Multiple Imputation and its Application

Statistics in Practice

Statistics in Practice is an important international series of texts which provide detailed coverage of statistical concepts, methods and worked case studies in specific fields of investigation and study.

With clear explanations and many worked practical examples, the books show in down-to-earth terms how to select and use an appropriate range of statistical techniques in a particular practical field within each title's special topic area.

The books provide statistical support for professionals and research workers across a range of fields of employment and research environments. Subject areas covered include medicine and pharmaceuticals; industry, finance and commerce; public services, and the earth and environmental sciences.

The books also provide support to students studying applied statistics courses in these areas. The demand for applied statistics graduates in these areas has led to such courses becoming increasingly prevalent at universities and colleges.

It is our aim to present judiciously chosen and well-written textbooks to meet everyday practical needs. Feedback from readers will be valuable in monitoring our success.

A complete list of titles in this series appears at the end of the volume.

Multiple Imputation and its Application

James R. Carpenter

and

Michael G. Kenward

Department of Medical Statistics
London School of Hygiene and Tropical Medicine, UK

WILEY

A John Wiley & Sons, Ltd., Publication

This edition first published 2013

Registered office John Wiley & Sons Ltd, The Atrium, Southern Gate, Chichester, West Sussex, PO19 8SQ, United Kingdom

For details of our global editorial offices, for customer services and for information about how to apply for permission to reuse the copyright material in this book please see our website at www.wiley.com.

Reprinted with corrections March 2014.

Library of Congress Cataloging-in-Publication Data

Carpenter, James R.
Multiple imputation and its application / James R. Carpenter, Michael G. Kenward. – 1st ed.
p. ; cm.
Includes bibliographical references and index.
ISBN 978-0-470-74052-1 (hardback)
I. Kenward, Michael G., 1956- II. Title.
[DNLM: 1. Data Interpretation, Statistical. 2. Biomedical Research–methods. WA 950]
610.72′4–dc23

2012028821

A catalogue record for this book is available from the British Library.

ISBN: 978-0-470-74052-1

Cover photograph courtesy of Harvey Goldstein

Set in 10/12pt Times by Laserwords Private Limited, Chennai, India

Contents

Preface

No study of any complexity manages to collect all the intended data. Analysis of the resulting partially collected data must therefore address the issues raised by the missing data. Unfortunately, the inferential consequences of missing data are not simply restricted to the proportion of missing observations. Instead, the interplay between the substantive questions and the reasons for the missing data is crucial. Thus, there is no simple, universal, solution.

Suppose, for the substantive question at hand, the inferential consequences of missing data are nontrivial. Then the analyst must make a set of assumptions about the reasons, or mechanisms, causing data to be missing, and perform an inferentially valid analysis under these assumptions. In this regard, analysis of a partially observed dataset is the same as any statistical analysis; the difference is that when data are missing we cannot assess the validity of these assumptions in the way we might do in a regression analysis, for example. Hence, sensitivity analysis, where we explore the robustness of inference to different assumptions about the reasons for missing data, is important.

Given a set of assumptions about the reasons data are missing, there are a number of statistical methods for carrying out the analysis. These include the EM algorithm, inverse probability weighting, a full Bayesian analysis and, depending on the setting, a direct application of maximum likelihood. These methods, and those derived from them, each have their own advantages in particular settings. Nevertheless, we argue that none shares the practical utility, broad applicability and relative simplicity of Rubin's Multiple Imputation (MI).

Following an introductory chapter outlining the issues raised by missing data, the focus of this book is therefore MI. We outline its theoretical basis, and then describe its application to a range of common analysis in the medical and social sciences, reflecting the wide application that MI has seen in recent years. In particular, we describe its application with nonlinear relationships and interactions, with survival data and with multilevel data. The last three chapters consider practical sensitivity analyses, combining MI with inverse probability weighting, and doubly robust MI.

Self-evidently, a key component of an MI analysis, is the construction of an appropriate method of imputation. There is no unique, ideal, way in which this should be done. In particular, there there has been some discussion in the literature about the relative merits of the joint modelling and full conditional specification approaches. We have found that thinking in terms of joint models is both natural and convenient for formulating imputation models, a range of which can then be (approximately) implemented using a full conditional specification approach. Differences in computational speed between joint modelling and full conditional specification are generally due to coding efficiency, rather than intrinsic superiority of one method over the other.

Throughout the book we illustrate the ideas with several examples. The code used for these examples, in various software packages, is available from the book's home page, which is at `http://www.wiley.com/go/multiple_imputation`, together with exercises to go with each chapter.

We welcome feedback from readers; any comments and corrections should be e-mailed to mi@lshtm.ac.uk. Unfortunately, we cannot promise to respond individually to each message.

Data acknowledgements

We are grateful to the following:

AstraZeneca for permission to use data from the 5-arm asthma study in examples in Chapters 1, 3, 7 and 10;

GlaxoSmithKline for permission to use data from the dental pain study in Chapter 4, and the RECORD study in Chapter 12;

Mike English (Director, Child and Newborn Health Group, Kemri-Wellcome Trust Research Programme, Nairobi, Kenya) for permission to use data from a multifaceted intervention to implement guidelines and improve admission paediatric care in Kenyan district hospitals, in Chapter 9;

Peter Blatchford for permission to use data from the Class Size Study (Blatchford *et al*, 2002) in Chapter 9, and

Sarah Schroter for permission to use data from the study to improve the quality of peer review in Chapter 10.

In Chapters 1, 5, 8, 10 and 11 we have analysed data from the Youth Cohort Time Series for England, Wales and Scotland, 1984-2002 First Edition, Colchester, Essex, published by and freely available from the UK Data Archive, Study Number SN 5765. We thank Vernon Gayle for introducing us to these data.

In Chapter 6 we have analysed data from the Alzheimer's Disease Neuro-imaging Initiative (ADNI) database (adni.loni.ucla.edu). As such, the investigators within the ADNI contributed to the design and implementation of ADNI and/or provided data but did not participate in the analysis or in the writing of this book. A complete listing of ADNI investigators can be found at: `http://adni.loni.ucla.edu/wp-content/uploads/how_to_apply/ADNI_Acknowledgement_List.pdf`.

The ADNI was launched in 2003 by the National Institute on Aging (NIA), the National Institute of Biomedical Imaging and Bioengineering (NIBIB), the Food and Drug Administration (FDA), private pharmaceutical companies and nonprofit organisations, as a $60 million, five-year public-private partnership. The primary goal of ADNI has been to test whether serial magnetic resonance imaging (MRI), positron emission tomography (PET), other biological markers, and clinical and neuropsychological assessment can be combined to measure the progression of mild cognitive impairment (MCI) and early Alzheimer's disease (AD). Determination of sensitive and specific markers of very early AD progression is intended to aid researchers and clinicians to develop new treatments and monitor their effectiveness, as well as lessen the time and cost of clinical trials.

The Principal Investigator of this initiative is Michael W. Weiner, MD, VA Medical Center and University of California San Francisco. ADNI is the result of the efforts of many co-investigators from a broad range of academic institutions and private corporations, and subjects have been recruited from over 50 sites across the US and Canada. The initial goal of ADNI was to recruit 800 adults, ages 55 to 90, to participate in the research, with approximately 200 cognitively normal older individuals to be followed for 3 years, 400 people with MCI to be followed for 3 years and 200 people with early AD to be followed for 2 years. For up-to-date information, see `www.adni-info.org`.

Data collection and sharing for this project was funded by the Alzheimer's Disease Neuroimaging Initiative (ADNI) (National Institutes of Health Grant U01 AG024904). ADNI is funded by the National Institute on Aging, the National Institute of Biomedical Imaging and Bioengineering, and through generous contributions from the following: Abbott; Alzheimer's Association; Alzheimer's Drug Discovery Foundation; Amorfix Life Sciences Ltd.; AstraZeneca; Bayer HealthCare; BioClinica, Inc.; Biogen Idec, Inc.; Bristol-Myers Squibb Company; Eisai, Inc.; Elan Pharmaceuticals, Inc.; Eli Lilly and Company; F. Hoffmann-La Roche Ltd and its affiliated company Genentech, Inc.; GE Healthcare; Innogenetics, N.V.; IXICO Ltd.; Janssen Alzheimer Immunotherapy Research & Development, LLC; Johnson & Johnson Pharmaceutical Research & Development, LLC; Medpace, Inc.; Merck & Co., Inc.; Meso Scale Diagnostics, LLC; Novartis Pharmaceuticals Corporation; Pfizer, Inc.; Servier; Synarc, Inc.; and Takeda Pharmaceutical Company. The Canadian Institutes of Health Research is providing funds to support ADNI clinical sites in Canada. Private sector contributions are facilitated by the Foundation for the National Institutes of Health (`www.fnih.org`). The grantee organisation is the Northern California Institute for Research and Education, and the study is coordinated by the Alzheimer's Disease Cooperative Study at the University of California, San Diego. ADNI data are disseminated by the Laboratory for Neuro-imaging at the University of California, Los Angeles. This research was also supported by NIH grants P30 AG010129 and K01 AG030514.

In Chapter 7 we have analysed data from the 1958 National Childhood Development Study. This is published, and freely available from the UK Data Archive, Study Number SN 5565 (waves 0–3) and SN 5566 (wave 4). We thank Ian Plewis for introducing us to these data.

Acknowledgements

No book of this kind is written in a vacuum, and we are grateful to many friends and colleagues for research collaborations, stimulating discussions and comments on draft chapters.

In particular we would like to thank members of the Missing Data Imputation and Analysis (MiDIA) group, including (in alphabetical order) Jonathan Bartlett, John Carlin, Rhian Daniel, Dan Jackson, Shaun Seaman, Jonathan Sterne, Kate Tilling and Ian White.

We would also like to acknowledge many years of collaboration with Geert Molenberghs, James Roger and Harvey Goldstein.

James would like to thank Mike Elliott, Rod Little, Trivellore Raghunathan and Jeremy Taylor for facilitating a visit to the Institute for Social Research and Department of Biostatistics at the University of Michigan, Ann Arbor, in Summer 2011, when the majority of the first draft was written.

Thanks to Tim Collier for the anecdote in §1.3.

We also gratefully acknowledge funding support from the ESRC (3-year fellowship for James Carpenter, RES-063-27-0257, and follow-on funding RES-189-25-0103) and MRC (grants G0900724, G0900701 and G0600599).

We would also like to thank Richard Davies and Kathryn Sharples at Wiley for their encouragement and support.

Lastly, thanks to our families for their forbearance and understanding over the course of this project.

Despite the encouragement and support of those listed above, the text inevitably contains errors and shortcomings, for which we take full responsibility.

James Carpenter and Mike Kenward
London School of Hygiene & Tropical Medicine

Glossary

Indices and symbols

i	indexes units, often individuals, unless defined otherwise
j	indexes variables in the data set, unless defined otherwise
n	total number of units in the data set, unless defined otherwise
p	depending on context, number of variables in a data set or number of parameters in a statistical model
X, Y, Z	random variables
$Y_{i,j}$	i^{th} observation on j^{th} variable, $i = 1, \ldots, n$, $j = 1, \ldots, p$.
θ	generic parameter
$\boldsymbol{\theta}$	generic parameter column vector, typically $p \times 1$
β, γ, δ	regression coefficients
$\boldsymbol{\beta}$	column vector of regression coefficients, typically $p \times 1$.

Matrices

$\mathbf{\Omega}$	matrix, typically of dimension $p \times p$.
$\mathbf{\Omega}_{i,j}$	i, j^{th} element of $\mathbf{\Omega}$
$\mathbf{\Omega}^T$	transpose of $\mathbf{\Omega}$, so that $\mathbf{\Omega}^T_{i,j} = \mathbf{\Omega}_{j,i}$.
$\mathbf{Y}_j = (Y_{1,j}, \ldots, Y_{n,j})^T$	$n \times 1$ column vector of observations on variable j.
$\mathrm{tr}(\mathbf{\Omega})$	sum of diagonal elements of $\mathbf{\Omega}$, *ie* $\sum \mathbf{\Omega}_{i,i}$ known as the trace of the matrix.

Abbreviations

AIPW	Augmented Inverse Probability Weighting
CAR	Censoring At Random
CNAR	Censoring Not At Random
EM	Expectation Maximisation
FCS	Full Conditional Specification
FEV_1	Forced Expiratory Volume in 1 second (measured in litres)
FMI	Fraction of Missing Information
IPW	Inverse Probability Weighting

MAR	Missing At Random
MCAR	Missing Completely At Random
MI	Multiple Imputation
MNAR	Missing Not At Random
POD	Partially Observed Data
POM	Probability Of Missingness
S.E.	Standard error

Probability distributions

$f(.)$	probability distribution function
$F(.)$	cumulative distribution function
'|'	to be verbalised 'given', as in $f(Y\|X)$
	'the probability distribution function of Y given X'

PART I

FOUNDATIONS

1

Introduction

Collecting, analysing and drawing inferences from data are central to research in the medical and social sciences. Unfortunately, for any number of reasons, it is rarely possible to collect all the intended data. The ubiquity of missing data, and the problems this poses for both analysis and inference, has spawned a substantial statistical literature dating from 1950s. At that time, when statistical computing was in its infancy, many analyses were only feasible because of the carefully planned balance in the dataset (for example, the same number of observations on each unit). Missing data meant the available data for analysis were unbalanced, thus complicating the planned analysis and in some instances rendering it unfeasible. Early work on the problem was therefore largely computational (e.g. Healy and Westmacott, 1956; Afifi and Elashoff, 1966; Orchard and Woodbury, 1972; Dempster *et al.*, 1977).

The wider question of the consequences of nontrivial proportions of missing data for inference was neglected until a seminal paper by Rubin (1976). This set out a typology for assumptions about the reasons for missing data, and sketched their implications for analysis and inference. It marked the beginning of a broad stream of research about the analysis of partially observed data. The literature is now huge, and continues to grow, both as methods are developed for large and complex data structures, and as increasing computer power and suitable software enable researchers to apply these methods.

For a broad overview of the literature, a good place to start is one of the recent excellent textbooks. Little and Rubin (2002) write for applied statisticians. They give a good overview of likelihood methods, and give an introduction to multiple imputation. Allison (2002) presents a less technical overview. Schafer (1997) is more algorithmic, focusing on the EM algorithm and imputation using the multivatiate normal and general location model. Molenberghs and Kenward (2007)

Multiple Imputation and its Application, First Edition. James R. Carpenter and Michael G. Kenward.

focus on clinical studies, while Daniels and Hogan (2008) focus on longitudinal studies with a Bayesian emphasis.

The above books concentrate on parametric approaches. However, there is also a growing literature based around using inverse probability weighting, in the spirit of Horvitz and Thompson (1952), and associated doubly robust methods. In particular, we refer to the work of Robins and colleagues (e.g. Robins *et al.*, 1995; Scharfstein *et al.*, 1999). Vansteelandt *et al.* (2009) give an accessible introduction to these developments. A comparison with multiple imputation in a simple setting is given by Carpenter *et al.* (2006). The pros and cons are debated in Kang and Schafer (2007) and the theory is brought together by Tsiatis (2006).

This book is concerned with a particular statistical method for analysing and drawing inferences from incomplete data, called *Multiple Imputation (MI)*. Initially proposed by Rubin (1987) in the context of surveys, increasing awareness among researchers about the possible effects of missing data (e.g. Klebanoff and Cole, 2008) has led to an upsurge of interest (e.g. Sterne *et al.*, 2009; Kenward and Carpenter, 2007; Schafer, 1999a; Rubin, 1996).

Multiple imputation (MI) is attractive because it is both practical and widely applicable. Recently developed statistical software (see, for example, issue 45 of the *Journal of Statistical Software*) has placed it within the reach of most researchers in the medical and social sciences, whether or not they have undertaken advanced training in statistics. However, the increasing use of MI in a range of settings beyond that originally envisaged has led to a bewildering proliferation of algorithms and software. Further, the implication of the underlying assumptions in the context of the data at hand is often unclear.

We are writing for researchers in the medical and social sciences with the aim of clarifying the issues raised by missing data, outlining the rationale for MI, explaining the motivation and relationship between the various imputation algorithms, and describing and illustrating its application to increasingly complex data structures.

Central to the analysis of partially observed data is an understanding of why the data are missing and the implications of this for the analysis. This is the focus of the remainder of this chapter. Introducing some of the examples that run through the book, we show how Rubin's typology (Rubin, 1976) provides the foundational framework for understanding the implications of missing data.

1.1 Reasons for missing data

In this section we consider possible reasons for missing data, illustrate these with examples, and draw some preliminary implications for inference. We use the word 'possible' advisedly, since with partially observed data we can rarely be sure of the mechanism giving rise to missing data. Instead, a range of possible mechanisms are consistent with the observed data. In practice, we therefore wish to analyse the data under different mechanisms, to establish the robustness of our inference in the face of uncertainty about the missingness mechanism.

All datasets consist of a series of *units* each of which provides information on a series of *items*. For example, in a cross-sectional questionnaire survey, the units would be individuals and the items their answers to the questions. In a household survey, the units would be households, and the items information about the household and members of the household. In longitudinal studies, units would typically be individuals while items would be longitudinal data from those individuals. In this book, units therefore correspond to the highest level in multilevel (i.e., hierarchical) data, and unless stated otherwise data from different units are statistically independent.

Within this framework, it is useful to distinguish between units where all the information is missing, termed *unit nonresponse* and units who contribute partial information, termed *item nonresponse*. The statistical issues are the same in both cases, and both can in principle be handled by MI. However, the main focus of this book is the latter.

Example 1.1 Mandarin tableau

Figure 1.1, which is also shown on the cover, shows part of the frontage of a senior mandarin's house in the New Territories, Hong Kong. We suppose interest focuses on characteristics of the figurines, for example their number, height, facial characteristics and dress. Unit nonresponse then corresponds to missing figurines, and item nonresponse to damaged – hence partially observed – figurines. □

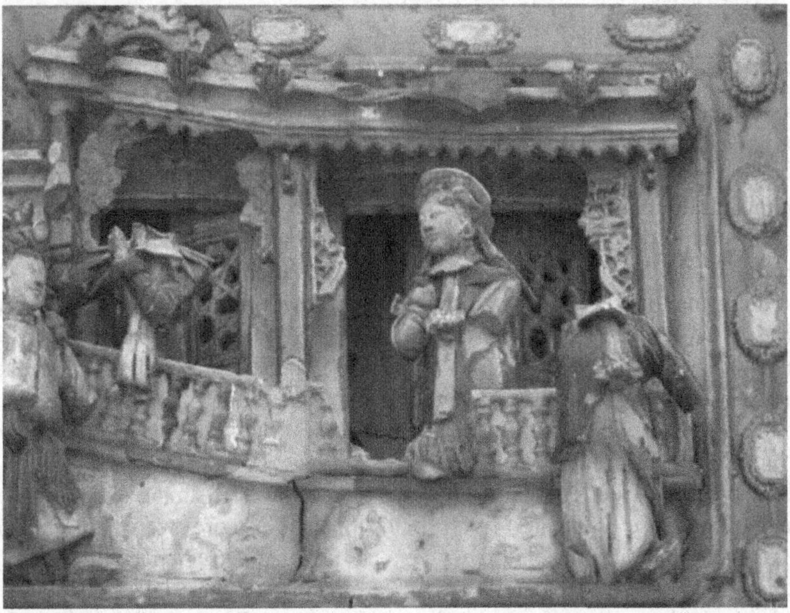

Figure 1.1 Detail from a senior mandarin's house front in New Territories, Hong Kong. Photograph by H. Goldstein.

1.2 Examples

We now introduce two key examples, which we return to throughout the book.

Example 1.2 Youth Cohort Study (YCS)

The Youth Cohort Study of England and Wales (YCS) is an ongoing UK government funded representative survey of pupils in England and Wales at school-leaving age (School year 11, age 16–17) (UK Data Archive, 2007). Each year that a new cohort is surveyed, detailed information is collected on each young person's experience of education and their qualifications as well as information on employment and training. A limited amount of information is collected on their personal characteristics, family, home circumstances, and aspirations.

Over the life-cycle of the YCS, different organisations have had responsibility for the structure and timings of data collection. Unfortunately, the documentation of older cohorts is poor. Croxford *et al.* (2007) have recently deposited a harmonised dataset that comprises YCS cohorts from 1984 to 2002 (UK Data Archive Study Number 5765). We consider data from pupils attending comprehensive schools from five YCS cohorts; these pupils reached the end of Year 11 in 1990, 1993, 1995, 1997 and 1999.

We explore relationships between Year 11 educational attainment (the General Certificate of Secondary Education) and key measures of social stratification. The units are pupils and the items are measurements on these pupils, and a nontrivial number of items are partially observed. □

Example 1.3 Randomised controlled trial of patients with chronic asthma

We consider data from a 5-arm asthma clinical trial to assess the efficacy and safety of budesonide, a second-generation glucocorticosteroid, on patients with chronic asthma. 473 patients with chronic asthma were enrolled in the 12-week randomised, double-blind, multi-centre parallel-group trial, which compared the effect of a daily dose of 200, 400, 800 or 1600 mcg of budesonide with placebo.

Key outcomes of clinical interest include patients' peak expiratory flow rate (their maximum speed of expiration in litres/minute) and their Forced Expiratory Volume, FEV_1, (the volume of air, in litres, the patient with fully inflated lungs can breathe out in one second). In summary, the trial found a statistically significant dose-response effect for the mean change from baseline over the study for both morning peak expiratory flow, evening peak expiratory flow and FEV_1, at the 5% level.

Budesonide treated patients also showed reduced asthma symptoms and bronchodilator use compared with placebo, while there were no clinically significant differences in treatment related adverse experiences between the treatment groups. Further details about the conduct of the trial, its conclusions and the variables collected can be found elsewhere (Busse *et al.*, 1998). Here, we focus on FEV_1 and confine our attention to the placebo and lowest active dose arms. FEV_1 was collected at baseline, then 2, 4, 8 and 12 weeks after randomisation. The intention was to compare FEV_1 across treatment arms at 12 weeks. However, excluding 3 patients whose participation in the study was intermittent, only 37 out of 90 patients in the placebo arm, and 71 out of 90 patients in the lowest active dose arm, still remained in the trial at twelve weeks. □

1.3 Patterns of missing data

It is very important to investigate the patterns of missing data before embarking on a formal analysis. This can throw up vital information that might otherwise be overlooked, and may even allow the missing data to be traced. For example, when analysing the new wave of a longitudinal survey, a colleague's careful examination of missing data patterns established that many of the missing questionnaires could be traced to a set of cardboard boxes. These turned out to have been left behind in a move. They were recovered and the data entered.

Most statistical software now has tools for describing the pattern of missing data. Key questions concern the extent and patterns of missing values, and whether the pattern is *monotone* (as described in the next paragraph), as if it is, this can considerably speed up and simplify the analysis.

Missing data in a set of p variables are said to follow a *monotone missingness pattern* if the variables can be re-ordered such that, for every unit i and variable j,

1. if unit i is observed on variable j, where $j = 2, \ldots, p$, it is observed on all variables $j' < j$, and
2. if unit i is missing on variable j, where $j = 2, \ldots, p$, it is missing on all variables $j' > j$.

A natural setting for the occurrence of monotone missing data is a longitudinal study, where units are observed either until they are lost to follow-up, or the study concludes. A monotone pattern is thus inconsistent with interim missing data, where units are observed for a period, missing for the subsequent period, but then observed. Questionnaires may also give rise to monotone missing data patterns when individuals systematically answer each question in turn from the beginning till they either stop or complete the questionnaire. In other settings it may be possible to re-order items to achieve a monotone pattern.

Example 1.2 Youth Cohort Study *(ctd)*

Table 1.1 shows the covariates we consider from the YCS. There are no missing data in the variables *cohort* and *boy*. The missingness pattern for GCSE score and the remaining two variables is shown in Table 1.2. In this example it is not possible to re-order the variables (items) to obtain a monotone pattern, due for example, to pattern 3 (N = 697). □

Table 1.1 YCS variables for exploring the relationship between Year 11 attainment and social stratification.

Variable name	Description
cohort	year of data collection: 1990, 93, 95, 97, 99
boy	indicator variable for boys
occupation	parental occupation, categorised as managerial, intermediate or working
ethnicity	categorised as Bangladeshi, Black, Indian, other Asian, Other, Pakistani or White

Table 1.2 Pattern of missing values in the YCS data.

Pattern	GCSE score	Occupation	Ethnicity	No.	% of total
1	✓	✓	✓	55145	87%
2	✓	·	✓	6821	11%
3	·	✓	✓	697	1%
4	✓	·	·	592	1%

Example 1.3 Asthma study *(ctd)*

Table 1.3 shows the withdrawal pattern for the placebo and lowest active dose arms (all the patients are receiving their randomised medication). We have removed three patients with unusual interim missing data from Table 1.3 and all our analyses. The remaining missingness pattern is monotone in both treatment arms. □

Table 1.3 Asthma study: withdrawal pattern by treatment arm.

Dropout pattern	Placebo arm						
	Mean FEV_1 (litres) measured at week					Number	Percent
	0	2	4	8	12		
1	✓	✓	✓	✓	✓	37	41
2	✓	✓	✓	✓	·	15	17
3	✓	✓	✓	·	·	22	24
4	✓	✓	·	·	·	16	18
	Lowest Active arm						
1	✓	✓	✓	✓	✓	71	79
2	✓	✓	✓	✓	·	8	9
3	✓	✓	✓	·	·	8	9
4	✓	✓	·	·	·	3	3

1.3.1 Consequences of missing data

Our focus is the practical implications of missing data for both parameter estimation and inference. Unfortunately, the two are often conflated, so that a computational method for parameter estimation when data are missing is said to have 'solved' or 'handled' the missing data issue. Since, with missing data, computational methods only lead to valid inference under specific assumptions, this attitude is likely to lead to misleading inferences.

In this context, it may be helpful to draw an analogy with the sampling process used to collect the data. If an analyst is presented with a spreadsheet containing columns of numerical data, they can analyse the data (calculate means of variables, regress variables on each other and so forth). However, they cannot draw any inferences unless they are told how and from whom the data were collected. This information is external to the numerical values of the variables.

We may think of the missing data mechanism as a second stage in the sampling process, but one that is not under our control. It acts on the data we intended to collect and leaves us with a partially observed dataset. Once again, the missing data mechanism cannot usually be definitively identified from the observed data, although the observed data may indicate plausible mechanisms (e.g. response may be negatively correlated with age). Thus we will need to make an assumption about the missingness mechanism in order to draw inference. The process of making this assumption is quite separate from the statistical methods we use for parameter estimation etc. Further, to the extent that the missing data mechanism cannot be definitively identified from the data, we will often wish to check the robustness of our inferences to a range of missingness mechanisms that are consistent with the observed data. The reason this book focuses on the statistical method of MI is that it provides a computationally feasible approach to the analysis for a wide range of problems under a range of missingness mechanisms.

We therefore begin with a typology for the mechanisms causing, or generating, the missing data. Later in this chapter we will see that consideration of these mechanisms in the context of the analysis at hand clarifies the assumptions under which a simple analysis, such as restriction to complete records, will be valid. It also clarifies when more sophisticated computational approaches such as MI will be valid and informs the way they are conducted. We stress again that the mechanism causing the missing data can rarely be definitively established. Thus we will often wish to explore the robustness of our inferences to a range of plausible missingness mechanisms – a process we call *sensitivity analysis*.

From a general standpoint, missing data may cause two problems: loss of efficiency and bias.

First, loss of efficiency, or information, is an inevitable consequence of missing data. Unfortunately, the extent of information loss is not directly linked to the proportion of incomplete records. Instead it is intrinsically linked to the analysis question. When crossing the road, the rear of the oncoming traffic is hidden from view – the data are missing. However, these missing data do not bear on the question at hand – will I make it across the road safely? While the proportion of missing data about each oncoming vehicle is substantial, information loss is negligible. Conversely, when estimating the prevalence of a rare disease, a small proportion of missing observations could have a disproportionate impact on the resulting estimate.

Faced with an incomplete dataset, most software automatically restricts analysis to complete records. As we illustrate below, the consequence of this for loss of information is not always easy to predict. Nevertheless, in many settings it will be important to include the information from partially complete records. Not least of the reasons for this is the time and money it has taken to collect even the partially complete records. Under certain assumptions about the missingness mechanism, we shall see that MI provides a natural way to do this.

Second, and perhaps more fundamentally, the subset of complete records may not be representative of the population under study. Restricting analysis to complete records may then lead to biased inference. The extent of such bias depends on the statistical behaviour of the missing data. A formal framework to describe this behaviour is thus fundamental. Such a framework was first elucidated in a seminal paper by Rubin (1976). To describe this, we need some definitions.

1.4 Inferential framework and notation

For clarity we take a frequentist approach to inference. This is not essential or necessarily desirable; indeed we will see that MI is essentially a Bayesian method, with good frequentist properties. Often, as Chapter 2 shows, formally showing these frequentist properties is most difficult theoretically.

We suppose we have a sample of n units, which will often be individuals, from a population that for practical inferential purposes can be considered infinite. Let $\mathbf{Y}_i = (Y_{i,1}, Y_{i,2}, \ldots, Y_{i,p})^T$ denote the p variables we intended to collect from the ith unit, $i = 1 \ldots, n$. We wish to use these data to make inferences about a set of p population parameters $\boldsymbol{\theta} = (\theta_1, \ldots, \theta_p)^T$.

For each unit $i = 1, \ldots, n$ let $\mathbf{Y}_{i,O}$ denote the subset of p variables that are observed, and $\mathbf{Y}_{i,M}$ denote the subset that are missing. Thus, for different individuals, $\mathbf{Y}_{i,O}$ and $\mathbf{Y}_{i,M}$ may well be different subsets of the p variables. If no data are missing, $\mathbf{Y}_{i,M}$ will be empty.

Next, again for each individual $i = 1, \ldots, n$ and variable $j = 1, \ldots, p$, let $R_{i,j} = 1$ if $Y_{i,j}$ is observed and $R_{i,j} = 0$ if $Y_{i,j}$ is missing. Let $\mathbf{R}_i = (R_{i,1}, \ldots, R_{i,p})^T$. Consistent with the definition of monotone missingness patterns on p. 10, the pattern is monotone if the p variables can be re-ordered so that for each unit i,

$$R_{i,j} = 0 \implies R_{i,j'} = 0 \text{ for } j' = j + 1, \ldots, p. \tag{1.1}$$

The missing value mechanism is then formally defined as

$$\Pr(\mathbf{R}_i | \mathbf{Y}_i), \tag{1.2}$$

that is to say the probability of observing unit i's data given their potentially unseen values $\mathbf{Y}_i$. It is important to note that, in what follows, we assume that unit i's data exist (or at least existed). In other words, if it had been possible for us to be in the right place at the right time, we would have been able to observe the complete data. What (1.2) describes therefore, is the probability that the data collection we were able to undertake on unit i yielded values of $Y_{i,O}$. Thus, (at least until we consider sensitivity analysis for clinical trials in Chapter 10) the missing data are not counter-factual, in the sense of what might have happened if a patient had taken a different drug from the one they actually took, or a child had gone to a different school from the one they actually attended.

Example 1.1 Mandarin tableau *(ctd)*

Here, $\mathbf{Y}_i$ take the form of observations on the $n = 4$ figurines, describing for example their size and dress. $R_{i,j}$ indicates those observations that are missing on figurine i because its head is missing. Originally, of course, all the heads were present, so we can refer to the underlying values of the unobserved variables. □

Example 1.2 Youth Cohort Study (YCS) *(ctd)*

Here, underlying values of missing GCSE score, parental occupation and ethnicity exist, and given sufficient time and money we would be able to discover many of them. □

Example 1.3 Asthma study *(ctd)*

Were resources not limited, researchers could have visited each patient in their home at each of the scheduled follow-up times to record their data. □

We now come to the three classes of missing data mechanism. These describe how the probability of seeing the data depends on the observed, and unobserved (but potentially observable, or underlying) values. In general, depending on the context, we will think of the same mechanism applying either to all $i = 1, \ldots, n$ units in the data set, or to an independent subset of them.

1.4.1 Missing Completely At Random (MCAR)

We say data are *Missing Completely At Random (MCAR)* if the probability of a value being missing is unrelated to the observed and unobserved data on that unit. Algebraically,

$$\Pr(\mathbf{R}_i|\mathbf{Y}_i) = \Pr(\mathbf{R}_i). \tag{1.3}$$

Since, when data are MCAR, the chance of the data being missing is unrelated to the values, the observed data are therefore representative of the population. However, relative to the data we intended to collect, information has been lost.

Example 1.1 Mandarin tableau *(ctd)*

Suppose we wish to summarise facial characteristics of the figurines, e.g. average head circumference. If the missing heads are MCAR, a valid estimate is obtained from the observed heads. Although valid, it is imprecise relative to an estimate based on all the heads.

Before moving on, note that the MCAR assumption is made for a specific analysis. It is not a property of the tableau. It may be plausible to assume that headgear is MCAR, while heads may systematically be missing because of racial characteristics. Further, if we step back from the tableau, we may see that missing heads correspond to missing, or recently replaced, roof tiles. If so, the mechanism causing the missing data is clear: however the assumption of MCAR is still likely to be appropriate, because the mechanism causing the missing data is unlikely to bear on (i.e., is likely statistically independent of) the analysis question.

Similarly, in certain settings we may find that the variables predictive of missing data are independent of the substantive analysis at hand. This is consistent with the MCAR assumption: analysis of the complete records will be unbiased, but some precision is lost. □

Example 1.2 Youth Cohort Study *(ctd)*

If data are MCAR in the YCS study, valid inference would be obtained from the 55145 complete records (Table 1.2). However, omitting the 8110 individuals with partial information means inferences are less precise than they could be. □

Example 1.3 Asthma study *(ctd)*

Assuming data are MCAR, a valid estimate of the overall mean in each group at 12 weeks is obtained by simply averaging the 37 available observations in the placebo group and the 71 available observations in the active group. This gives, respectively 2.05 l (s.e. 0.09) and 2.23 l (s.e. 0.10). □

1.4.2 Missing At Random (MAR)

We say data are *Missing At Random (MAR)* if *given, or conditional on, the observed data* the probability distribution of $\mathbf{R}_i$ is independent of the unobserved data. Recalling that for individual i we can partition $\mathbf{Y}_i$ as $(\mathbf{Y}_{i,O}, \mathbf{Y}_{i,M})$ we can express this mathematically as

$$\Pr(\mathbf{R}_i|\mathbf{Y}_i) = \Pr(\mathbf{R}_i|\mathbf{Y}_{i,O}). \tag{1.4}$$

This does not mean – as is sometimes supposed – that the probability of observing a variable on an individual is independent of the value of that variable. Quite the contrary: under MAR the chance of observing a variable will depend on its value. Crucially though, given the observed data this dependence is broken. Consider the following example.

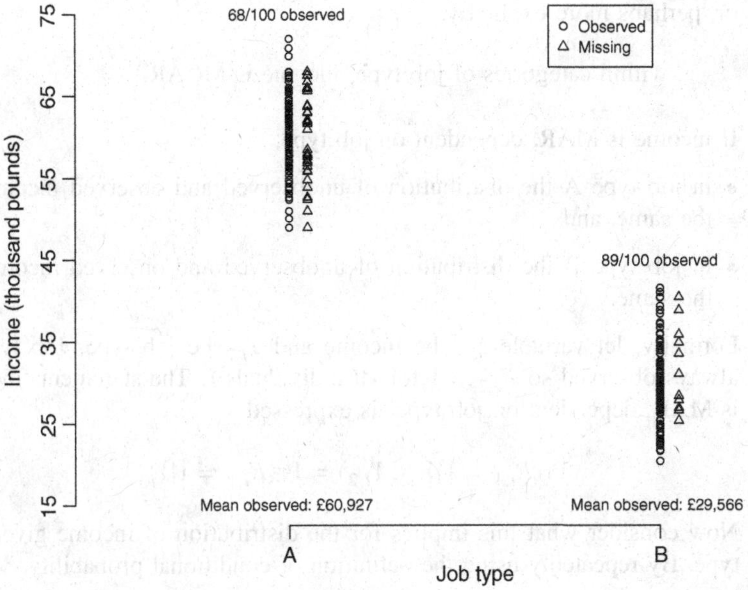

Figure 1.2 Plot of 200 hypothetical incomes against job type.

Example 1.4 Income and job type

Suppose we survey 100 employees of job type A and B for their income. Only 157 reveal their income, as shown in Figure 1.2. The figure shows that employees with higher incomes are less likely to divulge them: the probability of observing a variable depends on its value. However, if within job type A the probability of observing income does not depend on income, and within job type B the probability of observing income does not depend on income, then income is missing at random dependent on job type. □

The immediate consequence of this is that the mean of the observed incomes, marginal to (or aggregating over) job type is biased downwards. The data were generated with a mean income of £60,000 in job type A and £30,000 in job type B, so that the true mean income is £45,000. Contrast the observed mean income of

$$(68 \times 60927 + 89 \times 29566)/157 = £43,149.$$

We note three further points. First, if within job type the probability of observing income does not depend on income, it follows that:

1. To say 'income is MAR' is incomplete; we need instead to specify the variable which we assume makes income conditionally independent of job type. We could say

   'income is MAR, dependent on job type'

or, perhaps more explicitly,

'within categories of job type, income is MCAR.'

2. If income is MAR, dependent on job type,
   - in job type A the distribution of unobserved and observed incomes is the same, and
   - in job type B the distribution of unobserved and observed incomes is the same.

   Formally, let variable $Y_{i,1}$ be income and $Y_{i,2}$ be job type. Job type is always observed so $R_{i,2} = 1$ for all individuals i. The statement 'income is MAR, dependent on job type' is expressed

$$\Pr(R_{i,1} = 1|Y_{i,1}, Y_{i,2}) = \Pr(R_{i,1} = 1|Y_{i,2}). \tag{1.5}$$

   Now consider what this implies for the distribution of income given job type. By repeatedly using the definition of conditional probability

$$\begin{aligned}\Pr(Y_{i,1}|Y_{i,2}, R_{i,1} = 1) &= \frac{\Pr(Y_{i,1}, Y_{i,2}, R_{i,1} = 1)}{\Pr(Y_{i,2}, R_{i,1} = 1)} \\ &= \frac{\Pr(R_{i,1} = 1|Y_{i,1}, Y_{i,2})\Pr(Y_{i,1}, Y_{i,2})}{\Pr(R_{i,1} = 1|Y_{i,2})\Pr(Y_{i,2})} \\ &= \Pr(Y_{i,1}|Y_{i,2}),\end{aligned} \tag{1.6}$$

   where the last step follows from MAR, i.e., (1.5). The argument (1.6) holds if income is not observed, $R_{i,1} = 0$. Thus under MAR the distribution of income within job type is the same in the observed data, the unobserved data, and the population.
   In this case, to estimate the marginal income we average the observed income in each job type and then scale up:

$$(100 \times 60927 + 100 \times 29566)/200 = £45{,}247. \tag{1.7}$$

   Notice that to obtain this estimate we did not need to explicitly specify how the probability of observing income depends on job type; merely that given job type it does not depend on income.

3. The statement 'income is MAR, dependent on job type' is an untestable assumption. The data we would need to test it (represented by the triangles in Figure 1.2) is missing!

Of course, were it observed, we could 'test the MAR assumption' in two ways: first a logistic regression, for example:

$$\operatorname{logit} \Pr\{(R_{i,1} = 1)\} = \alpha_0 + \alpha_1 Y_{i,1} + \alpha_2 Y_{i,2} + \alpha_3 Y_{i,1} Y_{i,2};$$

if MAR is true then the hypothesis $\alpha_1 = \alpha_3 = 0$ is true. Or, we could fit a corresponding regression:

$$\mathrm{E}(Y_{i,1}) = \beta_0 + \beta_1 Y_{i,2} + \beta_2 R_{i,1} + \beta_3 Y_{i,2} R_{i,1};$$

If MAR is true then the hypothesis $\beta_2 = \beta_3 = 0$ is true.

This simple example draws out the following general points:

1. statements relating the probability of observing data to the values of data have direct consequences for conditional distributions of the data, and
2. under the MAR assumption, the precise missing data mechanism need not be specified; indeed the precise form can be different for different individuals.

These two points together mean that the MAR mechanism is much more subtle than might at first appear; these subtleties can manifest themselves unexpectedly.

Example 1.4 Income and job type *(ctd)*

Suppose the mechanism causing the missing income differed for each of the 200 individuals, that is

$$\operatorname{logit} \Pr(R_{i,1} = 1) = \alpha_{0,i} + \alpha_{1,i} Y_{i,2}.$$

Then missing data are still MAR, and (1.7) is still a valid estimate. □

Of course, it may be as contrived to think each individual has their own MAR mechanism as to think that the same mechanism holds for all. In a simple example this is not important, but in real applications a blanket assumption of MAR may be very contrived.

Example 1.5 Subtlety of MAR assumption

Suppose we have three variables, $Y_{i,1}, Y_{i,2}, Y_{i,3}$, and we are unfortunate, so that our dataset contains nontrivial numbers of all possible missingness patterns, as shown in Table 1.4.

If the same missingness mechanism applies to all the units, and it is either MAR or MCAR, then it must be MCAR. If we wish to assume data are MAR, we are forced to split the data into groups among which different MAR mechanisms are operating. These groups need not necessarily be defined by the missing data

Table 1.4 Three variables: all possible missing value patterns.

Pattern	Y_1	Y_2	Y_3
1	✓	✓	✓
2	✓	✓	·
3	✓	·	✓
4	·	✓	✓
5	✓	·	·
6	·	✓	·
7	·	·	✓

patterns; they could be defined by characteristics of the units. Settings like this are considered by Harel and Schafer (2009). To illustrate, though, we define groups by the missing data patterns.

For a MAR mechanism, we might assume the following:

- in patterns (1, 2) $Y_{i,3}$ is MAR given $Y_{i,1}$, $Y_{i,2}$;
- in patterns (3, 4, 7) $Y_{i,1}$ and/or $Y_{i,2}$ is MAR given $Y_{i,3}$, and
- in patterns (5, 6) data are MCAR.

In practice, often a relatively small number of the possible missingness patterns predominate, and it is assumptions about these that are important for any analysis. The remaining – relatively infrequent – patterns can often be assumed MCAR, with little risk to the final inference if this assumption is in fact wrong. □

Faced with complex data, there is a temptation to invoke the MAR assumption too readily, especially as this simplifies any analysis using MI. To guard against this, analysts need to be satisfied that any associations assumed to justify the MAR assumption are at least consistent with the observed data. Since consideration of selection mechanisms may not be as straightforward as might first appear, it can also be worth considering the plausibility of MAR from the point of view of the joint and conditional distribution of the data. As (1.6) illustrates, for MAR we need to be satisfied

1. that conditional distributions of partially observed variables given fully observed variables do not differ depending on whether the data are observed, and
2. in consequence the joint distribution of the data can be validly estimated by piecing together the marginal distributions of the observed patterns.

The above discussion explains why we do not regard the MAR assumption as a panacea, but nevertheless often both a plausible and practical starting point for the analysis of partially observed data. In particular, the points drawn out of Example 1.4 are not specific to either the number or type of variables (categorical or quantitative).

Example 1.1 Mandarin tableau *(ctd)*

Here the MAR assumption says that the distribution of head characteristics given body characteristics (i.e., dress, height, etc.) does not depend on whether the head is present. Thus, under MAR we can estimate the distribution of characteristics of figurines with missing heads from figurines with similar body characteristics.

Notice the two rightmost figurines in Figure 1.1 share the same necktie. Assuming headdress is MAR given necktie, the missing headdress on the rightmost figurine is similar to that on the second rightmost figurine.

Clearly this assumption cannot be checked from the tableau (data) at hand. However it might be possible to explore it using other tableaux (i.e., other datasets). If MAR is plausible for headdress given necktie, it does not mean it is plausible for skin colour given necktie. In other words MAR is an assumption we make for the analysis, not a characteristic of the dataset. For some analyses of partially observed data it may be plausible; for others not. □

1.4.3 Missing Not At Random (MNAR)

If the mechanism causing missing data is neither MCAR nor MAR, we say it is Missing Not At Random (MNAR). Under a MNAR mechanism, the probability of an observation being missing depends on the underlying value, and this dependence remains even given the observed data. Mathematically,

$$\Pr(\mathbf{R}_i|\mathbf{Y}_i) \neq \Pr(\mathbf{R}_i|\mathbf{Y}_{i,O}). \tag{1.8}$$

While in some settings MNAR may be more plausible than MAR, analysis under MNAR is considerably harder. This is because under MAR, equation (1.6) showed that conditional distributions of partially observed variables given fully observed variables are the same in units who do, and do not, have the data observed. However (1.6) does not hold if (1.8) holds.

It follows that inference under MNAR involves an explicit specification of either the selection mechanism, or how conditional distributions of partially observed variables given fully observed variables differ between units who do, and do not, have the data observed.

Formally, we can write the joint distribution of unit i's variables, $\mathbf{Y}_i$, and the indicator for observing those variables, $\mathbf{R}_i$ as

$$\Pr(\mathbf{R}_i|\mathbf{Y}_i)\Pr(\mathbf{Y}_i) = \Pr(\mathbf{R}_i, \mathbf{Y}_i) = \Pr(\mathbf{Y}_i|\mathbf{R}_i)\Pr(\mathbf{R}_i). \tag{1.9}$$

In the centre is the joint distribution, and this can be written either as

1. a *selection model* – the LHS of (1.9), i.e., a product of (i) the conditional probability of observing the variables, given their values and (ii) the marginal distribution of the data, OR

2. a pattern mixture model – the RHS of (1.9), i.e., a product of (i) the probability distribution of the data within each missingness pattern and (ii) the marginal probability of the missingness pattern.

Thus we can specify a MNAR mechanism either by specifying the selection model (which implies the pattern mixture model) or by specifying a pattern mixture model (which implies a selection model). Depending on the context, both approaches may be helpful. Unfortunately, even in apparently simple settings, explicitly calculating the selection implication of a pattern mixture model, or vice versa, can be awkward. We shall see in Chapter 10 that an advantage of multiple imputation is that, given a pattern mixture model, we can estimate the selection model implications quite easily.

Once again, as the example below shows, MNAR is an assumption for the analysis, not a characteristic of the data.

Example 1.1 Mandarin tableau *(ctd)*

It may be that the figurines with missing heads were wearing a head dress that identified them as a member of a class, or group, that subsequently became very unpopular – causing the heads to be smashed. This MNAR selection mechanism means that we cannot say anything about the typical characteristics of head dress without making untestable assumptions about the characteristics of the missing head dresses. Further, the MNAR assumption implies that the distribution of head dress given body dress is different for figurines with missing and observed heads.

We reiterate, under MNAR any summary statistics, or analyses, require *either* explicit assumptions about the form of the distribution of the missing data given the observed *or* explicit specification of the selection mechanism and the marginal distribution of the full (including unobserved) data. Contrast this with analyses assuming MAR, where these assumptions are made implicitly.

We repeat a point from the tableau: if head dress was the trigger for missing heads, but the type of head dress worn is not related to physical characteristics of the heads, analyses concerning their physical characteristics could be validly performed under MAR. Just because the heads are MNAR does not mean all analyses require the MNAR assumption. This underlines that, in applications, it is crucial to think carefully about the selection mechanism, and how it affects the analysis question. □

Example 1.6 Income MNAR

To illustrate (1.9), consider a simplified version of the income example above. Suppose that of the 100 people surveyed, 50 have the same income θ_L, and 50 have the same higher income, θ_U. Suppose further that all those with income θ_L disclose it, but only a fraction π of those with income θ_U disclose it.

This is an example of pattern mixture model, i.e., the RHS of (1.9). Let $1[\,.\,]$ be 1 if the statement in brackets is true and 0 otherwise. Then, in this simple example, it is clear what the the selection counterpart is:

$$\Pr(\text{income observed}) = 1 + (\pi - 1) \times 1[\text{income} = \theta_U], \quad \text{and}$$
$$\text{mean income} = (\theta_L + \theta_U)/2.$$

The pattern mixture model implies a selection model.

We now illustrate the same point with a bivariate normal model. Let Y denote income; to keep the algebra simple suppose $Y \sim N(0, 1)$, and we drop the index i. Let $R = 1$ if Y is observed, but now let $X \sim N(\mu_x, 1)$ be a normally distributed variable, correlated with Y, which is positive if Y is observed, that is when $R = 1$. We specify the selection model, and derive the pattern mixture model.

Let $\Phi(.)$ be the cumulative distribution of the standard normal, and suppose we choose the selection model as

$$\Pr(R = 1|Y) = \Pr(X > 0|Y) = \Phi(\alpha_0 + \alpha_1 Y). \tag{1.10}$$

Equation (1.10) thus assumes a specific MNAR mechanism, for α_0 and α_1 cannot be estimated from the observed values of Y.

Given (1.10) and the marginal standard normal distribution of Y, the joint distribution of (Y, X) is bivariate normal:

$$\begin{pmatrix} Y \\ X \end{pmatrix} \sim N\left[\begin{pmatrix} 1 \\ \mu_x \end{pmatrix}, \begin{pmatrix} 1 & \rho \\ \rho & 1 \end{pmatrix}\right], \tag{1.11}$$

where $\rho = \text{corr}(Y, X)$. Thus we have the central term in (1.9). It follows that

$$\Pr(X_i|y_i) \sim N\{\mu_x + \rho Y_i, (1 - \rho^2)\}.$$

Thus

$$\Pr(X > 0|Y) = \Phi\left(\frac{\mu_x + \rho Y}{\sqrt{1 - \rho^2}}\right) = \Phi\left(\frac{\mu_x}{\sqrt{1 - \rho^2}} + \frac{\rho}{\sqrt{1 - \rho^2}} Y\right).$$

Comparing with (1.10) we see $\rho = g(\alpha_1)$ and $\mu_x = h(\alpha_0, \alpha_1)$. Hence (α_0, α_1) define μ_x, which in turn defines the marginal probability, $\Pr(X > 0)$, of observing Y.

From the bivariate normal (1.11) the distribution of observed income, Y given $R = 1$ is $Y|x > 0$ which is

$$\frac{\phi(Y)}{\Phi(\mu_x)} \Phi\left(\frac{\mu_x + \rho Y}{\sqrt{1 - \rho^2}}\right) = \frac{\phi(Y)}{\Phi\{h(\alpha_0, \alpha_1)\}} \Phi(\alpha_0 + \alpha_1 Y).$$

A similar result follows for the distribution of unobserved income. Putting this together, we have arrived at the pattern mixture model, the RHS of (1.9). Specification of the selection mechanism, through α_0, α_1, together with the marginal distribution of income, fixes both the marginal probability of observing income and the distribution of the two 'patterns' of data: the seen and unseen incomes.

This is a simple example of the Heckman selection model, which is further discussed in Little and Rubin (1987), Ch. 11. More recently, it has also been used as a model for publication bias in meta analysis (Copas and Shi, 2000a). □

The example above illustrates that when data are MNAR, instead of thinking about the selection mechanism, it is equally appropriate to consider differences between conditional distributions of partially observed given fully observed variables. Under MAR such distributions do not differ depending on whether data is missing or not; under MNAR they do. Considering the conditional distribution of the observed data, and then exploring the robustness of inference as it is allowed to differ in the unobserved data, is therefore a natural way to explore the robustness of inference to an assumption of MAR. From our perspective it has two further advantages: (i) the differences can be expressed simply and pictorially, and (ii) MI provides a natural route for inference. Unfortunately, the selection counterparts, or implications, of pattern mixture models are rarely easy to calculate directly, but again MI can help: after imputing missing data under a pattern mixture model, it is straightforward to explore implications for the implied selection model.

Example 1.3 Asthma study ***(ctd)***

We illustrate the above using the 12 week data from the asthma study. Suppose first that 12 week response is MAR given treatment group. Then, in each treatment group the mean of unobserved and observed data are the same, so the treatment effect is $2.23 - 2.05 = 0.18$ litres. Suppose we have a MNAR mechanism and we express this as a pattern mixture model. Let μ_P, μ_A be the mean response under placebo and active treatment. Then

$$\mu_P = 37 \times 2.05 + (90 - 37) \times (2.05 + \Delta_P), \text{ and}$$

$$\mu_A = 71 \times 2.23 + (90 - 71) \times (2.23 + \Delta_A),$$

where Δ_P, Δ_A are respectively the mean differences between observed and unobserved response in the placebo and active group.

Figure 1.3 shows how the estimated treatment effect varies as we move away from the assumption of MAR, i.e., that $\Delta_p = \Delta_A = 0$. Since many more patients are missing in the placebo group, the treatment estimate is much more sensitive to departures from MAR in this group.

Notice the inherently arbitrary nature of MNAR: because we cannot estimate Δ_A, Δ_P from the data at hand, all possible values are – in general – equally plausible. This issue is the motivation for our proposed approach to sensitivity analysis in clinical trials of this type in Section 10.4. □

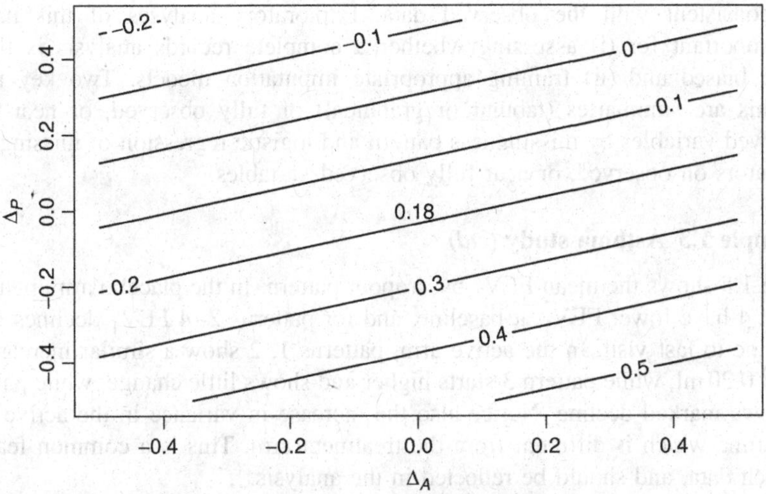

Figure 1.3 Contour plot of the difference in average FEV_1 (litres) between active and placebo groups, as Δ_P, Δ_A, vary. Under MAR, $\Delta_P = \Delta_A = 0$, and the difference is 0.18 litres.

1.4.4 Ignorability

If, under a specific assumption about the missingness mechanism, we can construct a valid analysis that does not require us to explicitly include the model for that missing value mechanism, we term the mechanism, in the context of this analysis, *ignorable*.

A common example of this is a likelihood based analysis assuming MAR.

However, as we see below there are other settings, where we do not assume MAR, that do not require us to explicitly include the model for the missingness mechanism yet still result in valid inference. For example, as discussed in Section 1.6.2, a complete records regression analysis is valid if data are MNAR dependent only on the covariates.

1.5 Using observed data to inform assumptions about the missingness mechanism

We have already noted that, given the observed data, we cannot definitively identify the missingness mechanism. Nevertheless, the observed data can help frame plausible assumptions about this – in other words assumptions which are consistent with the observed data. Exploratory analyses of this nature are important for (i) assessing whether a complete records analysis is likely to be biased and (ii) framing appropriate imputation models. Two key tools for this are summaries (tabular or graphical) of fully observed, or near-fully observed variables by missingness pattern and logistic regression of missingness indicators on observed, or near-fully observed variables.

Example 1.3 Asthma study *(ctd)*

Table 1.5 shows the mean FEV_1 by dropout pattern. In the placebo arm, patterns 3 and 4 have lower FEV_1 at baseline, and for patterns 2–4 FEV_1 declines from baseline to last visit. In the active arm, patterns 1, 2 show a similar increase of about 0.20 ml, while pattern 3 starts higher and shows little change, while pattern 4 shows marked decline. Notice also the increase in variance in the active arm over time which is different from the treatment arm. This is a common feature of such data, and should be reflected in the analysis.

MAR mechanisms that are dependent on treatment and response are consistent with these data. However, there is a suspicion that further decline between the last observed and first missing visit triggered withdrawal, probably followed in the placebo arm by switching to an active treatment. Thus it would be useful to explore sensitivity of treatment inferences to MNAR, which we do in Chapter 10. □

Table 1.5 Asthma study: mean FEV_1 (litres) at each visit, by dropout pattern and intervention arm.

Dropout pattern	Placebo arm						
	Mean FEV_1 (litres) measured at week					No.	%
	0	2	4	8	12		
1	2.11	2.14	2.07	2.01	2.06	37	40
2	2.31	2.18	1.95	2.13	–	15	16
3	1.96	1.73	1.84	–	–	22	24
4	1.84	1.72	–	–	–	16	17
All patients (Mean)	2.06	1.97	1.98	2.04	2.06	90	100
All patients (Std.)	0.57	0.67	0.56	0.58	0.55		
	Lowest Active arm						
1	2.03	2.22	2.23	2.24	2.23	71	78
2	1.93	1.91	2.01	2.14	–	8	9
3	2.28	2.10	2.29	–	–	8	9
4	2.24	1.84	–	–	–	3	3
All patients (Mean)	2.03	2.17	2.22	2.23	2.23	90	100
All patients (Std.)	0.65	0.75	0.80	0.85	0.81		

Example 1.2 Youth Cohort Study *(ctd)*

In Table 1.2, we saw that the principal missing data pattern has missing parental occupation. Let $R_i = 1$ if parental occupation is observed, and zero otherwise. Table 1.6 shows the results of various logistic regressions of R on the remaining fully, or near fully observed, variables: GCSE score, ethnicity, gender and cohort. The Receiver Operating Characteristic (ROC) is an assessment of how well a model discriminates between the missing and observed parental occupation, with a minimum value of 0.5 (no discrimination) and a maximum of 1. Of course, even if the model discriminated perfectly, this would say nothing about differences between observed and unobserved data, that is, whether the data are MNAR.

We see that GCSE score is the strongest predictor of missing parental occupation (ROC of 0.68), followed by ethnicity (here simplified to white/non-white) and cohort. Gender is a relatively weak predictor. Nevertheless, due to the size of the cohort, all are significant at the 5% level in model 4, which has reasonable discrimination (ROC = 0.74).

Figure 1.4 confirms that GCSE score is substantially higher among those whose parental occupation is observed (mean of 39 vs 28 points respectively). Further, 10% of children with missing parental occupation have no GCSEs (score 0) compared with 3% who have parental occupation observed.

We conclude the data are consistent with parental occupation missing at random, dependent strongly on GCSE score and ethnic group, but also associated

Table 1.6 Coefficients (standard errors), and receiver operating characteristic (ROC), from logistic models for the probability of observing parental occupation.

Variable	Models				
	1	2	3	4	5
cohort '93	−0.085				−0.168
	(0.036)				(0.039)
cohort '95	0.044				−0.212
	(0.038)				(0.042)
cohort '97	0.178				−0.032
	(0.040)				(0.043)
cohort '99	0.135				−0.165
	(0.040)				(0.046)
boy		−0.053			0.079
		(0.024)			(0.026)
GCSE score			0.037		0.038
			(0.001)		(0.001)
non-white				−1.723	−1.698
				(0.0288)	(0.031)
ROC	0.53	0.51	0.68	0.62	0.74

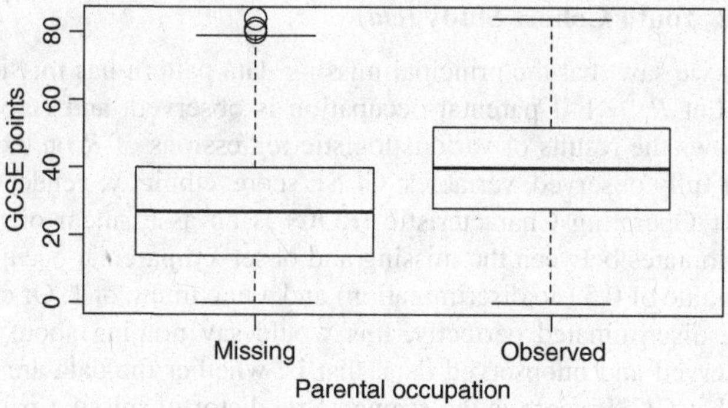

Figure 1.4 Boxplot of GCSE points by whether parental occupation is observed.

with cohort and weakly with gender. A relatively small number of values are missing for the other variables. It is plausible to assume these are either MCAR or perhaps MAR given observations on other variables; unless they are strongly MNAR this will have a negligible impact on subsequent inferences. □

1.6 Implications of missing data mechanisms for regression analyses

Usually, we will wish to fit some form of regression model to address our substantive questions. Here, we look at the implications, in terms of bias and loss of information, of missing data in the response and/or covariates under different missingness mechanisms. We first focus on linear regression; our findings there hold for most other regression models, including relative risk regression and survival analysis. Logistic regression is more subtle; we discuss this in Section 1.6.4.

1.6.1 Partially observed response

Suppose we wish to fit the model

$$Y_i = \beta_0 + \beta_1 x_i + e_i, \quad e_i \overset{i.i.d.}{\sim} N(0, \sigma^2), \quad i = 1, \ldots, n, \tag{1.12}$$

but Y is partially observed. Let R_i indicate whether Y_i is observed. For now assume that the x_i are known without error; for example it may be a design variable. Then the contribution to the likelihood for $\boldsymbol{\beta} = (\beta_0, \beta_1)$ from unit i, conditional on x_i, is

$$L_i = \Pr(R_i, Y_i | x_i) = \Pr(R_i | Y_i, x_i) \Pr(Y_i | x_i). \tag{1.13}$$

Assume, as will typically be the case, that the parameters of $\Pr(Y_i|x_i)$, $\boldsymbol{\beta}$, are distinct from the parameters of $\Pr(R_i|Y_i, x_i)$.

Figure 1.2 suggests that, provided Y is MAR given the covariates in the model, units with missing response have no information about $\boldsymbol{\beta}$. To see this formally, first observe that as Y_i is MAR given x_i, only the second term on the RHS of (1.13) involves Y.

The contribution to the likelihood for an individual with missing response is obtained by integrating (for discrete variables summing) over all possible values of the missing response variable Y_i, given x_i. This is

$$\int \Pr(Y_i|x_i)dY_i = 1,$$

because we are integrating (summing) over all possible values of Y_i given $\boldsymbol{\beta}, x_i$ so the total probability is 1. Conditional on x, all individuals with missing Y thus contribute 1 to likelihood for $\boldsymbol{\beta}$, and so have no effect on, or information about, the maximum likelihood estimate of $\boldsymbol{\beta}$.

This may feel counterintuitive, especially if we have a large number of units with Y missing but X observed. Do they really have no information on the regression?

For linear regression, the answer is yes (there is no information), because the parameter space of the conditional distribution of Y given X is separate from that of the marginal distribution for X. In other words, the mean and variance of X have no information on, and place no restriction on, the parameters of the distribution of $Y|X$. Equivalently, the conditional distribution of $\Pr(Y|X)$ has no information on, and places no restriction on, the marginal distribution of X.

Example 1.3 Asthma study *(ctd)*

To illustrate the above, consider estimating the effect of treatment on the 12 week response, adjusting for baseline, setting aside the measurements at 2, 4 and 8 weeks. If we assume that the 12 week response is MAR given treatment, then from the above argument it follows that fitting the regression model,

$$Y_i = \beta_0 + \beta_1 1[\text{treatment} = \text{active}_i] + e_i, \quad e_i \overset{i.i.d.}{\sim} N(0, \sigma^2), \tag{1.14}$$

using the complete records gives a valid estimate of the treatment effect (Table 1.7).

Now suppose, as Table 1.5 suggests, that baseline is also predictive of missing 12 week FEV_1; it is also strongly predictive of the actual 12 week FEV_1. Assuming 12 week FEV_1 is MAR given baseline and treatment, we can include baseline in the regression model (1.14). Again, the argument above shows that fitting this model to the observed data is valid and efficient; the results are in Table 1.7. Note that

Table 1.7 Asthma study: estimated treatment effect fitting treatment, and treatment and baseline. Inference is valid and fully efficient if assumption that data are MAR, dependent on the covariates in the model, is correct.

Covariates	n	Treatment estimate (s.e.)	p-value
Treat	108	0.172 L (0.149)	0.251
Treat & baseline	108	0.247 L (0.100)	0.016

(a) if baseline were predictive of underlying 12 week response, but given treatment not predictive of observing that response, we would still wish to include it, and

(b) in the unlikely case that baseline were predictive of missing 12 week response, but not related to the actual 12 week response value, there would be no benefit of including it.

We explore this study further, taking into account the longitudinal observations, in Chapters 3 and 7. □

The above argument extends naturally to partially observed multivariate responses. Suppose we have up to J observations on individual i, denoted $\mathbf{Y}_i = (Y_{i,1}, \ldots, Y_{i,j})$. Suppose they are MAR given X_i, and – whatever the pattern of missing data – we partition $\mathbf{Y}_i$ into $\mathbf{Y}_{i,O}$ and $\mathbf{Y}_{i,M}$. Then the contribution of individual i to the likelihood for the regression of $\mathbf{Y}$ on X is

$$\int \Pr(\mathbf{Y}_i | \boldsymbol{\beta}, X_i)\, d\mathbf{Y}_{i,M},$$

in other words, the marginal likelihood of the observed data. For the multivariate normal distribution, this is readily calculated; in fact most software fits the model to the observed pattern of data by default. Once again, in this setting there is no advantage to, or gain from, using multiple imputation.

The last setting we consider in this subsection is when we have missing response data, but these data are MNAR given the variables we wish to include in the model of interest. For a direct exposition we return to univariate Y_i; the extension to multivariate $\mathbf{Y}_i$ is immediate.

Consider (1.13) and let the parameters of $\Pr(R_i | Y_i, X_i)$ be η and distinct from those of $\Pr(Y_i | X_i)$, i.e., $\boldsymbol{\beta}$. The contribution to the likelihood from individual i is

$$\int \Pr(R_i, Y_i, X_i)\, dY_i = \Pr(X_i) \int \left\{\Pr(R_i | \eta, Y_i, X_i) \Pr(Y_i | \boldsymbol{\beta}, X_i)\right\} dY_i. \quad (1.15)$$

We see the likelihood contribution for $\boldsymbol{\beta}$ is now caught up with the selection mechanism; we have to evaluate the integral on the RHS of (1.15) to obtain the contribution of individual i to the likelihood. Failure to do this leads to biased inference for $\boldsymbol{\beta}$.

Example 1.7 Linear regression

To illustrate this, we generate a sample of 200 observations from the regression model

$$Y_i = \beta_0 + \beta_1 X_i + e_i, \quad e_i \overset{i.i.d.}{\sim} N(0, \sigma^2), \; i = 1, \ldots, n \tag{1.16}$$

with $(\alpha, \beta, \sigma^2) = (5, 1, 4^2)$. These data, together with the fitted regression, are shown in Figure 1.5(a), together with the least squares fitted line, which has estimated parameters $(\hat{\alpha}, \hat{\beta}) = (5.14, 1.01)$.

Now suppose that some of the Y values are MNAR, and $R_i = 1$ if Y_i is observed and 0 otherwise. Suppose

$$\Pr(R_i = 1) = \begin{cases} 0.8 & \text{if } Y_i > 18 \text{ and} \\ 0 & \text{otherwise} \end{cases} \tag{1.17}$$

Starting from the 200 observations shown in the left panel of Figure 1.5, the right panel plots a typical example of the complete records that remain under this mechanism. Fitting a regression line to the observed data gives $(\hat{\beta}_0, \hat{\beta}_1) = (5.75, 0.85)$. Because high values of Y, which correspond to high values of X, are likely to be missing, the intercept is biased slightly up and the slope down. □

Next, suppose that in addition to X, Y we have the fully observed variable Z. We suppose that Y is partially observed, we are interested in the regression of Y on X, that

$$\operatorname{logit} \Pr(R_i = 1) = \alpha_0 + \alpha_1 X_i + \alpha_2 Z_i, \tag{1.18}$$

and that Z is correlated with Y. Then, following from the discussion above, the regression of complete records Y_i on X_i will be biased, because setting Z aside

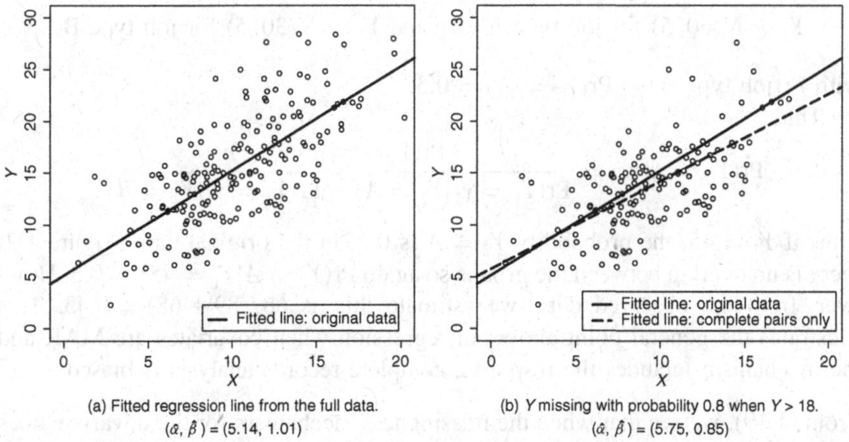

Figure 1.5 Regression lines for synthetic data. Left panel: fitted regression line to the full data, n = 200. Right panel, original and fitted line when Y is MNAR.

Y_i is MNAR. However, the regression of complete records Y_i on X_i, Z_i will be unbiased, and efficient, because given X and Z, Y is MAR.

1.6.2 Missing covariates

We now consider the regression of Y on X, when Y is fully observed and X is partially observed.

Let $R_i = 1$ if X_i is observed and $R_i = 0$ otherwise. Consider the regression of Y on X estimated from the complete records, i.e., given $R_i = 1$. Following (1.6), for each individual pair,

$$\begin{aligned} \Pr(Y_i|X_i, R_i = 1) &= \frac{\Pr(Y_i, X_i, R_i = 1)}{\Pr(X_i, R_i = 1)} \\ &= \frac{\Pr(R_i = 1|Y_i, X_i)\Pr(Y_i, X_i)}{\Pr(R_i = 1|X_i)\Pr(X_i)} \\ &= \left\{\frac{\Pr(R_i = 1|Y_i, X_i)}{\Pr(R_i = 1|X_i)}\right\}\Pr(Y_i|X_i). \end{aligned} \tag{1.19}$$

Thus, when the missingness mechanism for X, $\Pr(R_i = 1|Y_i, X_i)$, involves the response Y, restricting the analysis to the complete records gives biased point estimators and invalid inference. This holds whether the missingness mechanism only depends on Y, i.e., MAR, or whether it includes X as well, i.e., MNAR.

Example 1.6 Income *(ctd)*

Consider again the income example, but now suppose we wish to estimate the probability of job type given income, i.e., $\Pr(Y_{2,i}|Y_{1,i})$. As this is artificial data, we know the data generating mechanism:

$$Y_1 \sim N(60, 5) \text{ for job type A }, \quad \text{and } Y_1 \sim N(30, 5) \text{ for job type B},$$

with Pr(job type A) $= \Pr(Z_2 = A) = 0.5$.

Thus

$$\Pr(Y_2 = A|y_1) = \frac{\Pr(Y_1 = y_1|Y_2 = A)}{\Pr(Y_1 = y_1|Y_2 = A) + \Pr(Y_1 = y_1|Y_2 = B)}.$$

Thus if $Y_1 = 45$, the probability $Y_2 = A$ is 0.5. In the original data (Figure 1.2) there is no overlap between the groups so again $\Pr(Y_2 = A|Y_1 = 45) = 0.5$. However, from the observed data, we estimate this as $68/(89 + 68) = 0.43$. This illustrates the general point above: in regression when covariates are MAR and the mechanism includes the response, complete records analysis is biased. □

From (1.19), we see that when the missingness mechanism for the covariate does not depend on the response Y_i the probability of $Y|X$ among the complete records is the same as that in the population. In other words, although the covariate is MNAR, estimating the regression using complete records is unbiased and gives valid inference, although a full likelihood analysis with the correctly specified selection mechanism would be more efficient. Again, we note that the precise form of selection mechanism can vary between units or individuals; its precise form is not relevant to the argument.

Example 1.7 Linear regression *(ctd)*

Continuing with this example, suppose we take the original 100 pairs and set all X values greater than 12 to missing. This is a strong MNAR mechanism, but given the (possibly unobserved) X value, the probability of X being missing does not depend on Y. Figure 1.6(a) shows the regression of Y on X fitted to the remaining points and the fitted line to the original data. They are virtually indistinguishable. Indeed using the observed points, $(\hat{\beta}_0, \hat{\beta}_1) = (5.16, 1.00)$.

Thus, as (1.19) implies, there is no bias, but some information is lost. It is also important to note that (i) in this situation an analysis under MAR would be biased but (ii) given the observed data, we cannot conclude that X is MNAR dependent only on X; indeed it would be plausible to have X MAR, or MNAR dependent on Y and X. □

Now consider the setting where the covariate, X, is MNAR depending on both X and Y. In this setting, (1.19) implies regression using the complete records will be biased.

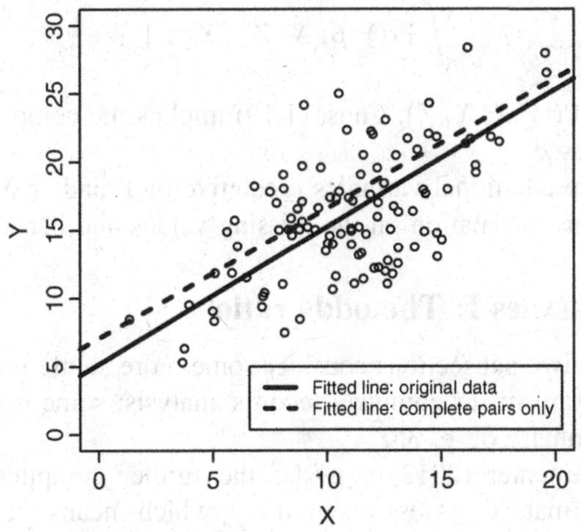

Figure 1.6 Missing covariates: effect of different mechanisms.

Example 1.7 Linear regression *(ctd)*

Continuing this example, suppose that

$$\Pr(X \text{ missing}) = \begin{cases} 0.8 \text{ if } Y < 15 \ \& \ X \ < 10 \\ 0.4 \text{ if } Y \geq 15 \ \& \ X \ \geq 10 \end{cases}$$

Figure 1.6(b) shows the results; the bias is clear. □

Lastly, consider the case where we have three variables (or sets of variables) X, Y, Z and we are interested in the regression of Y on X. Suppose X is MNAR given X, Z but that if we omit Z there is residual dependence of the missing mechanism on Y so that X is MNAR given X, Y.

In this setting, (1.19) shows us that using the complete records to regress Y on X will be biased; however, using the complete records to regress Y on X, Z will be unbiased for the latter, adjusted relationship. Unfortunately, unless Z is independent of X, so that including Z in the regression does not change the coefficient for X, it is not possible to use this to obtain a valid estimate of the regression of Y on X alone without making additional assumptions. Indeed, even if X is truly independent of Z, under a MNAR mechanism in the observed data they will typically be correlated.

1.6.3 Missing covariates and response

In our final, setting first suppose we have three variables, X, Y, Z and that Y and X are MAR given Z. Consider the linear regression of Y on X, Z. Units with X, Y missing contribute

$$\int \Pr(Y|\boldsymbol{\beta}; X, Z)\, dY = 1$$

to the likelihood $\Pr(Y|\boldsymbol{\beta}; X, Z)$. Thus, (1.19) implies the complete records analysis will be unbiased.

When we have additional variables predictive of Y and/or X then these may be used to recover information on the missing values and hence $\boldsymbol{\beta}$.

1.6.4 Subtle issues I: The odds ratio

This and the next two subsections consider some more subtle implications of the missingness mechanism for complete records analysis; some readers may prefer to skip to the summary on p. 35.

Harel and Carpenter (2012) consider the further complication that arises because some estimators possess a symmetry, which means they can be validly estimated from the complete records under a greater range of missing value mechanisms. The principal example is the odds ratio. Consider Table 1.8. We can either model A, C as binomial random variables with denominator $a + b$,

Table 1.8 Typical two-by-two table of counts relating outcome to exposure.

	Unexposed	Exposed
Good outcome	a	b
Poor outcome	c	d

$c + d$, or we can model A, B as binomial random variables with denominator $a + c$, $b + d$. In both cases estimates and inference for the odds ratio are identical. The first case corresponds to a case-control study, the latter to a cohort study.

Now suppose that the probability of outcome is MNAR dependent on only outcome. Consider the model

$$\text{logit}\,\Pr(\text{good outcome}) = \beta_0 + \beta_1 \times 1[\text{exposed}].$$

The preceding discussion would lead us to suppose that both β_0 and β_1 will be biased. In fact, β_1 will be unbiased. Symmetry of the odds ratio means inference for this is the same as if we performed a logistic regression of exposure on outcome where outcome was MNAR dependent only on outcome, However this is an example of a covariate MNAR, and (1.19) shows that inference using the complete records is valid in this case. The same argument applies if exposure is MAR given outcome. Bias will only occur when estimating β_1 if data are MNAR dependent on both the outcome and covariate.

More generally, we will wish to estimate the log-odds ratio relating outcome, Y, to X for various possible confounders, say Z. Applying the above argument, Y may be MNAR dependent on itself and Z, yet the OR relating X to Y will still be validly estimated from the complete records. Or, Y may be MNAR dependent on itself and X, and then the OR relating Z to Y estimated using the complete records is still valid. However, if the MNAR mechanism depends on Y, X, Z, inference from the complete records is generally biased. This argument extends naturally to log-linear models for multi-category, rather than just binary, classifications.

Example 1.8 Odds ratio

Consider synthetic data relating binary outcome, Y, to binary X and a continuous Z. We generate $1 = 1, \ldots, 20,000$ observations as follows:

$$x_i = \begin{cases} 1 \text{ for } i = 1, \ldots, 10000 \\ 0 \text{ for } i = 10001, \ldots, 20000 \end{cases},$$

$Z \sim N(0.5 \times (x_i - 0.5), 1)$ and

$$\text{logit}\,\Pr(Y_i = 1) = \beta_0 + \beta_1 X_i + \beta_2 Z_i. \tag{1.20}$$

where $(\beta_0, \beta_1, \beta_2) = (0, 1, 1)$.

Table 1.9 Missing data mechanisms, and bias of coefficient estimates with typical regression and logistic regression.

Mechanism depends on	Biased estimation of parameters using complete records					
	Typical regression			Logistic regression		
	constant	coeff. of X	coeff. of Z	constant	coeff. of X	coeff. of Z
Y	Yes	Yes	Yes	Yes	No	No
X	No	No	No	No	No	No
Z	No	No	No	No	No	No
X, Z	No	No	No	No	No	No
Y, X	Yes	Yes	Yes	Yes	Yes	No
Y, Z	Yes	Yes	Yes	Yes	No	Yes
Y, X, Z	Yes	Yes	Yes	Yes	Yes	Yes

We may consider either Z or X as the exposure. The relationship is confounded, so the unadjusted odds ratios are both biased.

Table 1.9 shows the mechanisms we consider, the bias we expect from a complete records analysis in a typical regression setting, and what we expect when using logistic regression (i.e., when we estimate log-odds ratios).

Notice that the bias does not depend on which variable has missing data, but instead on the mechanism that differentiates, or selects, the complete records from the rest of the sample. However, the appropriate approach for handling the bias (e.g. multiple imputation) will depend on the variable that is actually missing. For example, if the mechanism depends on Y and X is partially observed, data are MAR.

The results of fitting the logistic regression (1.20) for the seven scenarios in Table 1.9 are shown in Table 1.10. We see that when missing data depends on Y, odds ratios for coefficients are only biased if, in addition, the missingness mechanism depends on the covariates associated with those coefficients. This is a consequence of the symmetry of the logistic link. □

1.6.5 Implication for linear regression

Harel and Carpenter (2012) further show that, to first order approximation, the results for the odds ratio hold for linear and probit regression. In the case of linear regression of Y on X, Z, if missingness depends on Y and Z and the correlation between Y and X is moderate ($|\rho| < 0.75$), then when we estimate the regression using the complete records (i) the largest bias occurs for the coefficient for Z, but (ii) the coefficient for X is markedly less (but not completely) unbiased. As above, this applies even if the actual missing values occur in the variable Z.

Table 1.10 Empirical illustration of Table 1.9 using logistic regression.

Mechanism depends on	Probability of complete record	Estimated coefficients of		
		constant	X	Z
–	1	−0.03	1.03	1.03
Y	$[1+\exp(-y)]^{-1}$	0.34	0.99	1.01
X	$[1+\exp(-x)]^{-1}$	−0.04	1.02	1.00
Z	$[1+\exp(-z)]^{-1}$	−0.03	0.96	1.03
X, Z	$[1+\exp\{-(0.5(x-0.5)+z)\}]^{-1}$	−0.04	0.98	1.03
Y, X	$[1+\exp\{-(y+2(x-0.5))\}]^{-1}$	0.58	0.58	0.99
Y, Z	$[1+\exp\{-(y+z)\}]^{-1}$	0.38	0.96	0.82
Y, X, Z	$[1+\exp\{-(y+2(x-0.5)+z)\}]^{-1}$	0.63	0.58	0.81

This gives an informal guide to the difference between the coefficient estimates we might expect from a complete records analysis and those from an MAR analysis (typically obtained using MI). Because analysis under MAR, whether by MI or another route, is relatively complex – and thus relatively more prone to error – this provides a useful check on the plausibility of the results.

Related to this, Daniel *et al.* (2012) show how causal diagrams can be used to explore where bias due to missing data may arise. This can be a useful practical guide, both to whether it is worth using MI and to whether the results are consistent with the assumed missingness mechanisms.

Example 1.2 Youth Cohort Study *(ctd)*

Table 1.6 suggests that missing parental occupation depends on GCSE score and ethnicity. The above argument suggests that it is the coefficient for ethnicity that is most likely to be biased in the complete records analysis. After we have described MI for a range of data types, we return to this example at the end of Chapter 5. □

1.6.6 Subtle issues II: Subsample ignorability

Little and Zhang (2011) describe the related idea of subsample ignorable likelihood. Suppose we have four (sets of) variables, and the pattern of missing data shown in Table 1.11. We now make the *subsample ignorability*, that is:

1. within pattern 2, missing values of X and Y are MAR, and
2. within pattern 3, W is MNAR, with a mechanism that does not depend on Y.

Table 1.11 Missing data patterns for subsample ignorable likelihood. As before, '✓' denotes observed, '·' missing, and now '✓/·' denotes some observed and some missing.

Pattern	Variables				Number of observations
	Z	W	X	Y	
1	✓	✓	✓	✓	n_1
2	✓	✓	✓/·	✓/·	n_2
3	✓	·	✓/·	✓/·	n_3

Consider regression of Y on X, W, Z. Using the arguments developed earlier in this chapter, we see a complete records analysis will be invalid, because for observations in pattern 2 the missingness mechanism includes the response. Also, an analysis assuming MAR using observations from all three patterns will also be invalid, because data are MNAR in pattern 3. However, using only data from patterns 1 and 2, the missingness mechanism is MAR; therefore an appropriate analysis (e.g. using multiple imputation) in this setting gives valid inference. In essence this is a partial likelihood analysis, where the MNAR component is set aside.

Thus, by careful consideration of the reasons for missing data, we may be able to get valid inference via MI without recourse to a full MNAR analysis, even if a portion of the data are MNAR. A more formal justification of this approach is given by Little and Zhang (2011), who also present some simulations confirming the validity of inference when the subsample ignorability assumption holds, together with an example.

1.6.7 Summary: When restricting to complete records is valid

We have considered above the impact of various missing data mechanisms on regression analyses restricted to complete records. We note that restricting the regression analyses to complete records is generally invalid when the missingness mechanism includes the response. In establishing this, notice that what is important is the variables in the missingness mechanism, rather than variables with the missing data.

Consideration of the variables with missing data is important when deciding how to proceed beyond a complete records analysis. For instance, suppose the missingness mechanism depends on a covariate X and response Y but not on a third covariate, Z. Two possibilities are

1. Y partially observed, and

2. Z partially observed

In case (1) data are MNAR, so an analysis under the MAR assumption (e.g. using multiple imputation) will not be strictly valid. In case (2) we have a covariate MAR, so an analysis under MAR (e.g. using multiple imputation) will be valid.

In case (1), analysis under MAR may nevertheless be less biased, and the sensitivity to MNAR can be readily explored using multiple imputation, as we discuss in Chapter 10.

1.7 Summary

This chapter has introduced the central concepts involved in the analysis of partially observed data. These revolve around the 'reason for the data being missing' – more formally the missingness mechanism, and how this relates to the inferential question at hand. We have described Rubin's typology of missing data mechanisms (Rubin, 1976) and discussed these in the context of regression analysis.

We have stressed the importance of preliminary analysis of the data to identify the principal missingness patterns and elucidate plausible missingness mechanisms. Under particular missingness mechanisms, we have further explored when a regression restricted to complete records analysis is likely to give valid (if inefficient) inference.

The remainder of this book is concerned with using MI to obtain valid inference from partially observed data, predominantly the under assumption of MAR but also under the assumption of MNAR. However, there are a number of other methods that could be used to do this, for instance, the EM algorithm or a full Bayesian analysis (Clayton *et al.*, 1998). Why MI? The answer is because it is practical for applied researchers in a wide range of settings. The EM algorithm for parameter estimates is not computationally straightforward in general. Further it does not yield standard errors; a further step is required for this. A full Bayesian analysis usually requires specialist programming and will often be computationally demanding, particularly if a range of models have to be fitted.

By contrast, using multiple imputation, the researcher has to specify an appropriate imputation model. Robust software exists in many packages to fit (or approximately fit) this model, from which a series of say K imputed data sets are created. Assuming this has been done properly, the researcher can then fit their model of interest to each of the K imputed data sets in turn, obtaining K point estimates and standard errors. These are combined for final inference using Rubin's rules (Little and Rubin, 1987). These rules are relatively straightforward and perform remarkably well in a wide range of settings.

Thus, once the imputations have been created, inference proceeds using the usual software for fitting the model of interest to the complete records. It is therefore rapid. Further, analysis is not restricted to a single model: a range of models compatible with the imputation model can be explored. In addition, variables that the researcher does not wish to include in the model of interest (e.g. because they are on the causal path) can be included in the imputation model, improving both the plausibility of the MAR assumption and the imputation of the missing values.

The next chapter therefore introduces MI and sketches out its theoretical basis, illustrating this using linear regression. Subsequent chapters describe both algorithms for and application of MI to a broad range of social and medical data.

2

The multiple imputation procedure and its justification

2.1 Introduction

In this chapter we set out the Multiple Imputation (MI) procedure, initially from an intuitive standpoint in Section 2.2. We then give a more theoretical outline of MI from a Bayesian perspective in Section 2.3, before going on to consider its frequentist properties in so-called congenial (in the sense defined below) settings in Section 2.4. We discuss the choice of the number of imputations in Section 2.6. In Section 2.7 we consider some simple examples, deriving the frequentist variance of the MI estimator, and relating it to the estimator obtained using Rubin's MI variance formula. More general settings, where the imputation model and substantive model are uncongenial, are discussed in Section 2.8. In Section 2.10 we consider practical issues for formulating imputation models, and we conclude with a discussion in Section 2.11.

We do not provide a rigorous development. Instead, our aim is to highlight the main steps involved in justifying the MI procedure, together with how, and under what assumptions, these can be established. References are given for readers who wish to follow up the technical details. The principal goal is to draw attention to the aspects of the theoretical justification which have a bearing on the practical performance of MI, in particular to the several approximations that are employed. Understanding the role of these approximations sheds light on why MI works better in some settings than others, and on what we may do to improve its performance.

Multiple Imputation and its Application, First Edition. James R. Carpenter and Michael G. Kenward.

Rubin's original justification for MI is set out in Chapters 2–4 of Rubin (1987). Much of this is couched in the formalism of sample surveys, in particular in terms of design (or randomisation) based theory, although he extends the ideas to model based inference. This was a natural framework for Rubin's exposition, since at that time the primary intended application was to missing data in surveys, so that the aim was estimation of unknown observables rather than the parameters of hypothesised statistical models.

In this book we are primarily concerned with the analysis of data arising from randomised experiments or from observational studies that do not arise from a classical survey design, and for which the analysis will use conventional model based techniques in a frequentist paradigm. We therefore focus on the model based view of MI. In this context, in Section 2.8, we consider the pair of papers by Wang and Robins (1998) and and Robins and Wang (2000), which together with Nielsen (2003), provide important additional insights on the justification of the MI variance rules in a broad range of settings. These are highly technical papers, and a more accessible exposition of this material is given in Chapter 14 of Tsiatis (2006).

While it is clear that in a number of settings that inference from the MI procedure may be improved, nevertheless we will see that the over arching picture is one of the remarkable robustness of the MI procedure, especially if appropriate consideration is given to choice of the imputation model (see Section 2.10).

2.2 Intuitive outline of the MI procedure

Suppose we have two continuous variables, $(\mathbf{Y}_1, \mathbf{Y}_2)$, and we wish to estimate the regression of $\mathbf{Y}_1$ on $\mathbf{Y}_2$, but $\mathbf{Y}_2$ is MAR dependent on $\mathbf{Y}_1$. Then, as discussed in Section 1.6, the regression coefficients estimated from the complete records will be biased.

However, because $\mathbf{Y}_2$ is MAR dependent on $\mathbf{Y}_1$, the complete records give valid, efficient inference for the regression of $\mathbf{Y}_2$ on $\mathbf{Y}_1$. This suggests the following procedure:

1. Fit the regression of $\mathbf{Y}_2$ on $\mathbf{Y}_1$ to the complete records:

$$Y_{i,2} = \alpha_0 + \alpha_1 Y_{i,1} + e_i, \quad e_i \overset{i.i.d.}{\sim} N(0, \sigma^2_{2|1}), \tag{2.1}$$

obtaining $\hat{\alpha}_0, \hat{\alpha}_1, \hat{\sigma}^2_{2|1}$.

2. Impute the missing values of $\mathbf{Y}_2$ using (2.1), obtaining a 'completed' dataset.

3. Fit the substantive model, here the regression of $\mathbf{Y}_1$ on $\mathbf{Y}_2$, to the 'completed' data from step 2.

The problem with this strategy is that in step 3, the imputed values are given the same status as the actual observed values in fitting the substantive model. Further, as emphasised in Chapter 1, this strategy does not take into account the fact that we can never recover the missing data; the best we can do is to estimate the distribution of the missing data given the observed, under a specific assumption about the missingness mechanism. This distribution is not represented by a single draw from the distribution of the missing data given the observed, especially one taken assuming the estimated values of $\alpha_1, \alpha_2, \sigma^2_{2|1}$ are known without error.

Instead, we need to draw multiple times from the distribution of the missing data given the observed, taking full account of the uncertainty, to create say K imputed, i.e., 'complete' datasets. As we shall see later, we need these draws to be (at least approximately) Bayesian for Rubin's variance formula to work. Then, if we fit our substantive model to each of these, the K results together reflect the additional uncertainty induced by the missing data, while correcting the bias caused by the missing data. Rubin's rules are a general procedure for summarising these K results to obtain point estimates, associated estimates of variance, and to perform statistical tests.

Given a general data matrix $\mathbf{Y}$, write $\mathbf{Y}_O$ for the observed data and $\mathbf{Y}_M$ for the missing data. The general MI procedure is:

1. For $k = 1, \ldots, K$, taking full account of the uncertainty, impute the missing data from the distribution of the missing data given the observed, $f(\mathbf{Y}_M|\mathbf{Y}_O)$, to give K 'complete' datasets.
2. Fit the substantive model to each of the K imputed data sets (which are now 'complete' having no missing values), $k = 1, \ldots, K$. This gives K estimates of the parameters of the substantive model, say $\boldsymbol{\beta}_k$, and K estimates of their variance, $\text{Var}(\boldsymbol{\beta}_k)$.
3. Combine these for inference using Rubin's rules.

We elaborate step 1 in detail in a simple setting in the worked example below, and focus on step 3.

We denoted the vector of parameters in our substantive model by $\boldsymbol{\beta}$, and in general we may wish to apply Rubin's rules to all, or part, of this parameter vector. At this point, we suppose we are interested in a scalar element which we denote β, with associated variance σ^2. Let the estimates from imputed dataset k, obtained by fitting the substantive model to the 'completed' dataset exactly we would do if there were no missing data, be $\hat{\beta}_k, \hat{\sigma}^2_k$.

Rubin's rules for inference are as follows. The MI estimator of β is

$$\hat{\beta}_{\text{MI}} = \frac{1}{K}\sum_{k=1}^{K} \hat{\beta}_k, \tag{2.2}$$

with variance estimator

$$\widehat{V}_{\text{MI}} = \widehat{W} + \left(1 + \frac{1}{K}\right)\widehat{B}, \tag{2.3}$$

where

$$\widehat{W} = \frac{1}{K}\sum_{k=1}^{K} \hat{\sigma}_k^2, \text{ and } \widehat{B} = \frac{1}{K-1}\sum_{k=1}^{K}(\hat{\beta}_k - \hat{\beta}_{\mathrm{MI}})^2.$$

To test the hypotheses $\beta = \beta^0$, we refer

$$T = \frac{\hat{\beta}_{\mathrm{MI}} - \beta^0}{\sqrt{\widehat{V}_{\mathrm{MI}}}}$$

to a t-distribution with ν degrees of freedom, where

$$\nu = (K-1)\left[1 + \frac{\widehat{W}}{(1+1/K)\widehat{B}}\right]^2. \tag{2.4}$$

We use quantiles of the t_ν distribution to construct confidence intervals for $\hat{\beta}_{\mathrm{MI}}$.

Recall that the information on a parameter estimate is defined as the reciprocal of its variance; thus if the variance is small (because the parameter is precisely estimated) the information about the parameter value is large. Suppose the information about β in the complete data (were it available) is denoted I_C, and the information in the partially observed data is denote I_O. Then the percentage of information about β lost due to missing data is

$$\left(\frac{I_C - I_O}{I_C}\right) \times 100\%. \tag{2.5}$$

When there are no missing observations, then all the 'imputed' data sets are identical, so (2.5) is zero; were there no information in the partially observed data, it would be 100%.

From the definition of information, it follows that the information about β in the partially observed data is $I_O = 1/\widehat{V}_{\mathrm{MI}}$. As intuition suggests, it turns out that a reasonable estimate of the information in the complete data is $I_C = 1/\widehat{W}$. Thus (2.5) is

$$\left(\frac{(1+1/K)\widehat{B}}{\widehat{W} + (1+1/K)\widehat{B}}\right) \times 100\%. \tag{2.6}$$

Rubin (1987), p. 93 points out that a more accurate estimate of (2.6) is obtained by noting that minus the average second derivative of the log of the t_ν distribution (i.e., the information) is $(\nu+1)\{(\nu+3)(\widehat{W} + (1+1/K)\widehat{B})\}^{-1}$. If, as above, we estimate the information in the complete data by $\widehat{W}^{-1}$, then a better estimate of the fraction of missing information is

$$\frac{\widehat{W}^{-1} - (\nu+1)\{(\nu+3)(\widehat{W} + (1+1/K)\widehat{B})\}^{-1}}{\widehat{W}^{-1}} = \frac{r + 2/(\nu+3)}{1+r}, \tag{2.7}$$

where

$$r = \frac{(1 + 1/K)\widehat{B}}{\widehat{W}}.$$

This is the expression which many software packages calculate.

Example 2.1 Simple example of MI for a marginal mean

Let $X_i = i$, $1 = 1, \ldots, 10$ and generate Y as

$$Y_i = 1 + X_i + e_i, \quad e_i \overset{i.i.d.}{\sim} N(0, 1).$$

Suppose we wish to estimate the marginal mean of Y, but that we make Y MAR dependent on X, so that around half the observations on Y are missing if $X > 5$.

The resulting full set of 10 observations on Y are shown in the leftmost column of Table 2.1, and the observed values are shown in the second column. We see that the mean of the observed values is markedly below that of the full set of values, and the standard error is increased.

To impute the missing values, taking full account of the uncertainty, our imputation model is going to be the regression of Y on X,

$$Y_i = \beta_0 + \beta_1 X_i + e_i, \quad e_i \overset{i.i.d.}{\sim} N(0, \sigma^2).$$

Suppose we fit the model by least squares in the usual way, obtaining estimates $\hat{\beta}_0, \hat{\beta}_1, \hat{\sigma}^2$ and the estimated residuals $\hat{e}_i$, $i \in 1, \ldots n$. Consider the Bayesian posterior distribution (see Appendix A) of $\beta_0, \beta_1, \sigma^2$, and choose priors

Table 2.1 Simple example of MI; imputed values shown in bold.

	Y	Y_O	Values imputed in imputation			
			1	2	3	4
	2.23	2.23	2.23	2.23	2.23	2.23
	3.72	3.72	3.72	3.72	3.72	3.72
	3.54	3.54	3.54	3.54	3.54	3.54
	6.09	6.09	6.09	6.09	6.09	6.09
	6.53	6.53	6.53	6.53	6.53	6.53
	5.63	.	**7.08**	**8.13**	**6.98**	**7.08**
	8.28	8.28	8.28	8.28	8.28	8.28
	10.64	.	**8.68**	**9.25**	**9.68**	**10.49**
	10.74	10.74	10.74	10.74	10.74	10.74
	10.58	.	**10.87**	**10.86**	**11.74**	**13.96**
Mean	6.80	5.88	6.78	6.94	6.95	7.27
SE	1.00	1.13	0.94	0.96	1.01	1.16

so that this is equivalent to the usual frequentist sampling distribution, that is

$$f(\sigma^2|\mathbf{Y},\mathbf{X}) = \frac{\sum_{i=1}^{n} \hat{e}_i^2}{(n-2)X^2}, \tag{2.8}$$

where $X^2 \sim \chi^2_{n-2}$, and

$$\begin{pmatrix}\beta_0\\ \beta_1\end{pmatrix} \sim N_2\left[\begin{pmatrix}\hat{\beta}_1\\ \hat{\beta}_2\end{pmatrix}, \hat{\sigma}^2\begin{pmatrix} n & \sum_{i=1}^{n} X_i\\ \sum_{i=1}^{n} X_i & \sum_{i=1}^{n} X_i^2\end{pmatrix}^{-1}\right]. \tag{2.9}$$

To create the $K = 4$ imputed data sets shown in Table 2.1 we proceed as follows for $k = 1, \ldots, 4$:

1. draw $\tilde{\sigma}_k^2$ from distribution (2.8);
2. with $\sigma^2 = \tilde{\sigma}_k^2$, draw $(\tilde{\beta}_{0,k}, \tilde{\beta}_{1,k})$ from distribution (2.9);
3. for each of the missing observations, impute them as

$$Y_{i,k} = \tilde{\beta}_{0,k} + \tilde{\beta}_{1,k}X_i + \tilde{e}_{i,k}, \quad \tilde{e}_{i,k} \sim N(0, \tilde{\sigma}_k^2).$$

Notice that for imputation k we draw from the posterior (estimated) distribution of the parameters, and then impute the data; to create the second imputation we draw new parameters, and then impute the data. This is a vital part of the process, as it ensures that the imputed data is a Bayesian draw from the distribution of the missing data given the observed data.

Using this algorithm, we obtain the four imputed datasets shown in the right columns of Table 2.1, with the imputed values shown in bold. Our substantive model is simply the marginal mean of $\mathbf{Y}$. The bottom two rows of the table shows this for the full data, the observed data, and for each of the imputed datasets, together with the associated standard errors.

From (2.2) the MI estimate of the marginal mean is

$$(6.78 + 6.94 + 6.95 + 7.27)/4 = 6.99.$$

From (2.18), to calculate its standard error we first calculate

$$\widehat{W} = (0.94^2 + 0.96^2 + 1.01^2 + 1.16^2)/4 = 1.042725,$$

and

$$\widehat{B} = \left\{(6.78 - 6.99)^2 + (6.94 - 6.99)^2 + (6.95 - 6.99)^2 + (7.27 - 6.99)^2\right\}/3$$
$$= 0.0422,$$

so that the standard error is

$$\sqrt{\widehat{V}_{MI}} = \sqrt{1.042725 + (1 + 1/4) \times 0.0422} = 1.05.$$

In this very simple setting, MI has reduced the bias, and the standard error of the imputation estimate is smaller than that of the complete records analysis, while being larger than that of the original, full data (as must be the case). This is typical of what we should see in more general settings, subject to our (untestable) assumptions about the missingness mechanism, and an appropriate choice of imputation model.

Notice that $\widehat{B}$ is an order of magnitude less than $\widehat{W}$. This will typically be the case, and this relationship plays a role in some of the approximations that are used later on.

If desired, we could calculate a confidence interval for the MI estimate of the mean using the t-distribution with degrees of freedom given by (2.4). From (2.6) we can calculate the percentage of missing information in this example as $100 \times (0.0422/1.05^2) = 3.8\%$. □

This example highlights the following central points:

1. Rubin's rules are generic, requiring no substantive model specific or imputation model specific calculations. This is a key attraction of MI.

2. MI gives good frequentist properties for a remarkably small number of imputations.

3. Rubin's rules should be applied to estimators which are normally (or at least asymptotically normally) distributed. For example, for logistic regression we apply them on the log-odds ratio scale, not the odds-ratio scale, and analogously for other generalised linear models and hazard ratios from survival analysis.

Key to MI is that, under the assumed missingness mechanism, we can obtain a valid estimate of the parameters of the imputation model from the observed data. Typically, assuming MAR, this is achieved by the multivariate regression of the partially observed variables on the fully observed ones, or procedures that are approximately equivalent to this.

A important advantage of MI is that it can be applied in the same way whether the missing data are in the response of our substantive model, or its covariates, or any mixture of both. Further, MI lends itself to semi-automatic implementation. Given a substantive model, the analyst only has to specify the imputation model, and – given a method to fit this and impute the missing data – the computer can generate the imputed datasets, fit the substantive model to each and combine the results for inference using Rubin's rules. In practice, the greatest scope for error is thus inappropriate specification of the imputation model. We return to this in Section 2.10.

In the next sections, we consider the generic MI procedure from a more theoretical standpoint, and then go on to outline the steps required for its justification. Readers with an applied focus may prefer to skip to Section 2.6 and Section 2.10.

2.3 The generic MI procedure

Suppose that we are faced with an conventional estimation problem for a statistical model with a $(p \times 1)$ dimensional parameter vector $\boldsymbol{\beta}$. We call this the *substantive* model, and the aim is to make valid inferences about some or all of the elements of $\boldsymbol{\beta}$ from partially observed data. We assume that, if no data were missing, so the data were *complete*, a consistent estimator of $\boldsymbol{\beta}$ would be obtained as the solution to the estimating equation

$$\sum_{i=1}^{n} \mathbf{U}_i(\widehat{\boldsymbol{\beta}}; \mathbf{Y}_i) = \mathbf{U}(\widehat{\boldsymbol{\beta}}; \mathbf{Y}) = \mathbf{0}, \tag{2.10}$$

where the data represented by $\mathbf{Y}$ include both the outcome variable and covariates. Given complete data, we can calculate a consistent estimator of the covariance matrix of $\widehat{\boldsymbol{\beta}}$, denoted $\text{Var}(\widehat{\boldsymbol{\beta}})$, in the standard manner.

Suppose now that some data are missing, and define $\mathbf{R}$ to be the matrix of binary indicator random variables, taking the value 0 if the corresponding element of $\mathbf{Y}$ is missing and 1 otherwise. Denote by $\mathbf{Y}_M$, the set of elements of $\mathbf{Y}$ that are missing, *i.e.* for which the corresponding element of $\mathbf{R}$ is zero. The complement of $\mathbf{Y}_M$ in $\mathbf{Y}$ is the observed data, by $\mathbf{Y}_O$. A consistent estimator of $\boldsymbol{\beta}$ from the observed (incomplete) data can then be obtained from the estimating equation:

$$\text{E}_{f(\mathbf{Y}_M|\mathbf{Y}_O,\mathbf{R})} \left\{ \mathbf{U}(\widehat{\boldsymbol{\beta}}; \mathbf{Y}_O, \mathbf{Y}_M) \right\} = \mathbf{0}. \tag{2.11}$$

For the special case that $\mathbf{U}(\cdot)$ in (2.10) is the likelihood score function with the complete data, then the LHS of (2.11) similarly is the score function for the observed data. We call the conditional distribution over which the expectation is taken in (2.11), $f(\mathbf{Y}_M|\mathbf{Y}_O, \mathbf{R})$ the *conditional predictive distribution* of the missing data. Under the assumption of MAR it is not necessary to condition on the missingness indicator, so $f(\mathbf{Y}_M|\mathbf{Y}_O, \mathbf{R}) = f(\mathbf{Y}_M|\mathbf{Y}_O)$.

A consistent estimator of the covariance matrix of β from (2.11) is obtained using Louis's formula (Louis, 1982) which expresses the information matrix for the observed data in terms of expectations over complete data quantities:

$$I_O(\boldsymbol{\beta}) = I_C(\boldsymbol{\beta}) - \left[\text{E}\{\mathbf{U}(\widehat{\boldsymbol{\beta}}; \mathbf{Y})\mathbf{U}(\widehat{\boldsymbol{\beta}}; \mathbf{Y})^T\} - \text{E}\{\mathbf{U}(\widehat{\boldsymbol{\beta}}; \mathbf{Y})\} \text{E}\{\mathbf{U}(\widehat{\boldsymbol{\beta}}; \mathbf{Y})\}^T \right], \tag{2.12}$$

– that is, the observed information is the complete information minus the missing information – for $I_C(\cdot)$ the information matrix based on the complete data. All expectations are taken over the conditional predictive distribution $f(\mathbf{Y}_M \mid \mathbf{Y}_O, \mathbf{R})$. Although (2.11) and (2.12) provide a general scheme for dealing with standard regression models when data are missing, their practical value varies greatly from problem to problem. The expectations require the calculation of so-called *incomplete data* quantities for which there do not exist sufficiently straightforward and general methods of calculation. In such settings, one-off solutions, often quite complex, are required. Away from standard regression problems, the situation may be even more intractable.

One view of MI is that it provides an alternative, indirect route, to solving this problem which, most importantly, uses in the analysis phase only *complete date* quantities, *i.e.* those that arise in the solution to (2.10) and the accompanying estimator of precision. In applications, such quantities are typically readily available from model fitting software. Crudely stated, MI reverses the order of expectation and solution in (2.11). Thus the idea is to repeatedly:

1. draw $\tilde{\mathbf{Y}}_M$ from $f(\mathbf{Y}_M|\mathbf{Y}_O, \mathbf{R})$;
2. solve $\mathbf{U}(\beta; \tilde{\mathbf{Y}}_M, \mathbf{Y}_O) = \mathbf{0}$,

and combine the results in some way for inference.

Each $\tilde{\mathbf{Y}}_M$ is a *Bayesian* draw from the conditional predictive distribution of the missing observations, made in such a way that the set of imputations properly represents the information about the missing values that is contained in the observed data for the chosen model. Each draw of $\tilde{\mathbf{Y}}_M$ taken with $\mathbf{Y}_O$ gives a 'completed' dataset. Each of these is analysed using the method that would have been applied had no data been missing. The model used to produce the imputations, that is, to represent the conditional predictive distribution, is called the *imputation* model. One great strength of the MI procedure is that these two models, substantive and imputation, can be fitted quite separately, and also considered, to some extent, separately – although certain relationships between them do need to be observed.

Thus MI involves three distinct tasks:

1. The missing values are filled in K times to generate K complete data sets.
2. The K complete data sets are analyzed by using standard, complete data, procedures.
3. The results from the K analyses are combined to produce a single MI estimator and to draw inferences.

In more detail, the missing data are replaced by their corresponding imputation samples, producing K completed datasets. Denoting by $\widehat{\boldsymbol{\beta}}_k$ and $\widehat{\mathbf{V}}_k$ the estimate of $\boldsymbol{\beta}$ and its covariance matrix from the kth completed dataset, $k \in (1, \ldots, K)$, the MI estimate of $\boldsymbol{\beta}$ is the simple average of the estimates:

$$\widehat{\boldsymbol{\beta}}_{\mathrm{MI}} = \frac{1}{K} \sum_{k=1}^{K} \widehat{\boldsymbol{\beta}}_k. \tag{2.13}$$

We also need a measure of precision for $\widehat{\boldsymbol{\beta}}_{\mathrm{MI}}$ that properly reflects the between and within imputation variance. Rubin (1987) provides the following simple expression for the covariance matrix of $\widehat{\boldsymbol{\beta}}_{\text{MI}}$. It can be applied very generally and uses only complete data quantities. Define

$$\widehat{\mathbf{W}} = \frac{1}{K}\sum_{k=1}^{K}\widehat{\mathbf{V}}_k \tag{2.14}$$

to be the average within-imputation covariance matrix, and

$$\widehat{\mathbf{B}} = \frac{1}{K-1}\sum_{k=1}^{K}(\widehat{\boldsymbol{\beta}}_k - \widehat{\boldsymbol{\beta}}_{\text{MI}})(\widehat{\boldsymbol{\beta}}_k - \widehat{\boldsymbol{\beta}}_{\text{MI}})^T \tag{2.15}$$

to be the between-imputation covariance matrix of $\widehat{\boldsymbol{\beta}}_k$. Then an estimate of the covariance $\widehat{\boldsymbol{\beta}}_{\text{MI}}$ is given by

$$\widehat{\mathbf{V}}_{\text{MI}} = \widehat{\mathbf{W}} + \left(1 + \frac{1}{K}\right)\widehat{\mathbf{B}}. \tag{2.16}$$

Apart from an adjustment of $1/K$ to accommodate the finite number of imputations used, this is a very straightforward combination of between- and within-imputation variability.

2.4 Bayesian justification of MI

For simplicity, assume MAR, and suppose we obtain K imputed datasets from a Bayesian predictive distribution $f(\mathbf{Y}_M|\mathbf{Y}_O)$, fit our substantive model to each and combine the results for inference using Rubin's rules.

Separate to this, assume that there exists a full Bayesian procedure for obtaining the posterior of $\boldsymbol{\beta}$, such that, if – in addition – we were to use this full Bayesian procedure to impute the missing data, then the imputation distribution would be the same as the predictive distribution in the previous paragraph.

If this is the case, we say the imputation model and the substantive model are *congenial*, in the sense introduced by Meng (1994), noting that Meng's original definition extends to broader settings.

Given that the imputation model and substantive model are congenial, our substantive model can be derived from a likelihood model with parameters $\boldsymbol{\beta}$. In the Bayesian framework, the missing data, $\mathbf{Y}_M$, is equivalent to a set of additional parameters. Suppressing the parameters of the distribution of the observed data, $\mathbf{Y}_O$, the posterior distribution is therefore

$$f(\mathbf{Y}_M, \boldsymbol{\beta} \mid \mathbf{Y}_O).$$

Our focus is on $\boldsymbol{\beta}$, with $\mathbf{Y}_M$ being regarded as a nuisance. The posterior can be partitioned as:

$$f(\boldsymbol{\beta}, \mathbf{Y}_M \mid \mathbf{Y}_O) = f(\mathbf{Y}_M \mid \mathbf{Y}_O) f(\boldsymbol{\beta} \mid \mathbf{Y}_M, \mathbf{Y}_O),$$

so that the marginal posterior for $\boldsymbol{\beta}$ can be written

$$f(\boldsymbol{\beta} \mid \mathbf{Y}_O) = \mathrm{E}_{f(\mathbf{Y}_M|\mathbf{Y}_O)}\{f(\boldsymbol{\beta} \mid \mathbf{Y}_M, \mathbf{Y}_O)\}.$$

In particular, under regularity conditions which permit the order of integration to be exchanged, the posterior mean and variance for $\boldsymbol{\beta}$ can be expressed

$$\mathrm{E}(\boldsymbol{\beta} \mid \mathbf{Y}_O) = \mathrm{E}_{f(\mathbf{Y}_M|\mathbf{Y}_O)}\{\,\mathrm{E}_{f(\boldsymbol{\beta}|\mathbf{Y}_M,\mathbf{Y}_O)}(\boldsymbol{\beta})\} \tag{2.17}$$

$$\mathrm{Var}(\boldsymbol{\beta} \mid \mathbf{Y}_O) = \mathrm{E}_{f(\mathbf{Y}_M|\mathbf{Y}_O)}\{\mathrm{Var}_{f(\boldsymbol{\beta}|\mathbf{Y}_M,\mathbf{Y}_O)}(\boldsymbol{\beta})\} + \mathrm{Var}_{f(\mathbf{Y}_M|\mathbf{Y}_O)}\{\,\mathrm{E}_{f(\boldsymbol{\beta}|\mathbf{Y}_M,\mathbf{Y}_O)}(\boldsymbol{\beta})\}. \tag{2.18}$$

The posterior mean and variance can then be approximated empirically. Let $\widetilde{\mathbf{Y}}_{M,k}$ $k = 1, \ldots, K$, be draws from the Bayesian predictive distribution $f(\mathbf{Y}_M | \mathbf{Y}_O)$. Then from (2.17)

$$\mathrm{E}(\boldsymbol{\beta} \mid \mathbf{Y}_O) \simeq \frac{1}{K}\sum_{k=1}^{K}\{\mathrm{E}_{f(\boldsymbol{\beta}|\tilde{\mathbf{Y}}_{M,k},\mathbf{Y}_O)}(\boldsymbol{\beta})\} = \widehat{\boldsymbol{\beta}},$$

and from (2.18)

$$\mathrm{Var}(\boldsymbol{\beta} \mid \mathbf{Y}_O) \simeq \frac{1}{K}\sum_{k=1}^{K}\mathrm{Var}_{f(\boldsymbol{\beta}|\tilde{\mathbf{Y}}_{M,k},\mathbf{Y}_O)}(\boldsymbol{\beta})$$
$$+\frac{1}{K-1}\sum_{j=1}^{K}\{\,\mathrm{E}_{f(\boldsymbol{\beta}|\tilde{\mathbf{Y}}_{M,k},\mathbf{Y}_O)}(\boldsymbol{\beta}) - \widehat{\boldsymbol{\beta}}\}\{\,\mathrm{E}_{f(\boldsymbol{\beta}|\tilde{\mathbf{Y}}_{M,k},\mathbf{Y}_O)}(\boldsymbol{\beta}) - \widehat{\boldsymbol{\beta}}\}^T.$$

To use this in practice we need both Bayesian draws from the conditional predictive distribution, and a short cut to obtain the mean and variance of $\boldsymbol{\beta}$ over $f(\boldsymbol{\beta}|\tilde{\mathbf{Y}}_{M,k}, \mathbf{Y}_O)$. Without the latter, MI gains almost nothing in simplicity over a full Bayesian analysis. Thus, to use MI we need to assume that these can be approximated sufficiently well by the solution to, and accompanying variance estimator from, the full data estimating equations (i.e., fitting the substantive model to the imputed data set in the standard way).

When the full data estimating equations are likelihood score equations this approximation follows from the asymptotic property of joint Bayesian posteriors known as the Bernstein von-Mises theorem (Gelman et al., 1995). This states that, under standard regularity conditions, as the sample size n increases the joint posterior distribution tends to a multivariate normal. Moreover, as the sample size increases, the likelihood dominates the prior distribution and so the mode of the likelihood (the maximum likelihood estimator) and the inverse of the curvature of the likelihood (the information based covariance matrix) can be used to obtain the required moments. Additionally, the fact that after marginalising over $\mathbf{Y}_M$, only a relatively small marginal component of the full posterior is being approximated (i.e., that for $\boldsymbol{\beta}$, or more typically a subset of the elements of $\boldsymbol{\beta}$) potentially further improves the normal approximation.

We reiterate that two approximations are being used:

1. the asymptotic multivariate normal for the posterior, and

2. the estimator and covariance matrix from the full data estimating equations for the first two moments of this posterior.

Only when the substantive model gives rise to likelihood score equations does (2) have its usual justification. As usual, the approximations are not scale invariant. Thus, a scale should be chosen for the relevant elements of $\boldsymbol{\beta}$ that leads to the best approximation. For example, quantities like odds-ratios and hazard-ratios should be log-transformed before the MI procedure is applied. In the same vein, Gelman *et al.* (1995) p. 95–96 give an instructive example on the variance of a normal distribution, showing that a log transformation leads to a better approximation than the original scale.

The above discussion makes it clear why we need to impute from the full Bayesian predictive distribution. In the congenial setting, provided we have a method for generating Bayesian posterior draws from the conditional predictive distribution of the missing data, we see MI can be viewed as a three-step approximation to a full Bayesian analysis, in which in the second part we exploit the speed of computational algorithms for finding maximum likelihood estimates.

2.5 Frequentist inference

We now briefly discuss the additional considerations necessary for frequentist inference about $\boldsymbol{\beta}$, i.e., a valid estimate of the frequentist variance, the sampling distribution of pivotal quantities, and the resulting confidence intervals and tests. As before, we assume the imputation model and substantive model are congenial.

We begin by considering inference for a single parameter, β, from the parameter vector $\boldsymbol{\beta}$. We suppose we have drawn K imputations from the Bayesian predictive distribution, resulting in K completed datasets, and fitted the substantive model to each, giving estimates $\hat{\beta}_k$, $k = 1, \ldots, K$, with associated standard errors $\hat{\sigma}_k$.

We assume that the sample size, n, is large enough that the approximations described in the previous section hold. Then the mean of $\hat{\beta}_k$ is a consistent estimator of β, so we can set

$$\hat{\beta}_{\mathrm{MI}} = \frac{1}{K} \sum_{i=1}^{K} \hat{\beta}_k.$$

We also calculate the terms

$$\widehat{B} = \frac{1}{K-1}\sum_{k=1}^{K}(\hat{\beta}_k - \hat{\beta}_{\text{MI}})^2,$$

which is the sample variance of $\hat{\beta}_k$, and

$$\widehat{W} = \frac{1}{K}\sum_{k=1}^{K}\hat{\sigma}_k^2.$$

2.5.1 Large number of imputations

Suppose first that K is large, i.e., we have carried out a large number of imputations. Then $\widehat{W}$ will be a precise estimate of the first term in (2.18), and likewise $\widehat{B}$ will be a precise estimate of the second term in (2.18), so that, for practical purposes, denoting $\text{Var}(\hat{\beta}_{MI})$ by V_{MI}, we have

$$\widehat{V}_{MI} = \widehat{B} + \widehat{W}. \tag{2.19}$$

Because, under the assumptions in the previous section, n is large enough for $\hat{\beta}$ to be normally distributed if there are no missing data, we can interpret the Bayesian posterior from a frequentist viewpoint giving

$$\hat{\beta}_{\text{MI}} \sim N(\beta, \widehat{B} + \widehat{W}).$$

Thus we can test the hypothesis that $\beta = \beta_0$ by comparing

$$\frac{\hat{\beta}_{\text{MI}} - \hat{\beta}_0}{\sqrt{\widehat{V}_{\text{MI}}}}$$

to a standard normal distribution, and construct a $100(1-\alpha)\%$ confidence interval as

$$\left(\hat{\beta}_{\text{MI}} - z_{1-\alpha/2}\sqrt{\widehat{V}_{\text{MI}}},\ \hat{\beta}_{\text{MI}} - z_{\alpha/2}\sqrt{\widehat{V}_{\text{MI}}}\right),$$

where z is standard normal and $\Pr(z_\alpha < \alpha) = \alpha$.

In practice, of course, we need to know if K is large enough for the above results to hold; we shall see the development below will enable us to judge this.

2.5.2 Small number of imputations

We suppose now that, as may often be the case, we have carried out a relatively small number of imputations, say $K = 5$. How should we modify the above procedure? We first show that an additional term is needed in the variance formula (2.19), and then that for inference we need to replace the normal reference distribution by a t distribution. Our arguments are not rigorous; for more details see Rubin (1987) p. 87–93.

The idea is to condition the results for infinitely large K – essentially the results above – on the first few imputations. We therefore define

$$\hat{\beta}_{MI,\infty} = \lim_{K\to\infty} \frac{1}{K}\sum_{i=1}^{K} \hat{\beta}_k = \lim_{K\to\infty} \hat{\beta}_{\text{MI}}$$

$$\widehat{B}_\infty = \lim_{K\to\infty} \frac{1}{K-1}\sum_{k=1}^{K} (\hat{\beta}_k - \bar{\beta}_K)^2, \text{ where } \bar{\beta}_K = \frac{1}{K}\sum_{i=1}^{K} \hat{\beta}_k$$

and

$$\widehat{W}_\infty = \lim_{K\to\infty} \frac{1}{K}\sum_{k=1}^{K} \hat{\sigma}_k^2.$$

The posterior for β is

$$\beta \sim N(\hat{\beta}_\infty, \widehat{B}_\infty + \widehat{W}_\infty). \tag{2.20}$$

Now suppose that we have only performed a finite number of K imputations. As above, denote the average of the corresponding K estimates of β by $\overline{\beta}_K$. The expected value of $\overline{\beta}_K$ is $\hat{\beta}_\infty$. The variability of $\overline{\beta}_K$ about $\hat{\beta}_\infty/K$ is $\hat{\beta}_\infty/K$. Therefore, if we substitute $\hat{\beta}_{MI}$, based on K imputations, as an estiamtor of $\hat{\beta}_\infty$ in (2.20) we need to increase the variance by $\hat{\beta}_\infty/K$, giving

$$\beta \sim N\{\hat{\beta}_{\text{MI}}, \widehat{B}_\infty(K^{-1}+1) + \widehat{W}_\infty\}.$$

The extra term in the variance accounts for the increased uncertainty in the estimated mean of β when we take a finite number of imputations; it vanishes as K gets large.

Since, for a finite K, $\widehat{B}$ is unbiased for $\widehat{B}_\infty$, and likewise $\widehat{W}$ is unbiased for $\widehat{W}_\infty$ we have

$$\beta \approx \{\hat{\beta}_{\text{MI}}, (1+K^{-1})\widehat{B} + \widehat{W}\}. \tag{2.21}$$

Notice that we have dropped the 'N' from (2.21); since the variance parameters are estimated, the distribution can no longer be normal; instead it is likely to be approximately t_ν, for yet to be determined degrees of freedom ν. Note that the distribution will not be exactly t, because the variance estimator consists of the sum of two estimators; in this regard it resembles the distribution of the mean of observations from two groups with different variances – known as the Fisher-Behrens distribution.

Recall that the sample mean of $Z_1, \ldots, Z_K \overset{i.i.d.}{\sim} N(\mu, \sigma^2)$ is distributed as t_{K-1}, because

$$\hat{\sigma}^2 = \frac{1}{K-1}\sum_{k=1}^{K}(Z_i - \bar{Z})^2 \sim \frac{\sigma^2 \chi^2_{K-1}}{K-1}.$$

Thus, $\hat{\sigma}^2/\sigma^2$ has mean 1 and variance $2/(K-1)$.

Similarly, in our setting,

$$\frac{\widehat{B}}{\widehat{B}_\infty} \sim \frac{\chi^2_{K-1}}{K-1},$$

with mean 1 and variance $2/(K-1)$. Next notice that the MI variance estimator for finite K, divided by the same expression substituting the limiting values of the variance estimates, can be written as

$$\frac{\widehat{B}(1+K^{-1})+\widehat{W}}{\widehat{B}_\infty(1+K^{-1})+\widehat{W}_\infty} = \frac{\left\{\frac{\widehat{B}}{\widehat{W}}(1+K^{-1})+1\right\}\widehat{W}}{\left\{\frac{\widehat{B}_\infty}{\widehat{W}_\infty}(1+K^{-1})+1\right\}\widehat{W}_\infty}$$

Suppose we write $r = (\widehat{B}/\widehat{W})(1+K^{-1})$, and $A = \widehat{B}/\widehat{B}_\infty$. Then the above expression is

$$\left(\frac{\widehat{W}}{\widehat{W}_\infty}\right)\frac{r+1}{rA^{-1}(\widehat{W}/\widehat{W}_\infty)+1}.$$

Next, notice that in typical regression models with n observations and p parameters,

$$\frac{\widehat{W}}{\widehat{W}_\infty} \approx \frac{\chi^2_{n-p}}{n-p},$$

so that the expected value of $\widehat{W}/\widehat{W}_\infty$ is 1 with variance $O(n^{-1})$. Since we are assuming n is large, we can say $\widehat{W}/\widehat{W}_\infty \approx 1$. Also assume that $\widehat{B}_\infty/\widehat{W}_\infty$ is $O(n^{-l})$, $l > 0$, so that $\widehat{B}/\widehat{W}$ has variance $O(K^{-1}n^{-l})$. This is a less intuitive assumption, but is likely to be approximately true if there is relatively little missing information. Under this assumption, we can treat r as approximately constant, and to find the degrees of freedom ν of the approximating χ^2 distribution, we need to consider the mean and variance of

$$f(A) = \frac{r+1}{r/A+1}.$$

Recalling that $A \sim (1, 2/(K-1))$, we expand $f(A)$ about the mean of A to see

$$f(A) \approx f(1) + (A-1)f'(1),$$

where f' is the derivative of f. It follows that $\mathrm{E}\{f(A)\} \approx 1$ and

$$\mathrm{Var}\{f(A)\} \approx \frac{2}{K-1}\left(\frac{r}{r+1}\right)^2,$$

so that the distribution of W can be approximated by the χ^2_ν distribution where

$$\nu = (K-1)(1+r^{-1})^2 = (K-1)\left\{\frac{\widehat{W} + (1+K^{-1})\widehat{B}}{(1+K^{-1})\widehat{B}}\right\}^2. \tag{2.22}$$

In line with intuition, we see that, the smaller the between imputation variance, the larger ν, and likewise the greater the number of imputations the larger ν. If desired, in applications we can perform K imputations, evaluate (2.22) and increase the number of imputations till $\nu \approx 50$, say when the normal approximation is adequate for practical purposes.

Looking back to (2.21), we see one final step is needed, and this is to appeal to general results which allow us calibrate features of the posterior, such as credible intervals, from a frequentist repeated sampling perspective. Simply speaking, this allows us to interpret the posterior for β, with estimated mean $\hat{\beta}_{\mathrm{MI}}$, as a sampling distribution for $\hat{\beta}_{\mathrm{MI}}$, with population parameter value β. We therefore have that

$$\hat{\beta}_{\mathrm{MI}} \sim \beta + t_\nu \sqrt{\widehat{V}_{\mathrm{MI}}}, \tag{2.23}$$

where $\widehat{V}_{\mathrm{MI}} = \widehat{W} + (1+1/K)\widehat{B}$ and ν is given by (2.22). We can use (2.23) to test hypotheses and form confidence intervals in the usual way.

Notice that in the above derivation we repeatedly use the fact that, if there is no missing data, n (the sample size) is large enough that the estimator of the quantity of can be regarded as normally distributed. The case of small samples, so that with no missing data the estimator has a t-distribution, is considered by Barnard and Rubin (1999).

Inference for vector $\boldsymbol{\beta}$.

Inference for vector $\boldsymbol{\beta}$ and finite K is can be tackled along the same lines as above, as described by Li *et al.* (1991). They propose basing tests on the approximate pivot

$$F = (\hat{\boldsymbol{\beta}}_{\mathrm{MI}} - \boldsymbol{\beta})^T \widehat{\mathbf{V}}_{\mathrm{MI}}^{-1} (\hat{\boldsymbol{\beta}}_{\mathrm{MI}} - \boldsymbol{\beta}).$$

and referring $\{p(1+r)\}^{-1}F$ to an $F_{p,\nu'}$ reference distribution for the scaled statistic, where

$$\nu' = 4 + (t-4)\left[1 + \frac{(1-2t^{-1})}{r}\right]^2,$$

$$r = \frac{1}{p}\left(1+\frac{1}{K}\right)\mathrm{tr}(\mathbf{B}\mathbf{W}^{-1}), \text{ and}$$

$$t = p(K-1),$$

if $t > 4$, otherwise $\nu' = t(1 + p^{-1})(1 + r^{-1})^2/2$. Here, r is the average relative increase in variance due to missingness across the components of $\boldsymbol{\beta}$. As expected, the limiting distribution of F, as $K \to \infty$, is the χ_p^2 distribution. This procedure is applicable for any vector of parameters from the substantive model, or any linear combination of these. For inference about a scalar, this reduces in an obvious way to a t approximation for the ratio

$$\frac{\hat{\boldsymbol{\beta}}_{\text{MI}} - \boldsymbol{\beta}}{\sqrt{\hat{\mathbf{V}}_{\text{MI}}}}.$$

These results are derived under the strong assumption that the fraction of missing information for all elements of $\boldsymbol{\beta}$ are equal. In practice, this will not be true; nevertheless Li *et al.* (1991) report a simulation study in this setting which finds that performance is good, albeit a little conservative. If in doubt, in many settings it is simplest to perform more imputations, and use ν' as a guide to when variability in denominator of the F can be assumed negligible. The case of small samples is considered by Reiter (2007).

Combining likelihood ratio tests

Meng and Rubin (1992) extend the MI combination rules to likelihood ratio statistics. To simplify the exposition it is assumed that we wish to test the null hypothesis

$$H_0 : \boldsymbol{\beta}_2 = 0$$

for $\boldsymbol{\beta} = (\boldsymbol{\beta}_1, \boldsymbol{\beta}_2)^T$ with $\boldsymbol{\beta}_2$ of dimension $q < p$. Hence, under the null hypothesis, H_0, $\boldsymbol{\beta} = (\boldsymbol{\beta}_1, 0)^T = \boldsymbol{\beta}_{\underline{H}_0}$ say. From the kth completed data set we can obtain the unconstrained MLE, $\widehat{\boldsymbol{\beta}}_k$, and MLE under the null hypothesis, H_0, which we denote $\boldsymbol{\beta}_{k,H_0}$ Denote the corresponding log likelihood ratio statistic from the kth set as

$$D_k = 2\{\ell(\widehat{\boldsymbol{\beta}}_k) - \ell(\widehat{\boldsymbol{\beta}}_{k,H_0})\}.$$

We can then define three averages over the imputation sets:

$$\overline{D}_{\cdot} = \frac{1}{K}\sum_{i=1}^{K} D_k, \quad \bar{\boldsymbol{\beta}}_{\cdot} = \frac{1}{K}\sum_{i=1}^{K} \widehat{\boldsymbol{\beta}}_k \quad \text{and} \quad \bar{\boldsymbol{\beta}}_{\cdot,H_0} = \frac{1}{K}\sum_{i=1}^{K} \widehat{\boldsymbol{\beta}}_{k,H_0}.$$

Finally we define the average of the log likelihood ratios over the K imputed data sets *but with the parameters fixed at their average values*, that is

$$D_{\star} = \frac{1}{K}\sum_{i=1}^{K} 2\{\ell_k(\bar{\boldsymbol{\beta}}_{\cdot}) - \ell_k(\bar{\boldsymbol{\beta}}_{\cdot,H_0})\}.$$

where the subscript k indicates that the log likelihood is evaluated using the kth imputed data set. The MI likelihood ratio statistic due to Meng and Rubin

(1992) is

$$D_{\rm MI} = \frac{D^*}{q(1+r_*)}$$

for $r_* = (K+1)(\overline{D}_. - D_*)/\{q(K-1)\}$. The reference distribution for this is F_{q,v_*}, where

$$v_* = \begin{cases} 4+(a-4)\{1+(1-2/a)r_*^{-1}\}^2 & if\ \ a = q(K-1) > 4, \\ a(1+1/q)(1_1/r_*)^2/2 & \text{otherwise} \end{cases}$$

There is in addition a method for combining P-values over imputations, developed by Li *et al.* (1991). This does not appear to be used widely in practice, and its behaviour appears such that it should only be used as a rough guide.

Practical settings lend themselves naturally to Wald tests, so that the above rules have not seen wide use in applications.

2.6 Choosing the number of imputations

Multiple imputation is attractive because it can give valid inferences (that is, correct confidence interval coverage) even for small values of K. In some applications, merely 3–5 imputations are sufficient to obtain acceptable properties. From the discussion above, we see that the information on $\hat{\beta}_{\rm MI}$ based on K imputations, relative to that based on and infinite number, can be estimated by

$$\frac{I_K}{I_\infty} \approx \left\{\frac{\widehat{W} + (1+K^{-1})\widehat{B}}{\widehat{W}+\widehat{B}}\right\}^{-1} = \left\{1 + \frac{1}{K}\frac{\widehat{B}}{\widehat{B}+\widehat{W}}\right\}^{-1}.$$

Now, $\widehat{B}/(\widehat{B}+\widehat{W})$ is an estimate of the loss of information due to missing data, and from the discussion following (2.7) we have seen that a better estimate of this is

$$\gamma = \frac{r + 2/(v+3)}{r+1}.$$

Hence, the fraction of information lost for β using K rather than an infinite number of imputations is approximately $\gamma/(K+\gamma)$. The variance of an estimate from an infinite number of imputations, divided by that based on K imputations, i.e., the relative efficiency, is approximately

$$\left(\frac{I_K}{I_\infty}\right) = \left(1+\frac{\gamma}{K}\right)^{-1}, \tag{2.24}$$

as derived by Rubin (1987) p. 114. The efficiencies achieved for K versus an infinite number of imputations, for various γ, are shown in Table 2.2.

On the basis of Table 2.2, and the fact that MI inference works well for $K > 5$, it has been argued that a small number of imputations is sufficient for most applications.

Table 2.2 Table of relative efficiency ($\times 100$) from (2.24), for various values of K and γ.

	γ				
K	0.1	0.3	0.5	0.7	0.9
2	95	87	80	74	69
3	97	91	86	81	77
5	98	94	91	88	85
10	99	97	95	93	92
20	100	99	98	97	96

This is true, but it is not the whole story. While Table 2.2 applies to estimation of β, it does not carry over to estimation of p-values (see, for example, Carpenter and Kenward (2008), Chapter 4). If we want the error in estimating p-values to be small, say less than 0.005, then our experience is we will need to do at least $K = 100$ imputations. In a similar vein, Harel and Schafer (2003) report that the MI estimator of the fraction of missing information is considerably more noisy than the MI estimator of β.

This leads us to the following conclusions:

1. If, in the analysis at hand, inference is clear-cut after a small number of imputations, there is no need to perform more;

2. If inference is less clear-cut, and an accurate estimate of the p-value is required, or an accurate estimate of the fraction of missing information, take $K = 100$.

Since computing time is cheap relative to data collection, in applications we would err on a greater, rather than fewer, number of imputations. However, especially in large problems where imputation will be slower, pausing after a small number of imputations to check both that the results are plausible and whether more imputations are really required is sensible.

2.7 Some simple examples

Rubin's MI variance rules, described above, are both extremely general, and rely on a number of approximations. It is therefore interesting to examine them in some very simple settings, so simple in fact that imputation is strictly unnecessary. These settings allow us to derive exact expressions which add to our intuitive understanding of the procedure. We begin with arguably the simplest possible problem, the estimation of a simple mean under completely random missingness, with σ^2 first known, then unknown. Then we consider the general linear regression setting with σ^2 known.

Estimating the mean with σ^2 known

Suppose that we have a sample of n observations $Y_1, \ldots, Y_n$, drawn identically from a normal distribution with mean μ and known variance σ^2. Suppose that we are missing n_M of the observations in a completely random way, and set $n_O = n - n_M$ to be the number actually observed, with the sets of indices for the observed and missing observations denoted by $\mathcal{O}$ and $\mathcal{M}$ respectively. Define $\pi_M = n_M/n$ to be the proportion missing. Our aim is to estimate μ together with an appropriate measure of precision.

Given the MCAR assumption and lack of other relevant information, the obvious approach for this is to use the MLE

$$\hat{\mu} = \bar{Y}_O = \frac{1}{n_O}\sum_{i\in\mathcal{O}} Y_i,$$

the simple average of the observed data, with variance σ^2/n_O. In spite of this simple and obvious solution, we are nevertheless going to approach this problem using MI.

For this we need an appropriate imputation distribution for the missing data, which in turn requires a suitable posterior for the relevant parameters, in this case just μ. We assume flat, improper, priors for the missing observations themselves. Further we assume that whatever the distribution of the original data (in this case normal), the sample size is large enough for the posterior for μ to be approximately normal, and for the observed data to dominate the prior; that is the posterior mean and variance for $f(\mu \mid \mathbf{Y}_O)$ can be approximated by $\bar{Y}_O$ and σ^2/n_O respectively. As discussed on p. 47, although the MI procedure is derived using a proper Bayesian argument, it relies on the data dominating any prior. It is in this sense not a *general* Bayesian procedure in terms of the use of informative priors. The elegant simplicity of the variance formula derives from the use of the limiting form of the posterior that is obtained as n increases.

Given these priors, the posterior for the missing set of observations is

$$\mathbf{Y}_M \mid \mathbf{Y}_O \sim \mathrm{N}\left[\bar{Y}_O\mathbf{1}_{n_M}; \sigma^2\left(\boldsymbol{I}_{n_M} + \frac{1}{n_O}\mathbf{1}_{n_M}\mathbf{1}_{n_M}^T\right)\right],$$

for $\mathbf{1}_p$ the p-dimensional vector of ones. Hence we can draw the ith of n_M values from the kth of K imputation sets by using

$$\widetilde{Y}_{i,k} = \bar{Y}_O + e_{i,k} + s_k, \quad i \in \mathcal{M}, \tag{2.25}$$

where $e_{i,k} \sim \mathrm{N}(0, \sigma^2)$ and $s_k \sim \mathrm{N}(0, \sigma^2/n_O)$, noting that s_k is common to all draws from the kth imputation. We then have the following two complete data quantities from the kth imputation set: the sample mean,

$$\begin{aligned}\bar{Y}_k &= \frac{1}{n}\left(\sum_{i\in\mathcal{O}} Y_i + \sum_{i\in\mathcal{M}} \widetilde{Y}_{i,k}\right) \\ &= \bar{Y}_O + \pi_M(\bar{e}_{.k} + s_k).\end{aligned} \tag{2.26}$$

and the sample variance,

$$S_k^2 = \frac{1}{n-1}\left(\sum_{i\in\mathcal{O}}(Y_i - \bar{Y}_k)^2 + \sum_{i\in\mathcal{M}}(\widetilde{Y}_{i,k} - \bar{Y}_k)^2\right) \tag{2.27}$$

$$= \frac{1}{n-1}\left(\sum_{i\in\mathcal{O}}(Y_i - \bar{Y}_O)^2 + \sum_{i\in\mathcal{M}}(e_{i,k} - \bar{e}_{.k})^2 + n(1-\pi_M)\pi_M(\bar{e}_{.k} + s_k)^2\right).$$

From these we calculate the MI estimators of mean and precision using Rubin's rules. The MI estimator of μ is

$$\hat{\mu}_{\mathrm{MI}} = \frac{1}{K}\sum_{k=1}^{K}\bar{Y}_k$$

$$= \bar{Y}_O + \pi_M(\bar{e}_{..} + \bar{s})$$

and the MI variance estimator of this is

$$\mathrm{Var}(\hat{\mu}_{\mathrm{MI}}) = \frac{1}{nK}\sum_{k=1}^{K}S_k^2 + \left(1+\frac{1}{K}\right)\left(\frac{1}{K-1}\right)\sum_{k=1}^{K}(\bar{Y}_k - \hat{\mu}_{\mathrm{MI}})^2 \tag{2.28}$$

$$= \hat{W} + \left(1+\frac{1}{K}\right)\hat{B}.$$

The advantage of this very simple setting is that we can explore directly the exact sampling properties of these. The necessary expectations need to be taken in proper order, that is over the imputation distribution distribution first, then over the data. This is very straightforward here, and we find that the estimator, $\hat{\mu}_{\mathrm{MI}}$ is unbiased, and has exact variance

$$\mathrm{Var}(\hat{\mu}_{\mathrm{MI}}) = \frac{\sigma^2}{n_O}\left(1+\frac{\pi_M}{K}\right). \tag{2.29}$$

Note how, as K increases, $\hat{\mu}_{\mathrm{MI}}$ tends to $\bar{Y}_O$, and the expression in (2.29) tends to the exact variance of this, as we should expect. Our main goal however is to compare the finite (in terms of K) sampling properties of Rubin's variance estimator with the true variance (2.29). As the three components of (2.27) are independent, it follows that

$$\mathrm{E}(\hat{W}) = \frac{\sigma^2}{n}.$$

Similarly, we can rewrite $\hat{B}$ as

$$\frac{{\pi_M}^2}{K-1}\sum_{k=1}^{K}\left\{(\bar{e}_{.k} - \bar{e}_{..})^2 + (s_k - \bar{s}_{.})^2 + 2(\bar{e}_{.k} - \bar{e}_{..})(s_k - \bar{s}_{.})\right\}.$$

Noting that the third term inside the brackets has zero expectation (because the $e_{i,k}$ and s_k are uncorrelated), we get

$$\mathrm{E}(\hat{B}) = \frac{\pi_M \sigma^2}{n_O}.$$

Combining these gives

$$\mathrm{E}\{\mathrm{Var}(\hat{\mu}_{\mathrm{MI}})\} = \mathrm{E}(\hat{W}) + \left(1 + \frac{1}{K}\right) \mathrm{E}(\hat{B}) = \frac{\sigma^2}{n_O}\left(1 + \frac{\pi_M}{K}\right),$$

and comparing this with $\mathrm{Var}(\hat{\mu}_{\mathrm{MI}})$ we see that it is unbiased in terms of finite K, given the large n approximation being used for the posterior. In fact it is completely unbiased in a small sample sense (n and K) if we take a flat, improper, prior for μ.

This example illustrates that MI is not 'making up data'; no matter how many observations we might say are missing, MI gives a variance estimate that is bounded below by the standard error of the mean of the observed data.

Estimating the mean with σ^2 unknown

Keeping the same basic setup we now assume, more realistically, that σ^2 is unknown. We have the same priors for the unobserved values and for μ, and take the (improper) prior for σ^2 to be proportional to σ^{-2}. This is the limiting form of the conjugate scaled inverse-χ^2 prior (see for example Gelman *et al.* 1995, Section 2.8, and Appendix B). It follows that the posterior distribution for σ^2 has the form

$$\sigma^2 \mid \mathbf{Y}_O \sim \frac{(n_O - 1)S_O}{X^2} \tag{2.30}$$

for $X^2 \sim \chi^2_{n_O - 1}$ and S_O the sample variance of the observed data:

$$S_O = \frac{1}{n_O - 1} \sum_{i \in \mathcal{O}} (Y_i - \bar{Y}_O)^2.$$

The imputation proceeds as before, except that it begins, for each k, by taking a draw, $\tilde{\sigma}^2$ say, from the posterior (2.30), which is used in the imputation of the data through (2.25), that is:

$$f(e_{ik} \mid \mathbf{Y}_O) \sim \mathrm{N}(0, \tilde{\sigma}^2) \quad \text{and} \quad f(s_k \mid \mathbf{Y}_O) \sim \mathrm{N}(0, \tilde{\sigma}^2/n_O).$$

Again, because of the simplicity of the setup, we can derive exact properties of the multiple imputation quantities. The approach is exactly the same as above, except that expectations are taken in two steps, first conditional on the observed data $\mathbf{Y}_O$ and then with respect to this. As before it follows directly that $\hat{\mu}_{\mathrm{MI}}$ is unbiased for μ. Its variance can be obtained as follows. First we have

$$\mathrm{Var}(\hat{\mu}_{\mathrm{MI}} \mid \mathbf{Y}_O) = \frac{\pi_M}{n_O K^2} \sum_{k=1}^{K} \mathrm{E}_{\mathrm{I}}(\tilde{\sigma}^2)$$

where the expectations are taken over the imputation distribution. Given that the mean of the inverse χ^2_v distribution is $(v-2)^{-1}$,

$$\mathrm{E_I}(\tilde{\sigma}^2) = \left(\frac{n_O - 1}{n_O - 3}\right) S_O,$$

(where E_I denotes expectations over the imputation distribution) and so

$$\mathrm{Var}(\hat{\mu}_{\mathrm{MI}} \mid \mathbf{Y}_O) = \left(\frac{n_O - 1}{n_O - 3}\right) \frac{\pi_M}{n_O K} S_O,$$

giving, as S_O is unbiased for σ^2:

$$\mathrm{Var}(\hat{\mu}_{\mathrm{MI}}) = \frac{\sigma^2}{n_O} + \left(\frac{n_O - 1}{n_O - 3}\right) \frac{\pi_M}{n_O K} \sigma^2.$$

The expectation of the MI variance estimator (2.27) is obtained using similar two-stage arguments. Omitting details we find,

$$\mathrm{E}(\hat{W}) = \frac{\sigma^2}{n} \left(\frac{n - 3}{n - 1}\right) \left(\frac{n_O - 1}{n_O - 3}\right),$$

and

$$\mathrm{E}(\hat{B}) = \frac{\pi_M}{n_O} \left(\frac{n_O - 1}{n_O - 3}\right) \sigma^2,$$

from which we get

$$\mathrm{E}(\hat{V}_{\mathrm{MI}}) = \frac{\sigma^2}{n_O} \left(\frac{n_O - 1}{n_O - 3}\right) \left\{1 - \frac{2n_O}{n(n-1)} + \frac{\pi_M}{K}\right\}.$$

This bias in $\hat{V}_{\mathrm{MI}}$ is then

$$\mathrm{E}(\hat{V}_{\mathrm{MI}}) - \mathrm{V}(\hat{\mu}_{\mathrm{MI}}) = \frac{2\sigma^2}{n_O(n_O - 3)} \left\{1 - \frac{n_O(n_O - 1)}{n(n-1)}\right\}.$$

What is important here is the absence of K from this expression, implying that the bias does not depend on K, and so we do not need to rely on the number of imputations to ensure that the variance formula is working as we would wish. The bias that does exist disappears with increasing sample size n (assuming as usual, that the proportion of missing data is bounded), which is not an issue as we are anyway using large sample arguments to underpin the derivation of the MI procedure.

General linear regression with σ^2 known

Our final simple example is that of general linear regression with a known variance. We can infer from the relationships between the previous two settings that the additional complication of an unknown variance does not have a profound impact on the basic development: it essentially adds an additional step to the imputation process and hence to the derivation of the properties of the statistics. Hence, by keeping the known variance assumption, we can keep the basic simplicity of the development without serious loss of generality.

Our aim is to estimate the parameters of a simple linear regression model:

$$f(\mathbf{Y} \mid \mathbf{X}) \sim \mathrm{N}_n(\mathbf{X}\boldsymbol{\beta};\ \sigma^2 \boldsymbol{I}_n), \tag{2.31}$$

for $\mathbf{X}$ and $(n \times p)$ matrix of covariates, and σ^2 known. It is assumed that some of the outcomes in $\mathbf{Y}$ are MAR dependent on $\mathbf{X}$, which is assumed to be completely observed. As with estimating the simple mean above, we do not need MI here, the obvious, unbiased, estimator is given by

$$\widehat{\boldsymbol{\beta}}_O = (\mathbf{X}_O{}^T\mathbf{X}_O)^{-1}\mathbf{X}_O{}^T\mathbf{Y}_O,$$

for $\mathbf{Y}_O$ the observed outcomes and $\mathbf{X}_O$ the corresponding covariate matrix, with known covariance matrix $\mathbf{V}_O = \sigma^2(\mathbf{X}_O{}^T\mathbf{X}_O)^{-1}$. However, we again use MI for this, and it is instructive to see, in this simple setting, how this is related to the conventional approach.

Following the same basic steps as above, we assume that the large sample posterior for $\boldsymbol{\beta}$ is centred on the maximum likelihood estimator $\widehat{\boldsymbol{\beta}}_O$ with covariance matrix $\mathbf{V}_O$, that is,

$$\widetilde{\boldsymbol{\beta}} \mid \mathbf{Y}_O \sim \mathrm{N}_p(\widehat{\boldsymbol{\beta}}_O;\ \mathbf{V}_O).$$

The imputation model can therefore we expressed, for the kth imputation,

$$\widetilde{\mathbf{Y}}_{M,k} \mid \mathbf{Y}_O = \mathbf{X}_M(\widehat{\boldsymbol{\beta}}_O + \mathbf{b}_k) + \mathbf{e}_k$$

for $\mathbf{X}_M$ the covariate matrix for the missing outcomes, and

$$\mathbf{b}_k \sim \mathrm{N}_p(\mathbf{0};\ \mathbf{V}_O) \quad \text{and} \quad \mathbf{e}_k \sim \mathrm{N}(\mathbf{0};\ \sigma^2 \boldsymbol{I}_{n_M}).$$

The estimate of $\boldsymbol{\beta}$ from the kth imputation set is then

$$\widetilde{\boldsymbol{\beta}}_k = (\mathbf{X}^T\mathbf{X})^{-1}\mathbf{X}_O{}^T\mathbf{Y}_O + (\mathbf{X}^T\mathbf{X})^{-1}\mathbf{X}_M{}^T\widetilde{\mathbf{Y}}_{M,k}.$$

Using the fact that $\widetilde{\mathbf{Y}}_{M,k}$ can be written

$$\mathbf{X}_M(\widehat{\boldsymbol{\beta}}_O + \mathbf{b}_k) + \mathbf{e}_k = \mathbf{X}_M\left\{(\mathbf{X}_O{}^T\mathbf{X}_O)^{-1}\mathbf{X}_O{}^T\mathbf{Y}_O + \mathbf{b}_k\right\} + \mathbf{e}_k$$

since $\mathbf{X}^T\mathbf{X} = \mathbf{X}_O^T\mathbf{X}_O + \mathbf{X}_M^T\mathbf{X}_M$, we see that $\widetilde{\boldsymbol{\beta}}_k$ can be written as a sum of $\widehat{\boldsymbol{\beta}}_O$ (which depends only on $\mathbf{Y}_O$) and terms involving the imputed random variables:

$$\widetilde{\boldsymbol{\beta}}_k = \widehat{\boldsymbol{\beta}}_O + (\mathbf{X}^T\mathbf{X})^{-1}\mathbf{X}_M{}^T(\mathbf{X}_M\mathbf{b}_k + \mathbf{e}_k)$$

It is then simple to average these over the imputation sets to obtain the MI estimator:

$$\widehat{\boldsymbol{\beta}}_{\mathrm{MI}} = \widehat{\boldsymbol{\beta}}_O + (\mathbf{X}^T\mathbf{X})^{-1}\mathbf{X}_M{}^T(\mathbf{X}_M\bar{\boldsymbol{b}}_. + \bar{\boldsymbol{e}}_.),$$

using obvious notation.

To find the mean of $\widetilde{\boldsymbol{\beta}}_k$ we need to first take expectations over the imputation distribution (denoted I), given $\mathbf{Y}_O$ and then over $\mathbf{Y}_O$ itself, that is,

$$\mathrm{E}(\widehat{\boldsymbol{\beta}}_{\mathrm{MI}}) = \mathrm{E}_{\mathbf{Y}_O}\{\,\mathrm{E}_{\mathrm{I}|\mathbf{Y}_O}(\widehat{\boldsymbol{\beta}}_O)\}$$

which reduces to $\mathrm{E}_{\mathbf{Y}_O}(\widehat{\boldsymbol{\beta}}_O) = \boldsymbol{\beta}$. Hence the MI estimator of $\boldsymbol{\beta}$ is unbiased. We also see that it tends to the ML (or OLS) estimator as K increases. The latter property holds more generally for missing outcomes when estimation is based on score equations and the imputation model is congenial.

Similar arguments can be used to obtain the variance of $\widehat{\boldsymbol{\beta}}_{\mathrm{MI}}$:

$$\mathrm{Var}(\widehat{\boldsymbol{\beta}}_{\mathrm{MI}}) = \mathrm{E}_{\mathbf{Y}_O}\{\mathrm{Var}_{\mathrm{I}|\mathbf{Y}_O}(\widehat{\boldsymbol{\beta}}_{\mathrm{MI}})\} + \mathrm{Var}_{\mathbf{Y}_O}\{\,\mathrm{E}_{\mathrm{I}|\mathbf{Y}_O}(\widehat{\boldsymbol{\beta}}_{\mathrm{MI}})\},$$

which reduces to

$$\mathbf{V}_O + \frac{1}{K}\{\mathbf{V}_O - \sigma^2(\mathbf{X}^T\mathbf{X})^{-1}\}. \tag{2.32}$$

The matrix inside the braces is positive definite, so we see that the MI estimator is always less precise than the ML estimator $\widehat{\boldsymbol{\beta}}_O$, but the difference disappears as K increases. Again we expect to see this in general for missing outcomes with ML estimation and a congenial imputation model.

Our final step is to compare the behaviour of the MI variance estimator (2.27) with this exact value in (2.32). For this we need the expectation of

$$\widehat{\mathbf{V}}_{\mathrm{MI}} = \frac{1}{K}\sum_{k=1}^{K}\widetilde{\sigma}_k^2(\mathbf{X}^T\mathbf{X})^{-1} + \left(\frac{K+1}{K}\right)\left(\frac{1}{K-1}\right)\sum_{k=1}^{K}(\widetilde{\boldsymbol{\beta}}_k - \widehat{\boldsymbol{\beta}}_{\mathrm{MI}})(\widetilde{\boldsymbol{\beta}}_k - \widehat{\boldsymbol{\beta}}_{\mathrm{MI}})^T \tag{2.33}$$

for $\widetilde{\sigma}_k^2$ the residual variance from the analysis of the kth imputation set:

$$\widetilde{\sigma}_k^2 = \frac{1}{n-p}\Big\{(\mathbf{Y}_O - \mathbf{X}_O\widetilde{\boldsymbol{\beta}}_k)^T(\mathbf{Y}_O - \mathbf{X}_O\widetilde{\boldsymbol{\beta}}_k) + (\widetilde{\mathbf{Y}}_{M,k} - \mathbf{X}_M\widetilde{\boldsymbol{\beta}}_k)^T(\widetilde{\mathbf{Y}}_{M,k} - \mathbf{X}_M\widetilde{\boldsymbol{\beta}}_k)\Big\}.$$

By decomposing the two-right hand components separately it can be shown that

$$\mathrm{E}_{\mathbf{Y}_O}\{\,\mathrm{E}_{\mathrm{I}|\mathbf{Y}_O}(\widetilde{\sigma}_k^2)\} = \sigma^2,$$

and so the first term on the right-hand side of (2.33) is unbiased for

$$\sigma^2(\mathbf{X}^T\mathbf{X})^{-1}.$$

Noting that

$$\widetilde{\boldsymbol{\beta}}_k - \widehat{\boldsymbol{\beta}}_{\mathrm{MI}} = (\mathbf{X}^T\mathbf{X})^{-1}\mathbf{X}_M{}^T\left\{\mathbf{X}_M(\mathbf{b}_k - \bar{\boldsymbol{b}}_.) + (\mathbf{e}_k - \bar{\boldsymbol{e}}_.)\right\}$$

and using the independence of $\mathbf{b_k}$ and $\mathbf{e}_k$, it can also be shown that

$$\mathrm{E}_{\mathrm{I},\mathbf{Y}_O}\left[\left(\frac{1}{K-1}\right)\sum_{k=1}^{K}(\widetilde{\boldsymbol{\beta}}_k - \widehat{\boldsymbol{\beta}}_{\mathrm{MI}})(\widetilde{\boldsymbol{\beta}}_k - \widehat{\boldsymbol{\beta}}_{\mathrm{MI}})^T\right] = \mathbf{V}_O - \sigma^2(\mathbf{X}^T\mathbf{X})^{-1}.$$

Combining these two results we have

$$\begin{aligned}\mathrm{E}_{\mathrm{I},\mathbf{Y}_O}(\widehat{\mathbf{V}}_{\mathrm{MI}}) &= \sigma^2(\mathbf{X}^T\mathbf{X})^{-1} + \left(1+\frac{1}{K}\right)\left\{\mathbf{V}_O - \sigma^2(\mathbf{X}^T\mathbf{X})^{-1}\right\}\\ &= \mathbf{V}_O + \frac{1}{K}\left\{\mathbf{V}_O - \sigma^2(\mathbf{X}^T\mathbf{X})^{-1}\right\} \qquad (2.34)\\ &= \mathrm{Var}(\widehat{\boldsymbol{\beta}}_{\mathrm{MI}}).\end{aligned}$$

The MI variance estimator is exactly unbiased for the true variance of $\widehat{\boldsymbol{\beta}}_{\mathrm{MI}}$.

Again, in this simple setting we have been able to derive an exact result, which does not rely on asymptotics. This provides us with some insight into the behaviour of the MI variance estimator. For realistic problems, however, we must resort to asymptotic arguments, but interestingly we find that the structure observed here reflects the structure observed in the general case under congeniality when our substantive model is fitted by maximum likelihood. Specifically, let $\boldsymbol{I}(\boldsymbol{\beta})$ and $\boldsymbol{I}_O(\boldsymbol{\beta})$ be the expected Fisher information matrices for the complete data, here $\mathbf{Y}$, and observed data, here $\mathbf{Y}_O$, respectively. Then under congeniality and suitable regularity conditions, the MI variance estimator $\widehat{\mathbf{V}}_{\mathrm{MI}}$ has a limiting distribution, as the sample size increases, that has mean equal to

$$\boldsymbol{I}_O(\boldsymbol{\beta})^{-1} + \frac{1}{K}\left\{\boldsymbol{I}_O(\boldsymbol{\beta})^{-1} - \boldsymbol{I}(\boldsymbol{\beta})^{-1}\right\}.$$

It is easy to see how this reduces to (2.34) for the simple regression example. This result is most succinctly derived in Nielsen (2003), but is also given by Wang and Robins (1998). Another interesting feature of the MI variance estimator, as noted by both Wang and Robins (1998) and Nielsen (2003) is that the estimator is not actually consistent as the sample size increases; we also require $K \to \infty$. Nielsen (2003) shows that its limiting distribution is Wishart with $K - 1$ DF, with a mean that is shifted to the required value.

2.8 MI in more general settings

In the previous section we have assumed that MI is applied under congeniality, with maximum likelihood estimation of the parameters of the substantive model in each imputed dataset. There we saw that we can view MI as an approximate

Bayesian procedure, with frequentist inference obtained by appealing to general asymptotic results which calibrate features of the posterior from a repeated sampling perspective.

However, MI is used in settings which relax these restrictions. In particular other forms of estimation are used, such as those employing generalised estimating equations. Further, uncongenial imputation models, where typically the imputation model contains more variables than the substantive model, are common. Indeed, MI would lose much of its practical value if it were restricted to strict congeniality. However, the justification for the use of MI in this broader setting is less clear-cut. There are general arguments to suggest that its behaviour can remain, in many examples, good enough for practical purposes, with many simulation studies supporting this view. But set against this are specific theoretical and practical counter-examples. There are two main issues. First, does the procedure produce, at least approximately, consistent estimators of the parameters of interest and, second, does Rubin's variance formula produce acceptable inferential behaviour. The theoretical arguments can become very technical, and it is not our aim to attempt to reproduce these here. Rather we set out what general guidance can be taken from the many theoretical and simulation results that have been obtained.

In his original book, Rubin, (Rubin, 1987, p. 119) defines conditions for so-called 'proper' imputation in terms of the complete-data statistics which we denote, for a scalar problem, $\widehat{\beta}_{\text{C}}$ and $\widehat{V}_{\text{C}}$. These are the estimate of the parameter of the substantive model and associated variance respectively calculated using the intended, *complete* data. Rubin gives three conditions that need to be satisfied to justify the frequentist properties of the MI procedure. These are expressed in terms of the MI quantities defined in Section 2.5, and are needed to derive more rigorously the results presented there. The first two conditions are expressed in terms of repeated sampling of the missing value process R, given the complete data $\mathbf{Y}$ as fixed: first,

$$\frac{\widehat{\beta}_{\text{MI}} - \widehat{\beta}_{\text{C}}}{\sqrt{\widehat{B}}} \overset{K\rightarrow\infty}{\sim} \text{N}(0, 1)$$

and second, $\widehat{W}$ is consistent for $\widehat{V}_{\text{C}}$ as $K \to \infty$. The third condition is that as $K \to \infty$, $\widehat{B}$ is of lower order than $\widehat{W}$. How useful a guide these three conditions are in practice is hard to say. Apart from the simplest settings it is difficult to justify them rigorously. For further details we refer to Rubin (1987) Section 4.2 and Schafer (1997) Section 4.5.5.

Wang and Robins (1998) and Robins and Wang (2000) approach the problem in terms of the properties of regular asymptotic linear estimators and compare the properties of multiple imputation estimators under both proper Bayesian and improper imputation schemes. Improper imputation is defined as repeated imputation using *fixed* consistent estimators of the parameters of the imputation model, that is, when new draws of these parameters are *not* made for each set of imputations. They show that although, for finite K, the 'improper' estimators are the more efficient, Rubin's variance estimator, (2.16) is an overestimate of the variability of these. Unfortunately it appears that no such simple and generally applicable variance expression, akin to Rubin's variance estimator, exists for the 'improper' estimators. Instead, their variance formula requires the score equations of both the imputation model and the substantive model. A more accessible account of these developments is provided by Tsiatis (2006), Chapter 14.

Uncongenial imputation models

We suppose now that the imputation model is uncongenial. A common source of this is the incorporation of so-called auxiliary variables that provide information about the missing data and/or missing data mechanism but which are not in the substantive model. At the risk of oversimplification, we can think of two settings. In the first the imputation model is *richer* than the the substantive model. This would require considerable detail to formalise properly, but intuitively we could think of this as meaning that there is at least one congenial imputation model nested within it. This will often be the case. By contrast, in our second setting, the imputation model is *poorer* than the substantive model, *i.e.*, there exists structure and/or variables missing from the imputation model that is present in the substantive model and so there is no congenial imputation model nested within it. This latter case should be avoided, as it generally results in both inconsistent estimators of the substantive model parameters and invalidity of the Rubin's variance estimator (Robins and Wang, 2000). For example, in Chapter 9 we show how the omission of multilevel structure in the imputation model can lead to biases in both MI estimators and their variances when using a multilevel substantive model.

However, there are many situations when the first setting, that of a richer but uncongenial imputation model, may be highly desirable for use in practice. To provide an intuitive view of this setting we return to the simple regression example with known variance. We assume the same substantive model considered in Section 2.7 but assume now that the imputation model has additional variables, which are in this case redundant, that is their true regression coefficients in the imputation model are equal to zero. Thus we have a richer imputation model. The substantive model is then as (11.5):

$$f(\mathbf{Y} \mid \mathbf{X}) \sim \mathrm{N}_n(\mathbf{X}\boldsymbol{\beta};\, \sigma^2 \boldsymbol{I}_n).$$

but now assume we also have an additional q redundant auxiliary covariates in $\mathbf{V}$ $(n \times q)$ such that

$$\mathrm{E}(\mathbf{Y}) = \begin{bmatrix} \mathbf{X} & \mathbf{V} \end{bmatrix} \begin{bmatrix} \boldsymbol{\beta} \\ \mathbf{0} \end{bmatrix} = \mathbf{U}\boldsymbol{\alpha},$$

and this will be used as the imputation model. Partitioning $\mathbf{U}$ in the same way as $\mathbf{X}$, and following the same development as in Section 2.7 we have the posterior for $\boldsymbol{\alpha}$:

$$f(\widetilde{\boldsymbol{\alpha}} \mid \mathbf{Y}_O) \sim \mathrm{N}_p(\widehat{\boldsymbol{\alpha}}_O;\, \mathbf{W}_O),$$

for $\widehat{\boldsymbol{\alpha}}_O = (\mathbf{U}_O^T\mathbf{U}_O)^{-1}\mathbf{U}_O^T\mathbf{Y}_O$ and $\mathbf{W}_O = \sigma^2(\mathbf{U}_O^T\mathbf{U}_O)^{-1}$. Hence the imputation step can be expressed

$$\widetilde{\mathbf{Y}}_{M,k} \mid \mathbf{Y}_O = \mathbf{U}_M(\widehat{\boldsymbol{\alpha}}_O + \mathbf{a}_k) + \mathbf{e}_k,$$

for

$$\mathbf{a}_k \sim \mathrm{N}_p(\mathbf{0};\ \mathbf{W}_O) \quad \text{and} \quad \mathbf{e}_k \sim \mathrm{N}(\mathbf{0};\ \sigma^2\boldsymbol{I}_{n_M}).$$

The original model of interest (11.5) is fitted to each imputed data set, so that as in Section 2.7

$$\widetilde{\boldsymbol{\beta}}_k = (\mathbf{X}^T\mathbf{X})^{-1}\mathbf{X}_O{}^T\mathbf{Y}_O + (\mathbf{X}^T\mathbf{X})^{-1}\mathbf{X}_M{}^T\widetilde{\mathbf{Y}}_{M,k},$$

which can be written

$$\widetilde{\boldsymbol{\beta}}_k = \mathbf{H}\mathbf{Y}_O + (\mathbf{X}^T\mathbf{X})^{-1}\mathbf{X}_M{}^T(\mathbf{U}_M\mathbf{a}_k + \mathbf{e}_k),$$

for

$$\mathbf{H} = (\mathbf{X}^T\mathbf{X})^{-1}\left\{\mathbf{X}_O{}^T + \mathbf{X}_M{}^T\mathbf{U}_M(\mathbf{U}_M{}^T\mathbf{U}_M)^{-1}\mathbf{U}_O{}^T\right\}.$$

It follows that the MI estimator is

$$\widehat{\boldsymbol{\beta}}_{\mathrm{MI}} = \mathbf{H}\mathbf{Y}_O + (\mathbf{X}^T\mathbf{X})^{-1}\mathbf{X}_M{}^T(\mathbf{U}_M\bar{a}_. + \bar{e}_.),$$

As before we see the separation of the original data $\mathbf{Y}_O$ and the imputed variables $\mathbf{a}_k$ and $\mathbf{e}_k$. Because of the difference between the substantive and imputation models, however, this expression does not take the relatively simple form seen earlier. However the estimator remains unbiased for $\boldsymbol{\beta}$. To see this we merely need to note that $\mathbf{H}\mathbf{X}_O = \boldsymbol{I}_p$, from which $\mathrm{E}(\mathbf{H}\mathbf{Y}_O) = \mathbf{H}\mathbf{X}_O\boldsymbol{\beta} = \boldsymbol{\beta}$, and hence the result. In fact it is not hard to see, at least from an intuitive perspective, that we should expect consistency in more general settings with such richer uncongenial imputation models where the auxiliary variables are not redundant.

Similarly the variance of $\widehat{\boldsymbol{\beta}}_{\mathrm{MI}}$ can be shown to be

$$\mathrm{Var}(\widehat{\boldsymbol{\beta}}_{\mathrm{MI}}) = \sigma^2\left\{(\mathbf{X}_O{}^T\mathbf{X}_O)^{-1} + \mathbf{G}\right\} + \frac{\sigma^2}{K}\left\{(\mathbf{X}_O{}^T\mathbf{X}_O)^{-1} - (\mathbf{X}^T\mathbf{X})^{-1} + \mathbf{G}\right\} \tag{2.35}$$

where

$$\mathbf{G} = (\mathbf{X}^T\mathbf{X})^{-1}\mathbf{X}_M{}^T(\widehat{\mathbf{V}}_M - \mathbf{V}_M)^T\mathbf{Q}_O{}^{-1}(\widehat{\mathbf{V}}_M - \mathbf{V}_M)\mathbf{X}_M(\mathbf{X}^T\mathbf{X})^{-1}$$

for

$$\widehat{\mathbf{V}}_M = \mathbf{X}_M(\mathbf{X}_O{}^T\mathbf{X}_O)^{-1}\mathbf{X}_O{}^T\mathbf{V}_O$$

the predictor of $\mathbf{V}_M$ from the regression of $\mathbf{V}_O$ on $\mathbf{X}_O$, and

$$\mathbf{Q}_O = \mathbf{V}_O^T\left\{\boldsymbol{I}_{n_O} - \mathbf{X}_O(\mathbf{X}_O{}^T\mathbf{X}_O)^{-1}\mathbf{X}_O{}^T\right\}\mathbf{V}_O$$

the residual sum of squares and cross-products from the same regression.

It is instructive to compare (2.35) with the equivalent expression when there are no redundant covariates, as given in (2.32): the difference between these is equal to

$$\sigma^2 \left(\frac{K+1}{K} \right) \mathbf{G}.$$

By definition $\mathbf{G}$ is always positive definite, hence the addition of the redundant covariates has decreased the precision of the estimator by an amount proportional to $\mathbf{G}$, and this quantity does not disappear with increasing K. It can also be seen that the size of $\mathbf{G}$ depends on the predictive accuracy of the regression of $\mathbf{V}_O$ on $\mathbf{X}_O$ relative to the residual error from this regression.

We can also derive an exact expression for the expectation of the MI variance estimator of $\widehat{\boldsymbol{\beta}}_{\mathrm{MI}}$ in this setting:

$$\begin{aligned} \mathrm{E}(\widehat{\mathbf{V}}_{\mathrm{MI}}) &= \sigma^2 \left\{ (\mathbf{X}_O{}^T \mathbf{X}_O)^{-1} + \mathbf{G} \right\} + \frac{\sigma^2}{K} \left\{ (\mathbf{X}_O{}^T \mathbf{X}_O)^{-1} - (\mathbf{X}^T \mathbf{X})^{-1} + \mathbf{G} \right\} \\ &\quad + \left\{ \mathrm{E}(\tilde{\sigma}^2_{\mathrm{MI}}) - \sigma^2 \right\} (\mathbf{X}^T \mathbf{X})^{-1}, \end{aligned}$$

where

$$\tilde{\sigma}^2_{\mathrm{MI}} = \frac{1}{K} \sum_{k=1}^{K} \tilde{\sigma}^2_k$$

the average estimated residual variance over the imputations. Comparing this expression with the actual variance in (2.35) it can be seen that if $\tilde{\sigma}^2_{\mathrm{MI}}$ were unbiased, the MI variance estimator would itself be unbiased. However we find that

$$\mathrm{E}(\tilde{\sigma}^2_{\mathrm{MI}}) - \sigma^2 = \frac{2\sigma^2}{n-p} \left[\mathrm{tr} \left\{ (\boldsymbol{I}_{n_M} + \mathbf{C})(\boldsymbol{I}_{n_M} - \mathbf{D}) \right\} - n_M \right], \qquad (2.36)$$

where the two matrices $\mathbf{C}$ and $\mathbf{D}$ are defined as follows

$$\mathbf{C} = \boldsymbol{I}_{n_M} - \mathbf{K} + \mathbf{K}\mathbf{V}_M (\mathbf{V}_M{}^T \mathbf{K} \mathbf{V}_M)^{-1} \mathbf{V}_M{}^T \mathbf{K},$$

for

$$\mathbf{K} = \boldsymbol{I}_{n_M} - \mathbf{X}_M (\mathbf{X}_M{}^T \mathbf{X}_M)^{-1} \mathbf{X}_M{}^T$$

and $\mathbf{D} = \mathbf{X}_M (\mathbf{X}^T \mathbf{X})^{-1} \mathbf{X}_M{}^T$. Although it is not self-evident, it can be shown that the expression on the right-hand side of (2.36) is always positive, hence the MI variance estimator will always be conservative in this setting.

The most interesting feature of this result is that, as Meng (1994) shows, there is a sense in which this result holds generally, at least in so far as the behaviour is defined through the performance of the resulting confidence intervals. Unsurprisingly the precise result requires careful formulation, we refer to Meng (1994) for details. One important requirement is that the estimator from the substantive model is *self-efficient* in Meng's terms, which means, in the scalar setting, that the substantive analysis applied to the complete data delivers an estimator $\hat{\beta}(\mathbf{Y})$ say that has smaller MSE than any linear mixture with the incomplete data estimator $\hat{\beta}(\mathbf{Y}_O)$:

$$\lambda\hat{\beta}(\mathbf{Y}) + (1-\lambda)\hat{\beta}(\mathbf{Y}_O) \tag{2.37}$$

where the weight λ can take any value, including negative ones. This requirement excludes, for example, the rather artificial situation in which an estimator's efficiency can decrease with additional data. As indicated by Meng and Romero (2003), (2.37) is equivalent to the assumption that $\hat{\beta}(\mathbf{Y})$ is uncorrelated with the difference $\hat{\beta}(\mathbf{Y}) - \hat{\beta}(\mathbf{Y}_O)$. Hence, we see that the use of self-inefficient procedures, for which this correlation is not zero, will lead to bias in the MI variance estimator. It is the presence of this correlation, and related ones, that crops up repeatedly in establishing situations in which the MI variance formula fails in a survey sampling setting. We return to such settings briefly below. In the type of situations considered in this book we will typically be dealing with self-efficient estimators, and we note that this extends the estimation procedures we might use for the substantive model beyond maximum likelihood. It is interesting that counterexamples to the appropriateness of the MI procedure often use estimation procedures that are not self-efficient. See for example Fay (1993), Nielsen (2003) and the subsequent discussion in Meng and Romero (2003).

Hughes *et al.* (2012b) conducted a simulation study to examine the behaviour of the MI variance estimator, and to compare it with two other approaches: the estimator derived in Robins and Wang (2000) and a full mechanism bootstrap approach. They take as the substantive model a standard multiple linear regression with four continuous and one binary predictor variables. Only a single variable is partially observed, since the Robins and Wang variance estimator rapidly becomes very complex with more than one missing variable. In the simulation study one of the continuous predictors was chosen for this, and the missingness mechanism was MCAR.

Several different uncongenial scenarios were explored, with rather large proportions missing, 40% and 60%. The scenarios were

1. domain analysis, in which the imputations were constructed from the whole dataset, but the substantive model was fitted to one category of the binary predictor;
2. when the true error were heterogeneous, but homogeneous in the imputation model;
3. when an interaction was omitted from the imputation model that was present (although redundant) in the substantive model; and
4. non-normality of the true errors (both moderate and severe).

We summarise the results by focussing on the coverage of the 95% confidence intervals – the crucial operating characteristic in practice. With 60% average missingness, and a sample size of 1000, under scenarios (1) and (3) the coverage of the confidence intervals was conservative (99% and 98% respectively), and under under (2) anti-conservative (92%). For moderate non normality the coverage was close to nominal (95%), but strongly anti-conservative under severe non-normality (86%). Interestingly, the use of a robust/sandwich estimate of variance in the complete data analysis step improved the coverage (93%). The Robins and Wang variance estimator led to coverage closer to the nominal level in all scenarios (all 95% to two significant figure) except that of extreme non-normality, where it performed similarly to the Rubin's variance estimator with robust variance (92%). With $n = 100$ results were similar for the Rubin's variance estimator, but the Robins and Wang approach led to consistent under-coverage in all scenarios (ranging from 87% to 92%).

What should we conclude from these results? We know that when the imputation model is misspecified, the confidence interval coverage will not be exactly at the nominal level. It is thus very comforting to see that in the less extreme scenarios, the coverage is conservative, and is only anti-conservative in the extreme examples (heteroscedasticity and extreme non-normality) that should be spotted anyway at the stage at which the imputation model is being formulated. In none of these scenarios is the imputation model 'richer' (in the sense used earlier) than the substantive model, which is most commonly going to be the source of uncongeniality in practice, and there we expect mildly conservative coverage which will be unimportant in the vast majority of practical applications. As theory predicts, the Robins and Wang variance estimator provides better asymptotic coverage, although the consistent anti-conservative behaviour in the smaller sample size setting is worrying. We should note as well that these results have been obtained under very high missingness rates (60%).

The problem with the Robins and Wang procedure is its lack of generality; it is far more problem specific. To quote Hughes *et al*. (2012b)

> 'A major disadvantage of the Robins and Wang method is that calculation of the imputation variance estimate is considerably more complicated than for Rubin's MI and full mechanism bootstrapping, with a greater burden placed on both the imputer and the analyst. To our knowledge, there is no generally available software implementing the Robins and Wang method. The analyst must make available derivatives of the estimating equations for use in calculation of variance estimates, and these become harder to calculate as the complexity of the analysis procedure increases. Also, the complexity of the calculations conducted by the imputer increases when there are multiple incomplete variables with a general missing data pattern. For this reason, our simulation scenarios were restricted to data missing in a single variable, as were the scenarios considered in the papers proposing the approach.
>
> The Robins and Wang method requires the data to be imputed under a single imputation model. Therefore, currently, it cannot be applied

> if imputation is conducted using [full conditional specification, (see Chapter 3)], a flexible and commonly used method of imputation[...] By contrast, calculation of the variance of an imputation estimator by Rubin's MI method [...] is straightforward for more complex missing data patterns and analysis procedures, and can be applied when data are imputed using [full conditional specification]'

The two main messages that we take from these comparisons, and the theoretical results discussed earlier, is that first, appropriate care must be taken in constructing an imputation model that properly represents the structure of the data under analysis and the substantive model and, second, mildly conservative behaviour of the resulting inferences is an acceptable price to pay for the exceptional simplicity, flexibility and generality of the overall MI procedure. As Rubin (2003) writes

> 'In many fields, the collection of complete-data analyses that would be performed in the absence of missing data is often relatively fixed by tradition or the need to communicate clearly to an audience of non-statisticians and so these complete-data analyses [...] are not based on fully specified Bayesian or likelihood models. When confronted with missing data, it is a hopelessly daunting task to derive and implement new methods of data analysis, to validate their operating characteristics and to formulate ways to present them to an outside audience for each such situation compromised by the occurrence of missing data. For such problems, I believe that MI is a general solution because it allows the statistician to capitalize on what is already accepted – the complete – data analysis – and often avoid largely extraneous complications created by limited fractions of missing information.
>
> Also, MI allows the straightforward investigation of changes in the final completed-data inference resulting from changes in the assumed process for creating missing data, when there is a desire for such sensitivity analysis. In some cases, there will be a loss in efficiency, or in rare cases, even some validity, using MI, especially with large fractions of missing information, but this seems like a small price to pay relative to the practical benefits of MI in more realistic cases. [...] If statisticians do not provide solutions that are close to valid, users of data will not stop producing answers, but instead will turn to *ad hoc*, potentially entirely invalid methods, when approximately valid answers are readily available via MI. MI may not be the ideal solution for all missing data problems, but I now firmly believe it is as close as we have come to a general solution to them.'

A further implication of these results is that when building an imputation model it is better to err on the side of over-fitting rather than under-fitting. We see that the penalty for over-fitting, i.e., having a richer imputation model than strictly necessary, is some conservatism, probably slight, while omitting key variables can lead to inconsistent estimators. This advice has long history in the MI literature. For example, Section 2.6 of Rubin (1996):

> 'The possible lost precision when including unimportant predictors is usually viewed as a relatively small price to pay for the general validity of analyses of the resultant multiply-imputed data base.'

Collins *et al.* (2001) use a simulation study to compare restrictive 'minimal use of auxiliary variables' and inclusive 'liberal use of auxiliary variables' in the imputation model. Their conclusions are consistent with Rubin's advice: 'The simulation[s] showed that the inclusive strategy is much to be preferred'.

Our conclusion at this point is that, within our model-based framework, we can make use of uncongenial imputation models when convenient, provided that they are not lacking an essential aspect of the analysis procedure, and we should at worst expect some conservatism in the long-run properties of the MI based inferences.

2.8.1 Survey sample settings

Although we are not principally concerned in this book with the problems of applying multiple imputation in a survey sample context, we do touch on such issues when faced with estimators that require weighting. We summarise a few key points here before returning to the problem in Chapter 11. In the development so far in this chapter it has been assumed that that the complete data have been generated through random sampling from some population model which forms the basis of our substantive model. The behaviour of MI has been considered under such conditions. When this is not the case, and the sampling of the data from the population is not simple, as with most survey samples, the justification for the MI procedure raises addition issues, in particular, a naive application of Rubin's variance estimator is commonly inappropriate. One manifestation of this problem is the use of imputation procedures that are based on the entire sample, in conjunction with substantive models fitted to subsets of the data. Domain estimation is the common example of this. Again, a naive application of the MI variance in such settings will typically not be appropriate. Kott (1995) provides an early and clear description of the essential problem: the variance estimators derived from the the sets of multiply imputed data sets do not follow from the actual sampling mechanism and so do not condition appropriately.

2.9 Constructing congenial imputation models

Consider the linear regression model

$$f(\mathbf{Y} \mid \mathbf{X}) \sim \mathrm{N}_n(\mathbf{X}\boldsymbol{\beta};\ \sigma^2 \boldsymbol{I}_n), \tag{2.38}$$

for $\mathbf{X}$ an $(n \times p)$ matrix of covariates. Suppose that we have missing data in both response and covariates. Then, if we choose a distribution $g(\mathbf{X})$ for the covariates, the joint distribution for $(\mathbf{Y}, \mathbf{X})$ given by

$$f(\mathbf{Y}|\mathbf{X})g(\mathbf{X}) \tag{2.39}$$

gives an imputation model for the missing data which is congenial with (2.38) in the sense described in Section 2.4. If both f and g are correctly specified, then this congenial imputation model is correctly specified. However, it maybe that g is mis-specified, in which case the imputation model, though it remains congenial, will be mis-specified.

In passing, we note that the term incompatible is sometimes used in connection with the substantive model and the imputation model. We prefer to use this term for a set of conditional distributions which are *incompatible* with a common joint distribution.

By specifying a distribution for the covariates in the substantive model, it is therefore always possible to derive a congenial imputation model. However, to use MI, we need to draw from the distribution of the missing data given the observed. In order to do this in a way that is consistent with (2.39), it is simplest to derive the distribution of the partially observed variables given the fully observed variables from (2.39), fit this and impute from it. This is because, under MAR, valid inference for the parameters of this distribution can be obtained from the observed data. For example, if $\mathbf{X}$ is continuous and g the p-variate multivariate normal distribution, this will be a multivariate normal regression model.

This works well when the distribution of the partially observed variables given the fully observed variables derived from (2.39) has a known form, or is well approximated by a known form. However, with non-linear relationships (Chapter 6), interactions (Chapter 7) and in more complex settings (such as survival models, Chapter 8), this will generally not be the case. We then have a choice of either (i) approximating the joint distribution of the missing data given the observed with a distribution whose form we know, or (ii) using an appropriate MCMC sampler to fit (2.39) directly. We consider both approaches in Chapters 6–8.

2.10 Practical considerations for choosing imputation models

We summarise the above results as follows. When analysing a partially observed dataset by MI

1. Start by exploring the missing data patterns. Which variables have the most missing values?
2. Identify one or more substantive models, and fit these using the complete records, to become familiar with the data. Use the usual diagnostics to check for the plausibility of model assumptions.

3. The first analysis will usually be made under the MAR assumption. To this end, look for key predictors of missing values, noting that as discussed in Chapter 1:

   - variables not in the substantive model, but predictive of both the chance of missing values and the underlying values themselves, should be included in the imputation model to reduce the bias from a complete records analysis;
   - variables not in the substantive model, but predictive of only the underlying missing values, will improve efficiency but not address bias, and
   - variables only predictive of the chance of missing values will not add information, and should be omitted from the imputation model.

4. Choose the variables for the imputation model, which should include all the variables in the substantive model (including the response), together with the additional, *auxiliary variables* identified in the previous step.
5. Choose an appropriate imputation model, reflecting the data types, any interactions and non-linear structure, and multilevel structure if relevant. Such models are the focus of Chapters 3–9.
6. Fit the imputation model, and create a relatively small number of imputed data sets. Check the imputations are plausible, fit the substantive model to the imputed data and combine the results using Rubin's rules, as summarised on p. 52.
7. If the conclusions are clear, this small number of imputations should suffice; otherwise increase the number of imputations.
8. Explore the sensitivity of inferences to departure from MAR, as discussed in Chapter 10.

As the results of Hughes *et al.* (2012b) show, the extensive discussion in this chapter of various issues surrounding Rubin's rules must be kept in proportion. In applications, the issues concerning Rubin's rules considered in this chapter can be summarised as follows. Provided:

1. the imputation model contains within it a congenial imputation model;
2. the distributional assumptions of the imputation model are appropriate, e.g.:

   - the conditional mean of the variables to be imputed is appropriately specified;
   - the distributional assumptions are appropriate (e.g. if a – possibly transformed – variable is imputed from a conditional normal distribution, with constant variance, this assumption is plausible in the observed data), and

3. the substantive model is not fitted to a subset of the data (e.g. males) where covariates indicating this subset are not included in the imputation model,

then inference will be slightly conservative, typically to a practically negligible extent, and we may apply MI with confidence.

2.11 Discussion

It is probably true that in many missing data settings there are alternative approaches that can be taken to MI. These may be more efficient, and sometimes have a stronger justification in a strictly statistical sense. We have also seen that some care needs to be taken when using MI outside the congenial setting, for which a complete Bayesian framework exists, at least in principle. Following from this it has also been argued that having put so much effort into sampling from an approximately correct Bayesian posterior, it would be more sensible to follow a fully Bayesian route altogether. This is certainly true in some examples. However, in practice any statistical analysis is surrounded by less mathematical issues, which must be carefully balanced in the full picture. More efficient analyses, or more subtle precision estimators, for example, often require extensive bespoke theoretical and computational developments. MI is extraordinarily general and flexible in this respect, and represents a very successful practical compromise, provided due care is given to the broad requirements that justify its use. When in doubt the frequentist operating characteristic of a particular MI setup can be checked through simulation, and there are many extant examples of this that we quote throughout the following chapters. We close this chapter with a quote from Zaslavsky (1994) (also quoted by Meng and Romero (2003)) which is an excellent expression of these main ideas:

> 'Because it may be so difficult to specify fully a Bayesian analysis, in many problems the best strategy can be to use a model-based Bayesian inference for the part that requires it, in particular the imputation of missing data, and to use frequentist methods, relying on estimates of means and variances and approximate normality for the rest of the inference. Multiple imputation is a device for such a combined approach,[...] This strategy may engender uncongeniality of the analytic methods used in different parts of the inference, even though each is appropriate for its part of the inferential task, and even in cases in which the same organization carries out both parts of the analysis. Nonetheless, the mixed strategy is desirable when it is the most tractable valid approach.'

PART II

MULTIPLE IMPUTATION FOR CROSS SECTIONAL DATA

3

Multiple imputation of quantitative data

In this chapter we describe and illustrate multiple imputation for cross-sectional data whose joint distribution (possibly after appropriate transformation of one or more variables) can be considered to be multivariate normal. We begin, in Section 3.1, with the simplest computational approach, appropriate when the missingness pattern is monotone. In general, this will not be the case, and Section 3.2 describes imputation based on the joint multivariate normal distribution. Another option, equivalent for multivariate normal data, is the Full Conditional Specification (FCS) approach described in Section 3.3. We conclude with a brief review of software and a discussion in Sections 3.5 and 3.6.

3.1 Regression imputation with a monotone missingness pattern

Suppose we have $i = 1, \ldots, n$ units, on each of which we seek to measure variables $Y_{i,j}$, $j = 1, \ldots, p$. In other words, if no data are missing then the data set is rectangular, with dimension n by p. Let $\mathbf{Y}_j = (Y_{1,j}, \ldots, Y_{n,j})^T$ be the n by 1 column vector of the observations on variable j. We further suppose the data are well modelled by the multivariate normal distribution.

As usual, our substantive model is a regression; specifically in this chapter a linear regression. Our response is thus one of the p variables, and we impute assuming that the remaining $p - 1$ covariates are potentially important for the substantive model; having done so, if desired we can fit the substantive model to a reduced set of variables. At its simplest this means regressing the response on the constant alone, which estimates its marginal mean.

In this section we assume the missing data pattern is monotone (see page 10), with $\mathbf{Y}_1$ fully observed and most missing observations on $\mathbf{Y}_p$. We assume data are MAR with a mechanism which means that each of the regressions of $\mathbf{Y}_j$ on $\mathbf{Y}_1, \ldots, \mathbf{Y}_{j-1}$, $j = 2, \ldots, p$ is validly estimated from the set of complete records on $\mathbf{Y}_1, \ldots, \mathbf{Y}_j$. Suppose we fit each of these $(p-1)$ regression models, using the corresponding set of complete records for variables in each model, obtaining estimated vectors of regression coefficients $\widehat{\boldsymbol{\beta}}_2, \ldots, \widehat{\boldsymbol{\beta}}_p$ and residual variances $\hat{\sigma}^2{}_2, \ldots, \hat{\sigma}^2{}_p$. For example, the vector $\boldsymbol{\beta}_3 = (\beta_{0,3}, \beta_{1,3}, \beta_{2,3})^T$, which are the parameters in the linear regression

$$Y_{i,3} = \beta_{0,3} + \beta_{1,3} Y_{i,1} + \beta_{2,3} Y_{i,2} + e_{i,3}, \quad e_{i,3} \overset{i.i.d.}{\sim} N(0, \sigma_3^2).$$

Then, to impute the data set we impute missing values of each $\mathbf{Y}_j$, $j = 2, \ldots, p$ in turn using the following algorithm:

1. For variable j, suppose $i = 1, \ldots, n_j$ individuals have $Y_{i,j}$ observed; the monotone assumption means they have $Y_{i,1}, \ldots, Y_{i,j-1}$ observed. Using data from these n_j individuals, let $\mathbf{x}_{i,j} = (1, Y_{i,1}, Y_{i,2}, \ldots, Y_{i,j-1})^T$ so that

$$Y_{i,j} = \mathbf{x}_{i,j}^T \boldsymbol{\beta}_j + e_{i,j} \quad e_{i,j} \overset{i.i.d.}{\sim} N(0, \sigma_j^2). \tag{3.1}$$

   Fit this model, obtaining the ordinary least squares estimates of $\boldsymbol{\beta}_j$, σ_j^2, denoted $\widehat{\boldsymbol{\beta}}_j$, $\hat{\sigma}_j^2$ respectively.

2. Then:

   (a) draw z from the $\chi^2_{n_j - j}$ distribution and set

$$\tilde{\sigma}_j^2 = \frac{\hat{\sigma}_j^2 (n_j - j)}{z},$$

   and draw $\tilde{\boldsymbol{\beta}}$ from

$$\mathrm{N}(\widehat{\boldsymbol{\beta}}, \tilde{\sigma}_j^2 \mathbf{A}_j).$$

   where

$$\mathbf{A}_j = \left(\sum_{i=1}^{n_j} \mathbf{x}_{i,j} \mathbf{x}_{i,j}^T \right)^{-1}.$$

   (b) For each unobserved $Y_{i,j}$, $i = n_j + 1, \ldots, n$, draw $\tilde{e}_{i,j} \sim \mathrm{N}(0, \tilde{\sigma}_j^2)$ and impute by

$$(1, Y_{i,1}, \ldots, Y_{i,j-1}) \tilde{\boldsymbol{\beta}} + \tilde{e}_{i,j}, \tag{3.2}$$

   so that all the missing values of $\mathbf{Y}_j$ are imputed. We note that for $j = 3, \ldots, p$, there will be some units with $Y_{i,j}$ missing and with one or more of $Y_{i,2}, \ldots, Y_{i,j-1}$ missing, and imputed at previous steps. These previously imputed values are used in (3.2) when imputing $Y_{i,j}$.

Performing steps 1–2 above for $j = 2, \ldots, p$ gives the first imputed dataset; the whole sequence is repeated to generate successive imputed datasets.

3.1.1 MAR mechanisms consistent with a monotone pattern

With a monotone missingness mechanism, we can regard missingness as withdrawal; if a unit (typically individual) i has $Y_{i,j}$ missing, the observations $Y_{i,j+1}, \ldots, Y_{i,p}$ will be missing. Under MAR, we may envisage the probability that individual i withdraws at j, given observations up to that point, depends on the history $Y_{i,1}, \ldots, Y_{i,j-1}$, $j = 2, \ldots, p$. In other words, the conditional distribution of $Y_{i,j}, \ldots, Y_{i,p} | Y_{i,1}, \ldots, Y_{i,j-1}$ is the same whether or not $Y_{i,j}, \ldots, Y_{i,p}$ are observed. If appropriate in the context, the fully observed variables can include group indicators, such as treatment in a randomised controlled study.

Example 3.10 Asthma study

We continue with the 5-arm asthma clinical trial introduced in Chapter 1, p. 6. We consider the placebo arm. Clinic visits to record FEV_1 were scheduled at baseline, 2, 4, 8 and 12 weeks. The missingness pattern, which is monotone, is shown in Table 1.3. Histograms and Q-Q plots are consistent with the observed data following a multivariate normal distribution, so we can apply all the imputation algorithms discussed in this chapter.

In the placebo arm, let $\mathbf{Y}_1, \ldots, \mathbf{Y}_5$ denote the lung function measurements at baseline, weeks 2, 4, 8 and 12. Note there are no missing observations at baseline and week 2. Using all the observed data for each $j = 3, 4, 5$ we regress of $\mathbf{Y}_j$ on $\mathbf{Y}_1, \ldots, \mathbf{Y}_{j-1}$, giving the estimates in Table 3.1.

Using the above algorithm, we begin by imputing missing values on Y_3 (4 weeks):

1. Draw z from the χ^2_{71} distribution. Suppose we get 60.32, implying that the draw of $\tilde{\sigma}^2$ is $0.39^2 \times (74 - 3)/z = 0.39^2 \times 74/60.32 = 0.43^2$. Form $\mathbf{x}_{i,3} = (1, Y_{i,1}, Y_{i,2})$, $i = 1, \ldots n_3$, of dimension (74×3). Draw $\tilde{\boldsymbol{\beta}}_3 = (\tilde{\beta}_{0,3}, \tilde{\beta}_{1,3}, \tilde{\beta}_{2,3})^T$ from the $N(\hat{\boldsymbol{\beta}}_3, 0.43^2 \mathbf{A}_3)$ distribution where

$$\hat{\boldsymbol{\beta}}_3 = (0.52, 0.27, 0.44)^T$$

Table 3.1 Coefficient estimates from regressions on observed data in placebo arm of asthma study. There are no missing values on Y_1 (baseline) and Y_2 (week 2).

Response:	Regression on					Residual variance	n_j
	Intercept	Y_1	Y_2	Y_3	Y_4		
Y_3	0.52	0.27	0.44	–	–	0.39^2	74
Y_4	0.08	0.15	0.51	0.27	–	0.41^2	52
Y_5	0.49	−0.73	1.03	0.01	0.43	0.29^2	37

and

$$A_3 = \left(\sum_{i=1}^{74} \mathbf{x}_{i,3}\mathbf{x}_{i,3}^T\right)^{-1} = \begin{pmatrix} 0.15 & -0.06 & -0.01 \\ -0.06 & 0.07 & -0.05 \\ -0.01 & -0.05 & 0.06 \end{pmatrix}.$$

Suppose that this draw is equal to

$$\widetilde{\boldsymbol{\beta}}_3 = \begin{pmatrix} 0.33 \\ 0.56 \\ 0.20 \end{pmatrix}.$$

2. Then, for each individual i, with missing data at week 4, draw the imputed value of $Y_{i,3}$ from

$$N(0.33 + 0.56Y_{i,1} + 0.20Y_{i,2}, 0.43^2).$$

To impute missing data at week 8, we proceed in a similar way, but now, for individuals i missing both $Y_{i,3}$ and $Y_{i,4}$, we need the imputed data $Y_{i,3}$ in step 2. Lastly, we repeat the process again to impute missing values at week 12. Together this gives a single imputation of the whole dataset. The whole process is repeated to generate successive imputed datasets.

Applying this algorithm, we created 100 imputed datasets. For each we calculated the mean of $\mathbf{Y}_3$, $\mathbf{Y}_4$, $\mathbf{Y}_5$ and then combined the results using Rubin's rules. The results are shown in Table 3.2, where the top row shows the mean FEV_1

Table 3.2 Results of multiple imputation for the placebo arm of the asthma study, using the different algorithms described in this chapter. Mean FEV_1 (litres) and standard error at each follow-up visit. Each method used 100 imputations.

Analysis	Mean FEV_1 (litres) measured at week				
	0	2	4	8	12
Complete records	2.11	2.14	2.07	2.01	2.06
	(0.09)	(0.09)	(0.10)	(0.10)	(0.09)
All observed data	2.06	1.97	1.98	2.04	2.06
	(0.06)	(0.07)	(0.06)	(0.08)	(0.09)
REML	2.06	1.97	1.94	1.91	1.88
	(0.06)	(0.07)	(0.06)	(0.08)	(0.09)
Sequential MI	2.06	1.97	1.94	1.92	1.88
	(0.06)	(0.07)	(0.06)	(0.09)	(0.09)
Joint MI (Jeffreys prior)	2.06	1.97	1.94	1.91	1.88
	(0.06)	(0.07)	(0.07)	(0.08)	(0.09)
FCS MI	2.06	1.97	1.94	1.91	1.87
	(0.06)	(0.07)	(0.07)	(0.09)	(0.10)

at each follow-up visit estimated using the 37 patients who completed, the second row shows the estimates using all available data at each visit (respectively 90, 90, 74, 52, 37 patients), and the third row shows estimates obtained by fitting a saturated repeated measures model with an unstructured covariance matrix using REstricted Maximum Likelihood (REML). We see that the complete records and all observed data estimates (which assume data are MCAR) are markedly higher at the end of the study than the REML estimates, which are valid under the assumption data are MAR given earlier visits. As theory predicts, these agree very closely with the results using sequential MI. □

3.1.2 Justification

To see why this approach is valid note that the joint distribution

$$\begin{aligned} f(Y_{i,1}, Y_{i,2}, \ldots, Y_{i,p}) &= f(Y_{i,p} \mid Y_{i,1}, \ldots, Y_{i,p-1}) \\ &\times f(Y_{i,p-1} \mid Y_{i,1} \ldots, Y_{i,p-2}) \times \cdots \times f(Y_{i,2} | Y_{i,1}) \times f(Y_{i,1}). \end{aligned} \tag{3.3}$$

With a monotone missingness pattern, the assumption of MAR means that each of the conditional distributions on the right-hand side can be validly estimated from the observed data. Putting these together gives a valid estimate of the joint distribution. Therefore, imputing from each of the conditionals in turn gives a valid imputation from the joint distribution.

Of course, in many applications the missingness pattern will not be monotone. In that case, data may be MAR, although we cannot then assume the same mechanism applies to all units. Indeed the concept of MAR for nonmonotone missingness has been called into question by some authors (*e.g.* Robins and Gill 1997). We return to this issue in Section 12.2.2. More reasonably we might assume that MAR is a sufficiently good working assumption for the analysis. With nonmonotone missingness one or more of the distributions on the RHS of (3.3) will not be validly estimated from corresponding regression (as there will be units where $Y_{i,j}$ is observed but one or more of $Y_{i,1}, \ldots, Y_{i,j-1}$ will be missing). In this case, we need to model the joint distribution of the data explicitly in order to impute. We now describe how this is done.

3.2 Joint modelling

In this section, we make no assumptions about the missingness pattern, but assume that the missingness mechanism is MAR, so that we do not have to model it.

The imputation model, i.e., the joint model for the data, is then the multivariate normal model,

$$\mathbf{Y} \sim \mathrm{N}(\boldsymbol{\beta}, \boldsymbol{\Omega}) \tag{3.4}$$

for

$$\mathbf{Y} = \begin{pmatrix} Y_{i,1} \\ Y_{i,2} \\ \vdots \\ Y_{i,p} \end{pmatrix} \quad \text{and} \quad \boldsymbol{\beta} = \begin{pmatrix} \beta_{0,1} \\ \beta_{0,2} \\ \vdots \\ \beta_{0,p} \end{pmatrix},$$

where $\boldsymbol{\Omega}$ is the unstructured $p \times p$ covariance matrix with $p(p+1)/2$ parameters.

We now describe the use of the Gibbs sampler for imputation.

3.2.1 Fitting the imputation model

The Gibbs sampler allows us to both estimate the parameters in the joint imputation model (3.4) and impute the missing data. It is a special case of the more general Metropolis-Hastings sampler, which is described in Appendix A. For a fuller description of MCMC methods in the context of missing data, and specifically fitting the multivariate normal model, see Schafer (1997).

We show in Appendix B how, if there were no missing data, and we take a flat, improper, prior for the mean $\boldsymbol{\beta}$ of $\mathbf{Y}_i$, a $\mathrm{W}(\nu, \mathbf{S}_p)$ prior distribution for the inverse of the covariance matrix, $\boldsymbol{\Omega}^{-1}$, then the posterior distribution of $\boldsymbol{\beta}, \boldsymbol{\Omega}$ given $\mathbf{Y}$ can be written as the product of a normal distribution for $\boldsymbol{\beta}$ given $\boldsymbol{\Omega}^{-1}$ and marginal Wishart distribution for $\boldsymbol{\Omega}^{-1}$. This can be expressed

$$\begin{aligned} \boldsymbol{\beta} \mid \mathbf{Y}, \boldsymbol{\Omega} &\sim \mathrm{N}(\overline{\mathbf{Y}}, n^{-1}\boldsymbol{\Omega}), \quad \text{and} \\ \boldsymbol{\Omega}^{-1} \mid \mathbf{Y} &\sim \mathrm{W}\{n+\nu, (\mathbf{S}_p^{-1} + \mathbf{S})^{-1}\}, \end{aligned} \tag{3.5}$$

for $\overline{\mathbf{Y}} = (\overline{Y}_1, \ldots, \overline{Y}_p)^T$, $\overline{Y}_j = n^{-1} \sum_{i=1}^{n} Y_{i,j}$ and

$$\mathbf{S} = \sum_{i=1}^{n} (\mathbf{Y}_i - \overline{\mathbf{Y}})(\mathbf{Y}_i - \overline{\mathbf{Y}})^T,$$

that is, $\overline{\mathbf{Y}}$ and $(n-1)^{-1}\mathbf{S}$ are the sample mean and covariance matrix respectively.

Now suppose we have missing data, and we write $\mathbf{Y} = (\mathbf{Y}_O, \mathbf{Y}_\mathrm{M})$. As described in Appendix A, the Gibbs sampler proceeds by drawing each parameter (or set of parameters) in turn, conditional on all the others and the data. Further, in the Bayesian framework, missing data are treated as parameters. We could take a prior for the missing data, and in subsequent chapters we show this can be very useful in certain applications. For now, we assume the prior for the missing values is a flat, improper one.

To initialise the Gibbs sampler, we choose starting values for (i) $\boldsymbol{\beta}$, (ii) $\boldsymbol{\Omega}$ and (iii) $\mathbf{Y}_\mathrm{M}$. A natural choice is to estimate (i) and (ii) using the observed data. For (iii), we can draw a starting value for missing $Y_{i,j}$ by sampling with replacement from the observed values of the variable $\mathbf{Y}_j$. Denote these values by $\boldsymbol{\beta}^0$, $\boldsymbol{\Omega}^0$

and $\mathbf{Y_M}^0$. Form $\overline{\mathbf{Y}}^0$ as the sample mean calculated using $\mathbf{Y_M}^0$, $\mathbf{Y}_O$, and likewise calculate $\mathbf{S}^0$.

The algorithm then proceeds as follows. At iteration $r = 1, 2, \ldots,$

1. draw
$$\boldsymbol{\Omega}^{-1,r} \sim \mathrm{W}\{n + \nu, (\mathbf{S}_\mathrm{p}^{-1} + \mathbf{S}^{r-1})^{-1}\};$$
2. draw
$$\boldsymbol{\beta}^r \sim N(\overline{\mathbf{Y}}^{r-1}, n^{-1}\boldsymbol{\Omega}^r);$$
3. Draw, as detailed below, $\mathbf{Y_M}^r \sim f(\mathbf{Y_M} \mid \boldsymbol{\beta}^r, \boldsymbol{\Omega}^r, \mathbf{Y}_O)$;
4. Update the sample mean $\overline{\mathbf{Y}}^r$ using $(\mathbf{Y_M}^r, \mathbf{Y}_O)$;
5. Update the sample matrix of sums of squares and cross products, $\mathbf{S}^r$ using $(\mathbf{Y_M}^r, \mathbf{Y}_O$.) We thus have $\boldsymbol{\beta}^r, \boldsymbol{\Omega}^r, \overline{\mathbf{Y}}^r, \mathbf{S}^r, \mathbf{Y_M}^r$ completing iteration r, and
6. Return to step 1.

We next describe how to draw $\mathbf{Y_M}^r$. For each unit $i = 1, \ldots, n$, with missing data, let $\mathbf{Y}_{\mathrm{i,M}}$ denote the missing values and $\mathbf{Y}_{i,O}$ the observed data. We draw $\mathbf{Y}_{i,\mathrm{M}}{}^r$ from the conditional normal distribution given $\mathbf{Y}_{i,O}$ calculated from the joint multivariate distribution at the current draws,
$$\mathbf{Y}_i \sim N_p(\boldsymbol{\beta}^r, \boldsymbol{\Omega}^r).$$
As we have, potentially, a different missingness pattern for each unit, the appropriate conditional will have to be derived for each unit in turn, as follows. Re-order unit i's variables so that $Y_{i,1}, \ldots, Y_{i,p_1}$ are observed and $Y_{i,p_1+1}, \ldots, Y_{i,p}$ are missing. Correspondingly re-order $\boldsymbol{\beta}, \boldsymbol{\Omega}$ and partition $\boldsymbol{\beta} = (\boldsymbol{\beta}_1^T, \boldsymbol{\beta}_2^T)^T$ where $\boldsymbol{\beta}_1^T = (\beta_1, \ldots, \beta_{p_1})$, and $\boldsymbol{\beta}_2 = (\beta_{p_1+1}, \ldots, \beta_p)$. Likewise partition
$$\boldsymbol{\Omega} = \begin{pmatrix} \boldsymbol{\Omega}_{1,1} & \boldsymbol{\Omega}_{1,2} \\ \boldsymbol{\Omega}_{2,1} & \boldsymbol{\Omega}_{2,2} \end{pmatrix}$$
Then, at the current values of $\boldsymbol{\beta}$, $\boldsymbol{\Omega}$, in the Gibbs sampler, draw $\mathbf{Y}_{i,\mathrm{M}} = (Y_{i,p_1+1}, Y_{i,p_1+2}, \ldots, Y_{i,p})^T$ using
$$\mathrm{N}\left\{\boldsymbol{\beta}_2 + (\mathbf{Y}_{i,O} - \boldsymbol{\beta}_1)^T \boldsymbol{\Omega}_{11}^{-1}\boldsymbol{\Omega}_{12},\ \boldsymbol{\Omega}_{22} - \boldsymbol{\Omega}_{21}\boldsymbol{\Omega}_{11}^{-1}\boldsymbol{\Omega}_{12}\right\}. \quad (3.6)$$
This completes the Gibbs sampler for drawing from $f(\mathbf{Y_M}, \boldsymbol{\beta}, \boldsymbol{\Omega}|\mathbf{Y}_O)$, with prior $\mathrm{W}(\nu, \mathbf{S}_p)$. For MI we proceed as follows:

1. Start the sampler, and update it n_{burn} times to allow it to reach its stationary distribution.
2. Put the current draw of the missing data, $\mathbf{Y_M}^{n_{burn}}$, together with the observed data $\mathbf{Y}_O$ to form the first imputed dataset, denoted $\mathbf{Y}^1$.

3. Update the Gibbs sampler a further n_{between} times.

4. Put the current draw of the missing data together with the observed data to form the second imputed data set, $\mathbf{Y}^2$.

5. Repeat steps 3, 4 to create successive imputed datasets $\mathbf{Y}^k$, $k = 3, \ldots, K$.

As discussed in Chapter 2, we then fit the substantive model to each imputed data set, obtaining K point estimates and associated standard errors, which are combined for inference using Rubin's rules.

To start the algorithm, we need values for $\overline{\mathbf{Y}}$ and $\mathbf{S}$. As already mentioned, the simplest approach is to estimate each component of these using all the available data. A more sophisticated approach is to use the EM algorithm (Orchard and Woodbury, 1972; Dempster *et al.*, 1977) to estimate $\boldsymbol{\beta}, \boldsymbol{\Omega}$, then use these values to draw each unit's missing data from the appropriate conditional distributions, and then take these as starting values for the Gibbs sampler. Schafer (1997), p. 163, describes the appropriate EM algorithm in detail. The advantage of using the EM algorithm to provide initial values for the Gibbs sampler is (i) the Gibbs sampler starts from a converged state (or very close to it), so that limited burn in is needed, and (ii) it is obvious when the EM algorithm has not converged. If the EM algorithm fails to converge, this gives warning of a problem with the data. Such problems are much harder to detect from the output of the Gibbs sampler, which will continue to iterate whether or not the model is well specified.

Formal diagnostics for convergence of MCMC algorithms are discussed elsewhere (e.g. Gilks *et al.*, 1996), but for the multivariate normal model considered here, with starting values obtained from the observed data and of the order of 10 variables, we have found a burn-in of $n_{\text{burn}} = 1000$ iterations with $n_{\text{between}} = 500$ works well. The parameter chains should be checked for convergence, and more formal diagnostic tests may be appropriate. For larger datasets, the attraction of using the EM algorithm to obtain starting values increases, and more updates may be desirable, together with automating application of convergence diagnostics.

There are a number of other ways to obtain approximate samples from the Bayesian posterior distribution of $\boldsymbol{\beta}$, $\boldsymbol{\Omega}$. The most natural is to fit the multivariate normal model (3.4) to the observed data using maximum, or better restricted maximum, likelihood giving estimates $\widehat{\boldsymbol{\beta}}$, $\widehat{\boldsymbol{\Omega}}$ and create each imputed data set by:

1. drawing $\widetilde{\boldsymbol{\Omega}}^{-1} \sim \mathrm{W}\{n - p, (n\widehat{\boldsymbol{\Omega}})^{-1}\}$;

2. drawing $\widetilde{\boldsymbol{\beta}} \sim N(\widehat{\boldsymbol{\beta}}, n^{-1}\widetilde{\boldsymbol{\Omega}})$;

3. using $\widetilde{\boldsymbol{\beta}}$ and $\widetilde{\boldsymbol{\Omega}}$ to impute the missing data using (3.6).

Again, this has the advantage that lack of convergence of the REML algorithm is obvious, and warns of difficulties with the data. As the sample size increases, this algorithm will give very similar results to the full Gibbs sampler.

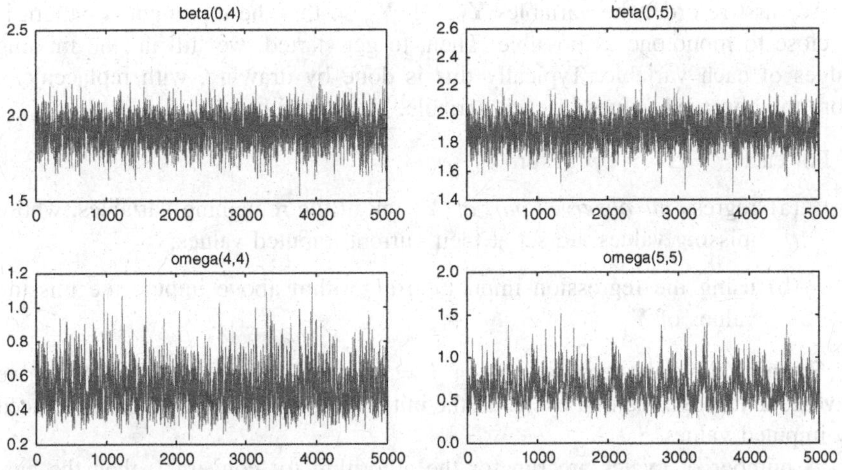

Figure 3.1 Post burn-in trace plots for $\beta_{0,4}$, $\beta_{0,5}$ and corresponding elements of the covariance matrix $\mathbf{\Omega}_{4,4}$, $\mathbf{\Omega}_{5,5}$, from the Gibbs sampler.

Example 3.10 Asthma study *(ctd)*

Continuing with the asthma data, we apply the Gibbs sampler, with prior $\propto 1$, to impute the placebo arm of the trial; we then calculate the sample means at each time point. Taking $n_{\text{burn}} = 5000$ and $n_{\text{between}} = 5000$, we created $K = 100$ imputations, then applied Rubin's rules to estimate the mean and standard error at each time point.

Figure 3.1 shows the chains for four of the parameters, which are typical of what we would expect if the sampler has reached its stationary distribution at the end of the burn in and is mixing (i.e., moving around the posterior distribution) well. The resulting estimates are shown in the fifth row of Table 3.2. As expected, they are virtually identical to both the estimates from REML and sequential MI. □

3.3 Full conditional specification

If the missing data pattern is monotone, the sequential regression approach above is relatively simple to program within most statistical software packages, as it uses the linear regression command. One would also expect it to be a good approximation if the missingness pattern were close to monotone. Specifically, we may consider relaxing the requirement that all covariate values in the sequential regressions are observed. Following this line of thought leads to the approach of *imputation using chained equations* (ICE), which is now more commonly referred to as *full conditional specification* (FCS). Early proponents were van Buuren *et al.* (1999) and, in the sample survey literature, Raghunathan *et al.* (2001). For a more recent review see van Buuren (2007).

We first re-order the variables $\mathbf{Y}_1, \ldots, \mathbf{Y}_p$ so that the missingness pattern is as close to monotone as possible. Then, to get started, we 'fill in' the missing values of each variable. Typically this is done by drawing, with replacement, from the observed values of each variable. The algorithm is:

For each $j = 1, \ldots, p$ in turn

(a) regress *the observed part of* $\mathbf{Y}_j$ on all the remaining variables, whose missing values are set at their current imputed values;

(b) using the regression imputation algorithm above impute the missing values of $\mathbf{Y}_j$.

Running through steps (a)–(b) for $j = 1, \ldots, p$ is termed a *cycle*. Once we have gone through the first cycle, all the initial starting values have been replaced by imputed values.

A number of cycles are run for the algorithm to 'converge', then the current values of $\mathbf{Y}_i$, $i = 1, \ldots, n$, form the first imputed dataset. The algorithm is then run for some more cycles, so that current imputed values are stochastically independent of the first imputation, and then second imputation is recorded. We proceed in this way until the desired number of imputed datasets has been created.

The name 'full conditional specification' was coined because each variable is imputed from its full conditional distribution on all the other variables.

3.3.1 Justification

We note that even if the missingness pattern is monotone, FCS is not transparently equivalent to sequential regression imputation. However, under the multivariate normal distribution, the joint distribution defines unique conditional distributions, and vice versa. So the two specifications are compatible.

Now consider the relationship between FCS and the standard Gibbs sampler (Appendix A, also Gilks *et al.* (1996), Ch. 1). To implement a Gibbs sampler, we start with the joint distribution, work out the conditional distributions of each parameter given the remainder and the data, and then draw from each conditional in turn.

Suppose we have no missing data, and for illustration $p = 2$. As discussed above, we have $f(\boldsymbol{\beta}, \boldsymbol{\Omega}|\mathbf{Y}) = f(\boldsymbol{\beta}|\boldsymbol{\Omega}, \mathbf{Y}) f(\boldsymbol{\Omega}|\mathbf{Y})$. Thus to fit the unstructured multivariate normal model using a Gibbs sampler at each iteration we draw a covariance matrix, then a mean given this covariance matrix.

An alternative approach would be to consider the conditional distribution (regression) of Y_1 on Y_2, and Y_2 on Y_1 :

$$\begin{aligned} Y_{1i} &= \alpha_{1|2} + \gamma_{1|2} Y_{2i} + e_{1i}, \quad e_{1i} \sim N(0, \sigma^2_{1|2}) \\ Y_{2i} &= \alpha_{2|1} + \gamma_{2|1} Y_{1i} + e_{2i}, \quad e_{2i} \sim N(0, \sigma^2_{2|1}) \end{aligned} \tag{3.7}$$

With a flat improper prior on all 6 parameters, we can draw from their posterior via the sampling distribution of the parameters (see the sequential regression imputation algorithm). Since the two conditional normal distributions define a unique joint normal distribution, this implies a draw from the posterior of $(\boldsymbol{\beta}, \boldsymbol{\Omega})$ given $\mathbf{Y}$. However, as we have drawn six parameters in (3.7), but the bivariate normal only has five parameters, we have sampled one parameter more than we need to; this is discarded before calculating $(\boldsymbol{\beta}, \boldsymbol{\Omega})$.

Now suppose we have $\mathbf{Y}_1$ and $\mathbf{Y}_2$ partially observed. To initialise the process, we fill in the missing values with some starting values. Once we have done this, given $\mathbf{Y}_1, \mathbf{Y}_2$ we can use the approach in the preceding paragraph to draw from the posterior of $(\alpha_{2|1}, \beta_{2|1}, \sigma^2_{2|1}; \alpha_{1|2}, \beta_{1|2}, \sigma^2_{1|2})$. Then, in turn, we can draw from the missing $\mathbf{Y}_1$ given $\mathbf{Y}_2$ and the current parameter draws, and vice versa. However, the FCS algorithm differs from this, because each regression is only fitted using data from units whose response is observed.

These two points together mean the FCS algorithm is not a true Gibbs sampler; it has been described as a 'poor man's Gibbs sampler', see for example Section 5.6 of Tanner (1996).

However, the multivariate normal distribution has a special property: any conditional distribution implies no constraint on the parameters of the corresponding marginal distribution. For instance, for the bivariate normal, the distribution of $\mathbf{Y}_1 \mid \mathbf{Y}_2$ (which we can estimate by linear regression) does not restrict in any way, or give any information on, the marginal distribution of $\mathbf{Y}_2$. Hughes *et al.* (2012a) use this result to show that – with appropriate choice of priors – for the multivariate normal, FCS is equivalent to the Gibbs sampler for the joint distribution. Therefore in the settings described in this chapter, there should be no inferential differences between results obtained from the two algorithms.

3.4 Full conditional specification versus joint modelling

Given the above, there are few substantive reasons for choosing between a joint modelling approach and the FCS approach for the multivariate normal setting considered in this chapter. In general, FCS will be slower than Gibbs sampling for the joint model, because of the existence of efficient algorithms for the latter, as discussed in Schafer (1997), Ch. 6. However, we have not experienced this as a practical issue with moderate datasets. If we wish to include prior information, whether on the parameters or the distribution of the missing values, this is usually more natural and computationally straightforward through the joint modelling approach. Further, initialising the joint model using the EM algorithm acts as a useful check that the model is appropriate for the data.

An additional complication arises if the number of variables, p, is large relative to the number of observations, n. In this case it may be useful to stabilise the covariance matrix using a ridge parameter. This is more naturally done using a joint modelling approach, and we return to this in Chapter 8.

3.5 Software for multivariate normal imputation

Software is constantly changing; nevertheless the packages we describe here are fairly well established, and will hopefully be available in a similar form for some time to come. Our choice reflects the packages we routinely use, and no criticism of other software is implied. Interested readers should also refer to issue 45 of the *Journal of Statistical Software* (2011) (http://www.jstatsoft.org/) which is devoted to software for multiple imputation.

Sequential regression imputation This can be readily programmed in any statistical software. It is available in SAS PROC MI (V9 onwards). Note that the software first checks if the missingness pattern is monotone, and will not run if this is violated. If desired, a few nonmonotone values can be imputed using a joint modelling approach in a preliminary step.

Joint modelling approach Perhaps the earliest widely used software implementing this approach is Shafer's standalone `NORM` package (http://sites.stat.psu.edu/~jls/misoftwa.html, accessed 14 April 2012). Details of the algorithm are presented in Schafer (1997). An EM algorithm is used to initiate the MCMC sampler. `NORM` has been ported to `R` and `S-plus`.

The `NORM` package is also the inspiration for multivariate normal imputation in SAS PROC MI (V9 onwards) and similar software in Stata (v10 onwards). The windows standalone `REALCOM-impute` (Carpenter *et al.*, 2011a) also imputes using the joint multivariate normal model. It is available from www.bristol.ac.uk/cmm/ (accessed 14 April 2012). Stata routines exporting and importing data to `REALCOM-impute` are available from www.missingdata.org.uk.

Full conditional specification A SAS macro implementing this approach, *IVEware*, is freely available from http://www.isr.umich.edu/src/smp/ive/. In Stata, the `ice` software (imputation using chained equations) (Royston, 2007) is well established and stable. In `R`, two packages are available: `mice` (Su *et al.*, 2011) and `mi` (van Buuren, 2007).

3.6 Discussion

In this chapter we have outlined how to impute data which can be modelled using the multivariate normal distribution. If the multivariate normal distribution is not appropriate, for example because the data are skewed, one can transform the data to approximate multivariate normality, then impute, then transform back. In practice, this is usually done by looking at univariate summaries of the variables, and transforming one or more of them as appropriate. Such an approach neither checks for, nor will ensure, multivariate normality. However, it does address obvious departures, and in simulations has been found essential to achieve good results (Lee and Carlin, 2010). These authors used the transformation $Z = \log_e(\pm Y - k)$, choosing the sign of Y, and k, so that Z has no skewness. Skew variables are transformed before imputation, and back transformed after imputation before fitting the model of interest.

In practice when using these methods, one should check for convergence of the stochastic algorithm. All the software packages allow output to be saved for this purpose, although with some it is easier than others. As with all statistical modelling, problems are likely to arise if variables are very highly correlated, and if the number of variables is large relative to the number of parameters.

Because, in practice, few examples involve only continuous variables, we consider in Chapters 4 and 5 imputation schemes for binary and categorical variables.

4

Multiple imputation of binary and ordinal data

In this chapter we extend the approaches described in Chapter 3 to handle first binary and then ordinal data, in other words to allow imputation of a mix of continuous and binary/ordinal variables. As before, we begin by considering the special case of a monotone missingness pattern in Section 4.1. We then consider the joint modelling approach, first using a the multivariate normal assumption in Section 4.2 and then using a latent normal model and the general location model in Sections 4.3 and 4.4. Full conditional specification is described in Section 4.5. We conclude by discussing issues with overfitting, the pros and cons of the various approaches, and software, in Sections 4.6, 4.7 and 4.8 respectively.

4.1 Sequential imputation with monotone missingness pattern

The monotone data pattern is defined on p. 7, and its implications for the missingness mechanism are elaborated on p. 79. A general justification of the sequential regression algorithm is given in Section 3.1.2.

Using the notation from Chapter 3, we suppose that $\mathbf{Y}_1$ is fully observed, and that the data are MAR with a monotone pattern. Suppose we apply the sequential imputation algorithm described on p. 78, and that as we work through $j = 2, \ldots, p$, $\mathbf{Y}_j$ is the first binary variable. In essence, we replace linear regression with logistic regression. The details are as follows:

1. For binary variable j, suppose $i = 1, \ldots n_j$ individuals have $Y_{i,j}$ observed. Using data from these n_j individuals, as before let $\mathbf{1}$ be a vector of n_j

Multiple Imputation and its Application, First Edition. James R. Carpenter and Michael G. Kenward.

1's and form $\mathbf{W} = (\mathbf{1}, \mathbf{Y}_1, \mathbf{Y}_2, \ldots, \mathbf{Y}_{j-1})$, say, so that $\mathbf{W}$ is the $n_j \times j$ regression matrix with rows $\mathbf{W}_i$, $i \in 1, \ldots n_j$.
Fit the model

$$\text{logit}\{\Pr(Y_{i,j} = 1)\} = \mathbf{W}_i \boldsymbol{\beta}_j \tag{4.1}$$

obtaining the maximum likelihood estimate $\hat{\boldsymbol{\beta}}_j$ with covariance matrix $\hat{\boldsymbol{\Sigma}}$ where $\hat{\boldsymbol{\Sigma}} = (\mathbf{W}^T \hat{\mathbf{V}}^{-1} \mathbf{W})^{-1}$, and $\hat{\mathbf{V}}$ is a matrix with diagonal elements $\widehat{\text{Var}}(\mathbf{Y}_{i,j}) = \hat{\pi}_{i,j}(1 - \hat{\pi}_{i,j})$, and all off diagonal elements 0, where

$$\hat{\pi}_{i,j} = \frac{1}{1 + \exp(-\mathbf{W}_i \hat{\boldsymbol{\beta}}_j)}.$$

2. Then

   (a) draw $\tilde{\boldsymbol{\beta}}_j$ from $N(\hat{\boldsymbol{\beta}}_j, \hat{\boldsymbol{\Sigma}})$

   (b) For each unobserved $Y_{i,j}$ calculate

   $$\tilde{\eta}_{i,j} = (1, Y_{i,1}, \ldots, Y_{i,j-1}) \tilde{\boldsymbol{\beta}}_j \tag{4.2}$$

   and draw $Y_{i,j}$ from the Bernoulli distribution with

   $$\tilde{\pi}_{i,j} = \frac{1}{1 + \exp(-\tilde{\eta}_{i,j})}$$

   so that all the missing values of $\mathbf{Y}_j$ are imputed. We note that for $j = 3, \ldots, p$ there will be some units with $Y_{i,j}$ missing and with one or more of $Y_{i,2}, \ldots, Y_{i,j-1}$ missing, and imputed at previous steps. These previously imputed values are used in (4.2) when imputing $Y_{i,j}$.

To impute a dataset with a monotone missingness pattern and a mix of binary and continuous data, we therefore begin by putting the variables in order to make a monotone missing pattern, with the fully observed variables first. Then we impute each partially observed variable in turn, conditional on previous variables, using steps 1–2 from p. 78 if the variable is continuous and steps 1–2 above if it is binary.

The whole sequence is repeated to generate successive imputed datasets.

The above algorithm can be readily adapted for binomial data, assuming the denominators $m_{i,j}$ are known; we replace (4.1) with a binomial regression, and likewise impute from a binomial, instead of a Bernoulli, distribution in step 2(b). If the data are ordinal, and satisfy the proportional odds model (McCullagh 1980), then we replace (4.1) with ordinal logistic regression, and impute from an ordinal logistic distribution in step 2(b).

In applications, for reasonably large j it is not uncommon to encounter difficulties with perfect or near-perfect prediction for some parts of the dataset in model (4.1). In this case, the corresponding coefficient estimates in $\hat{\boldsymbol{\beta}}$ will be large in absolute magnitude, and the corresponding estimates of $\widehat{\boldsymbol{\Sigma}}$ will also be large. This allows drawn values of the corresponding components of $\tilde{\boldsymbol{\beta}}_j$ to be large, and of *opposite sign* to $\hat{\boldsymbol{\beta}}_j$. This in turn means probabilities $\tilde{\pi}_{i,j}$ are close to the opposite of the fitted probabilities from (4.1), which leads to inappropriate imputations. We explore this issue further in Section 4.6, but note that it may be addressed by reducing the number of predictors in (4.1).

4.2 Joint modelling with the multivariate normal distribution

When we have a nonmonotone missingness pattern, an attractive approach is to treat binary, binomial and ordinal variables as continuous for the purpose of imputation, and then in the imputed data to round their imputed values to the nearest valid discrete value before continuing to fit the substantive model. If there are no missing observations in such variables, then treating them as continuous in a multivariate normal imputation implies that the distribution of other variables is conditioned on a linear function of them, just as when they are included as covariates in a regression imputation model. If, instead, we formally model fully observed binary variables using, say, the latent normal model described below, the results are likely to be indistinguishable in most applications.

If we adopt this approach, then we first apply the algorithm in Section 3.2 without modification to obtain the imputed datasets. Then we round the continuous imputed values for the discrete variables. Bernaards *et al.* (2007) consider the case of binary data, and use simulation to compare three ways this can be done:

1. *simple rounding*: round to the nearest of 0 or 1;
2. *coin flip*, and
3. *adaptive rounding*.

The *coin flip* algorithm is:

1. if the imputed value, $Y_{i,j}$, is ≤ 0 return 0; if ≥ 1 return 1; otherwise
2. impute a binary response taking 1 with probability $Y_{i,j}$.

The *adaptive rounding* algorithm is:

1. For binary variable j in imputed dataset $k = 1, \ldots, K$, let $\bar{\mathbf{Y}}_{j,k}$ denote the mean of the observed (binary) and imputed (continuous) values.
2. Construct the threshold $c_{j,k} = \bar{\mathbf{Y}}_{j,k} - \Phi^{-1}(\bar{\mathbf{Y}}_{j,k})\sqrt{\bar{\mathbf{Y}}_{j,k}(1 - \bar{\mathbf{Y}}_{j,k})}$
3. In imputed data set k, re-code continuous imputed values of the binary variable $\mathbf{Y}_j$ according to the following rule: $Y_{i,j} \leq c_{j,k}$ becomes $Y_{i,j} = 0$, and $Y_{j,k} > c_{j,k}$ becomes $Y_{i,j} = 1$.

The rationale for step 2 is the normal approximation to the binomial distribution, i.e.,

$$\frac{\bar{\mathbf{Y}}_{i,j} - c_{i,j}}{\sqrt{\bar{\mathbf{Y}}_{j,k}(1 - \bar{\mathbf{Y}}_{j,k})}} = z_{i,j},$$

say, where $\Phi(.)$ is the cumulative distribution function of the standard normal and we set $\Phi(z_{i,j}) = \bar{\mathbf{Y}}_{j,k}$.

Adaptive rounding is thus close to simple rounding, but now the threshold is adapted, as illustrated in Figure 4.1. Compared to simple rounding, the effect of this is that for $\bar{\mathbf{Y}}_j$ closer to 0 or 1, there will be more variability in the imputed binary values.

Horton *et al.* (2003) anticipate bias in parameter estimates when applying simple rounding. Bernaards *et al.* (2007) compare all three proposals in simulation studies looking at, among other things, bias and confidence interval coverage for a marginal (i.e., sample) proportion, odds ratio, difference in means of a continuous variable between groups defined by an imputed binary variable, and coefficients in a logistic regression. The results show that coin flipping performs worst, and adaptive rounding has a slight edge over simple rounding. Focusing on the results from adaptive rounding, aside from the intercept in logistic regression when the outcome is rare (odds 0.07 and bias is over 50%), bias is below 12%, and often much smaller. Coverage for nominal 95% intervals is above 90% in all simulations, but furthest from the nominal level when estimating, with 50% of the data imputed, a marginal proportion whose true value is below 0.1.

Thus, when adopting this approach adaptive rounding is the preferred method; this is likely to perform satisfactorily in applications if the underlying probability is between 0.1 and 0.9.

With binomial data, where each $Y_{i,j}$ is the number of successes out of say $m_{i,j}$ trials and $m_{i,j}$ is known, the most straightforward approach is to treat $Y_{i,j}$ as continuous, and round to the nearest integer in $0, \ldots, m_{i,j}$. An alternative,

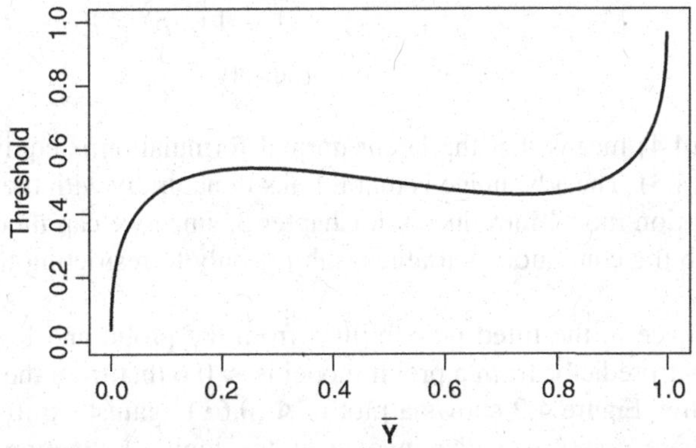

Figure 4.1 Adaptive rounding threshold, as $\bar{\mathbf{Y}}$ *varies.*

analogous to the coin flip method above, is also possible. We treat $p_{i,j} = Y_{i,j}/m_i$ as the response in imputation, and then for missing $Y_{i,j}$ round the imputed $p_{i,j}$ to lie in (0, 1) and then draw $Y_{i,j}$ from $\text{Bin}(m_{i,j}, p_{i,j})$. However, the simulation results discussed above for the coin flip approach with binary data provide little incentive to use it with binomial data.

While it is possible to see how to extend the adaptive rounding approach to ordinal data, given the relatively small advantage over simple rounding in the more difficult case of binary data, there appears no need in practice; simple rounding (back to the ordinal score) is likely to prove sufficient. As discussed in Chapter 3, if the variable has a skew distribution, transformation to approximate marginal normality before imputation, and back transformation afterwards, will often result a practically relevant improvement.

4.3 Modelling binary data using latent normal variables

An alternative approach is to use a latent normal variable for each binary $Y_{i,j}$. These latent normal variables and the other continuous variables can then be jointly modelled using the multivariate normal model, building on the approach set out in Section 3.2.

To describe how this approach works, consider a single binary variable $\mathbf{Y}$ and the probit regression on a constant:

$$\Phi^{-1}\{\Pr(Y_i = 1)\} = \beta, \quad i \in (1, \ldots n) \tag{4.3}$$

where $\Phi^{-1}(.)$ is the inverse cumulative density function of the standard normal. Define a latent normal variable $Z_i \sim N(\beta, 1)$ such that $Z_i > 0 \iff Y_i = 1$. Then[1]

$$\begin{aligned}\Pr(Y_i = 1) = \Pr(Z_i > 0) &= \Pr(Z_i - \beta > -\beta)\\ &= 1 - \Phi(-\beta)\\ &= \Phi(\beta).\end{aligned} \tag{4.4}$$

Equation (4.4) means that the latent normal formulation is equivalent to the probit model (4.3). The advantage is that it links in naturally with the multivariate normal imputation model introduced in Chapter 3, since we can model the latent Z's along with the continuous variables, subject only to restricting their variance to be 1.

The difference in the fitted probabilities from the probit and logit models is small; the linear predictor from a probit model is ≈ 0.6 that from the logit model. To illustrate this, Figure 4.2 shows a plot of $\Phi(0.6x)$ against $\text{expit}(x) = 1/\{1 + \exp(-x)\}$, where expit(.) is the inverse of the logit(.) function. The minor

[1] Recalling that $1 - \Phi(-x) = \Pr(Z > -x) = \Pr(Z < x) = \Phi(x)$.

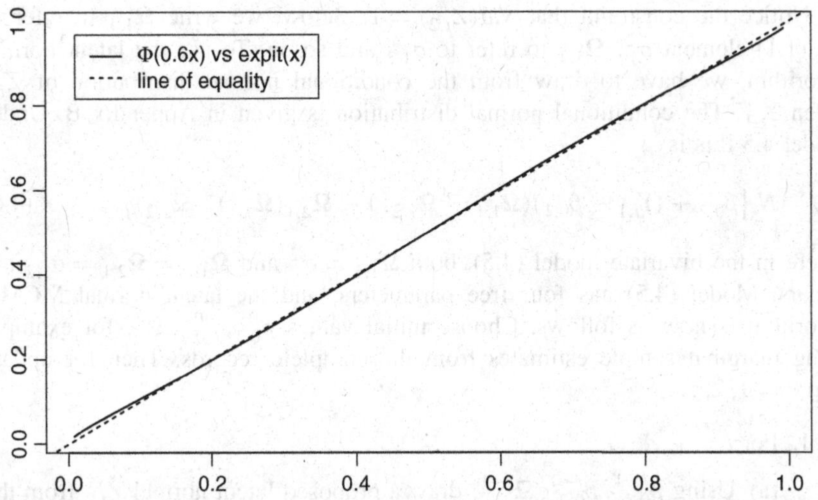

Figure 4.2 *Plot of* $\Phi(0.6\mathrm{x})$ *versus expit*(x) *and line of equality, when* x *runs between* -4 *and* 4.

departures from the line of equality are unlikely to be important in applications. Thus, although they are strictly uncongenial, in practice we can impute using a probit model and fit a logistic model of interest.

Albert and Chib (1993) give a Gibbs sampling algorithm for estimating β using the latent normal values explicitly. We first give this in the simplest case of fitting (4.3) (where it is of course not necessary) and then describe how it links in with the multivariate normal approach in the case of a binary and continuous variable. We proceed as follows: initialise $\beta^0 = 0$. At update step $r = 1, 2, \ldots$

1. For $i = 1, \ldots, n$
   (a) propose $\tilde{Z}_i \sim N(\beta^{r-1}, 1)$
   (b) if $Y_i = 1$ and $\tilde{Z}_i > 0$ or $Y_i = 0$ and $\tilde{Z}_i \leq 0$, accept the proposal, setting $Z_i^r = \tilde{Z}_i$; otherwise return to 1 (a).
2. Since the variance of Z is fixed to be 1, we update β by drawing $\beta^r \sim N(\bar{Z}^r, 1/n)$, where $\bar{Z}^r = \sum_{i=1}^n Z_i^r / n$.

Now suppose we have two variables, continuous $\mathbf{Y}_1$ and binary $\mathbf{Y}_2$. Using the latent normal approach, the joint model is:

$$\begin{aligned} Y_{i,1} &= \beta_{0,1} + e_{i,1} \\ \Pr(Y_{i,2} = 1) &= \Pr(Z_{i,2} > 0);\ Z_{i,2} = \beta_{0,2} + e_{i,2} \\ \begin{pmatrix} e_{i,1} \\ e_{i,2} \end{pmatrix} &\sim N_2 \left[\mathbf{0}, \mathbf{\Omega} = \begin{pmatrix} \sigma_1^2 & \sigma_{1,2} \\ \sigma_{1,2} & 1 \end{pmatrix} \right]. \end{aligned} \tag{4.5}$$

Notice the constraint that $\text{Var}(Z_{i,2}) = 1$. Below, we write $\boldsymbol{\Omega}_{1,1}$ to refer to the (1,1) element σ_1^2, $\boldsymbol{\Omega}_{1,2}$ to refer to $\sigma_{1,2}$ and so on. To use the latent normal algorithm, we have to draw from the conditional normal distribution of $Z_{i,2}$ given $Y_{i,1}$. The conditional normal distribution is given in Appendix B. Under model 4.5 this is

$$N\left\{\beta_{0,2} + (Y_{i,1} - \beta_{0,1})(\boldsymbol{\Omega}_{1,1})^{-1}\boldsymbol{\Omega}_{1,2},\ 1 - \boldsymbol{\Omega}_{2,1}(\boldsymbol{\Omega}_{1,1})^{-1}\boldsymbol{\Omega}_{1,2})\right\}, \tag{4.6}$$

where in the bivariate model (4.5), both $\boldsymbol{\Omega}_{1,1} = \sigma_1^2$ and $\boldsymbol{\Omega}_{1,2} = \boldsymbol{\Omega}_{2,1} = \sigma_{1,2}$ are scalars. Model (4.5) has four free parameters, and the latent normal MCMC algorithm is now as follows. Choose initial values $\beta_{0,1}^0, \beta_{0,2}^0, \boldsymbol{\Omega}^0$, for example using marginal sample estimates from the complete records. Then for update step $r = 1, 2, \ldots$

1. For $i = 1, \ldots, n$

   (a) Using $\beta_{0,1}^{r-1}, \beta_{0,2}^{r-1}, \boldsymbol{\Omega}^{r-1}$, draw a proposed latent normal $\tilde{Z}_{i,2}$ from the conditional normal (4.6) given $Y_{i,1}$.

   (b) If $Y_{i,2} = 1$ and $\tilde{Z}_{i,2} > 0$ or $Y_{i,2} = 0$ and $\tilde{Z}_{i,2} \leq 0$, accept the proposal, setting $Z_{i,2}^r = \tilde{Z}_{i,2}$; otherwise return to 1 (a).

2. Conditional on $(\mathbf{Y}_1, \mathbf{Z}_2^r)$, update the elements of $\boldsymbol{\Omega}$ to obtain $\boldsymbol{\Omega}^r$ as detailed below.

3. Draw $(\beta_{0,1}^r, \beta_{0,2}^r)$ from $N_2[(\bar{\mathbf{Y}}_1, \bar{\mathbf{Z}}_2^r)^T, n^{-1}\boldsymbol{\Omega}^r]$.

Comparing with the multivariate normal algorithm with no missing data in Section 3.2.1, the additional step we need is to draw the latent normals, conditional on continuous $\mathbf{Y}_1$ and binary $\mathbf{Y}_2$, which we do in step 1.

In fact, we can avoid the rejection step when drawing $Z_{i,2}$ in step 1. First, under the conditional normal distribution (4.6) we calculate the probability that $Z_{i,2} < 0$. Suppose this is p_i. Then if $Y_{i,2} = 0$ draw $u_i \sim \text{uniform}[0, p_i]$; otherwise draw $u_i \sim \text{uniform}[p_i, 1]$. Lastly, set $\tilde{Z}_{i,j} = \Phi_{c,i}^{-1}(u_i)$, where $\Phi_{c,i}^{-1}$ is the inverse cumulative distribution function for the conditional normal (4.6).

Updating elements of $\boldsymbol{\Omega}$

The complication is that because $\boldsymbol{\Omega}$ has a constraint ($\boldsymbol{\Omega}_{2,2} = 1$) we cannot directly update with a draw from the Wishart distribution in step 2. Instead, we update $\boldsymbol{\Omega}$ element-wise, as proposed by Browne (2006), using the Metropolis-Hastings algorithm below. In passing, notice that with more than two variables, we could bring together the continous and binary variables into two groups A and B respectively. We could then update $\boldsymbol{\Omega}_B$ element-wise (as below) and then update $\Omega_{A,B}$ from the appropriate multivariate normal distribution and $\boldsymbol{\Omega}_A$ from the appropriate conditional Wishart (Mardia *et al.* 1979). We do not pursue this further here.

Given $(\mathbf{Y}_1, \mathbf{Z}_1)$ the bivariate normal likelihood is

$$L(\boldsymbol{\beta}, \boldsymbol{\Omega}) \propto |\boldsymbol{\Omega}|^{-n/2} \times \exp\left\{-\frac{1}{2}\sum_{i=1}^{n}(Y_{i,1} - \beta_{0,1}, Y_{i,2} - \beta_{0,2})\boldsymbol{\Omega}^{-1}(Y_{i,1} - \beta_{0,1}, Y_{i,2} - \beta_{0,2})^T\right\}. \quad (4.7)$$

At update step r, a generic Metropolis-Hastings sampler for updating element $\boldsymbol{\Omega}_{k,l}$ of $\boldsymbol{\Omega}$ is:

1. draw a proposal $\tilde{\boldsymbol{\Omega}}_{k,l}$ from a symmetric proposal distribution;
2. check that $\boldsymbol{\Omega}$ is positive definite when $\boldsymbol{\Omega}_{k,l}$ is replaced by $\tilde{\boldsymbol{\Omega}}_{k,l}$; if not draw again, until it is;
3. accept $\tilde{\boldsymbol{\Omega}}_{k,l}$ with probability
$$\min\left(1, \frac{L(\boldsymbol{\beta}, \tilde{\boldsymbol{\Omega}}_{k,l}, \boldsymbol{\Omega}_{-k,l})p(\tilde{\boldsymbol{\Omega}}_{k,l}, \boldsymbol{\Omega}_{-k,l})}{L(\boldsymbol{\beta}, \boldsymbol{\Omega})p(\boldsymbol{\Omega})}\right), \quad (4.8)$$
where L is given by (4.7) and $\boldsymbol{\Omega}_{-k,l}$ refers to elements of $\boldsymbol{\Omega}$ *excluding* the $(k, l)^{th}$;
4. if $\tilde{\boldsymbol{\Omega}}_{k,l}$ is accepted, then set $\boldsymbol{\Omega}^r_{k,l} = \tilde{\boldsymbol{\Omega}}_{k,l}$, otherwise retain $\boldsymbol{\Omega}^r_{k,l} = \boldsymbol{\Omega}^r_{k,l}$.

In (4.8), $p(.)$ is the prior distribution for $\boldsymbol{\Omega}$. We discuss options for this at the end of Appendix B.

There are a number of possible choices for the proposal distribution. Since we assume a symmetric proposal, we omit the Hastings ratio (Appendix A) from (4.8). Browne (2006) compared various options and found good performance with a normal proposal, centred at the current value, with component specific variance $\gamma^2_{k,l}$, i.e., $\tilde{\boldsymbol{\Omega}}_{k,l} \sim N(\boldsymbol{\Omega}_{k,l}, \gamma^2_{k,l})$. The value of $\gamma_{k,l}$ may be chosen adaptively during the burn in. To maximise the efficiency of the MCMC sampler, Browne (2006) suggest aiming for a $\approx$50% acceptance rate.

The `REALCOM-impute` program (Carpenter *et al.*, 2011a) uses the following by default:

1. for the (l, l) variance term, draw proposals from $N(\boldsymbol{\Omega}_{l,l}, \gamma^2_{l,l})$, where $\gamma_{l,l} = \boldsymbol{\Omega}_{l,l}\sqrt{2 \times 5.8/n}$, where the proposal standard deviation is given by Gelman *et al.* (1996);
2. for the (k, l) covariance term, draw proposals from $N(\boldsymbol{\Omega}_{k,l}, \gamma^2_{k,l})$, where $\gamma_{k,l} = 0.1\sqrt{\boldsymbol{\Omega}_{k,k}\boldsymbol{\Omega}_{k,l}}$.

For variance parameters, negative proposals are immediately rejected, and a new value drawn.

Imputing missing values

Thus far we have assumed no missing data. Missing values are handled in the way described in Section 3.2.1. To initiate the MCMC sampler, we draw missing values on variables by sampling at random from the observed values. Then we modify step 1 of the sampler as follows:

1. If binary $Y_{i,2}$ is missing, draw $Z^r_{i,2}$ from the conditional normal distribution given $Y_{i,1}$, 4.6. If $Z^r_{i,2} > 0$ set $Y^r_{i,2} = 1$, otherwise set $Y^r_{i,2} = 0$.
2. If continuous $Y_{i,1}$ is missing, then in step 1(a) instead of drawing $Z^r_{i,2}$ from the conditional normal, draw it from the marginal normal $N(\beta^{r-1}_{0,2}, 1)$ Then accept or reject this draw usual in step 1(b).
   Then draw $Y^r_{i,1}$ from the conditional normal given $Z^r_{i,2}$,

$$N\left\{\beta^{r-1}_{0,1} + (Z^r_{i,2} - \beta^{r-1}_{0,2})(\mathbf{\Omega}^{r-1}_{2,2})^{-1}\mathbf{\Omega}^{r-1}_{2,1}, \mathbf{\Omega}^{r-1}_{1,1} - \mathbf{\Omega}^{r-1}_{1,2}(\mathbf{\Omega}^{r-1}_{2,2})^{-1}\mathbf{\Omega}^{r-1}_{2,1})\right\}.$$

As discussed in Chapter 3, we (i) burn in the sampler for n_{burn} updates, and if satisfied that convergence has been achieved, then keep the current draws of the missing data to form the first imputed dataset, then (ii) update the sampler $n_{between}$ times, and keep the current draws to form the second imputed dataset, and so on, until we reach desired number of imputed datasets, K.

A drawback of the probit model is that there are no sufficient statistics, and so implementing an EM algorithm is more awkward. Approximate starting values and a first test of the estimability of the model can be obtained by using the EM algorithm treating the binary responses as continuous, with 1 coded as 2.5 and 0 coded −2.5.

More than two variables; binomial data

Thus far we have only considered two variables, one continuous and one binary. With p variables, the conditional normal distribution (4.6) is calculated from the p-variate normal. Now $\mathbf{\Omega}_{1,2}$ is a vector, which we update element-wise using Metropolis Hastings steps as described above.

For binomial data, where $Y_{i,j}$ is the (possibly missing) number of successes out of a known $m_{i,j} > 1$ trials, the simplest approach is to use the variance stabilising transformation $Z_{i,j} = \arcsin(Y_{i,j}/m_{i,j})$ and treat $Z_{i,j}$ as normal responses in the imputation. Alternatively, one can draw a latent normal for each of the $m_{i,j}$ trials; these latent normals need to have covariance 0 to mimic the binomial being made up of $m_{i,j}$ independent draws. In practice, once the denominator of the binomial is greater than 3 or so, the discussion in Section 4.2 suggests the normal approximation followed by rounding will likely be adequate.

4.3.1 Latent normal model for ordinal data

Consider a single ordinal variable, Y_i, with M ordinal values, $m = 1, \ldots, M$. Let $\pi_{i,m} = \Pr(Y_i = m)$, and let $\gamma_{i,m} = \Pr(Y_i \leq m) = \sum_{l=1}^{m} \pi_{i,l}$. The proportional probit model (McCullagh, 1980) is

$$\text{probit}(\gamma_{i,m}) = \Phi^{-1}(\gamma_{i,m}) = \alpha_m, \quad m = 1, \dots, M \tag{4.9}$$

If we define $\alpha_0 = -\infty$ and $\alpha_M = \infty$, the above model implies

$$\pi_m = \int_{\alpha_{m-1}}^{\alpha_m} \phi(z)\, dz, \quad m = 1, \dots, M. \tag{4.10}$$

In other words, (4.9) is equivalent to a latent normal model, where $Z_i \sim N(0, 1)$ and

$$\begin{aligned} &Z_i \le \alpha_1 \text{ if } Y_i = 1 \\ &Z_i \in (\alpha_{m-1}, \alpha_m] \text{ if } Y_i = m, m \in (2, \dots, M-1) \\ &Z_i > \alpha_{M-1} \text{ if } Y_i = m. \end{aligned} \tag{4.11}$$

If $M = 2$ so that Y_i is a binary variable, then this is equivalent to (4.3) and (4.4), because:

- if $Z \sim N(\beta, 1)$ and $Y_i = 1 \iff Z_i > 0$ then

$$\Pr(Z > 0) = 1 - \Phi(-\beta) = \Phi(\beta)$$

  from (4.4), and
- if $Z \sim N(0, 1)$ and $Y_i = 1 \iff Z_i > -\beta$ then

$$\Pr(Z > -\beta) = 1 - \Phi(-\beta) = \Phi(\beta).$$

However, with $M > 2$, formulation (4.11) is easier to work with.

To estimate the cut points, $(\alpha_1, \dots, \alpha_{M-1})$ we could proceed as follows. Choose initial values $(\alpha_1^0, \dots, \alpha_{M-1}^0)$, and then at update step $r = 1, 2, \dots$

1. for $i \in 1, \dots, n$
   (a) draw $Z_i^r \sim N(0, 1)$ and recalling $\alpha_0 = -\infty, \alpha_M = \infty$,

$$\text{if } Y_i = m, \text{ accept } Z_i^r \text{ if } \alpha_{m-1}^{r-1} < Z_i^r \le \alpha_M^{r-1}, \quad m \in (1, \dots, M)$$

   (b) if Z_i^r is rejected, return to 1(a)
2. for each parameter α_m, $m \in (1, \dots, M-1)$,
   (a) find unit m_L such that $Z_{m_L}^r$ is the largest latent normal Z_i^r with $Z_i^r < \alpha_m^{r-1}$;
   (b) find unit m_U such that $Z_{m_U}^r$ is the smallest latent normal Z_i^r with $Z_i^r > \alpha_m^{r-1}$;
   (c) sample α_m^r as a random draw from the interval $(Z_{m_L}^r, Z_{m_U}^r)$.

This update procedure is essentially due to Albert and Chib (1993), Chib and Greenburg (1998). However, the parameters α_m only update slowly, especially if the dataset is large, as the update intervals in step 2(c) can be quite narrow.

Cowles (1996) proposed a Metropolis-Hastings algorithm for updating the parameters α_m, $m = 1, \ldots, M-1$ which we now describe. Let $1[\,.\,]$ be an indicator for the event in brackets, so that $1[Y_i = m]$ is 1 when Y_i takes on the value m, and 0 otherwise. The likelihood is proportional to

$$L(\alpha_1, \ldots, \alpha_M) = \prod_{i=1}^{n} \prod_{m=1}^{M} \pi_m^{1[Y_i=m]}, \tag{4.12}$$

and we proceed as follows. Take an improper prior $\propto 1$ for each α_m. At update step $r = 1, 2, \ldots$

1. for $m = 1$:
   (a) draw a proposal $\widetilde{\alpha} \sim N(\alpha^{r-1}, \nu^2)$
   (b) accept $\widetilde{\alpha}$ with probability
   $$\min\{1, L(\widetilde{\alpha}, \alpha_2^{r-1}, \ldots, \alpha_{M-1}^{r-1})/L(\alpha_1^{r-1}, \alpha_2^{r-1}, \ldots, \alpha_{M-1}^{r-1}\}$$
   (c) If $\widetilde{\alpha}$ is accepted, set $\alpha_1^r = \widetilde{\alpha}$, else $\alpha_1^r = \alpha_1^{r-1}$.
2. for $m = 2, \ldots, (M-2)$
   (a) draw a proposal $\widetilde{\alpha} \sim N(\alpha_m^{r-1}, \nu^2)$
   (b) accept $\widetilde{\alpha}$ with probability
   $$\min\left\{1, \frac{L(\alpha_1^r, \ldots, \alpha_{m-1}^r, \widetilde{\alpha}, \alpha_{m+1}^{r-1}, \ldots, \alpha_{M-1}^{r-1})}{L(\alpha_1^r, \ldots, \alpha_{m-1}^r, \alpha_m^{r-1}, \alpha_{m+1}^{r-1}, \ldots, \alpha_{M-1}^{r-1})}\right\}$$
   (c) if $\widetilde{\alpha}$ is accepted, set $\alpha_m^r = \widetilde{\alpha}$, else $\alpha_m^r = \alpha_m^{r-1}$;
3. for $m = (M-1)$
   (a) draw a proposal $\widetilde{\alpha} \sim N(\alpha_{M-1}^{r-1}, \nu^2)$
   (b) accept $\widetilde{\alpha}$ with probability
   $$\min\{1, L(\alpha_1^r, \ldots, \alpha_{M-2}^r, \widetilde{\alpha})/L(\alpha_1^r, \ldots, \alpha_{M-2}^r, \alpha_{M-1}^{r-1})\}$$
   (c) if $\widetilde{\alpha}$ is accepted, set $\alpha_{M-1}^r = \widetilde{\alpha}$, else $\alpha_{M-1}^r = \alpha_{M-1}^{r-1}$.

Following Gelman *et al.* (1996), we suggest taking $\nu^2 = 5.8/n$.

Continuous and ordinal variable

We now consider continuous $\mathbf{Y}_1$ and ordinal $\mathbf{Y}_2$. We can again use the latent normal structure to link into the multivariate normal model described in Section 3.2. The details are slightly different from the binary case, however. Let $\beta_{0,1}$ be the mean of $\mathbf{Y}_1$, and $\boldsymbol{\Omega}$ the covariance matrix of $\mathbf{Y}_1, \mathbf{Z}_2$. Define $\alpha_0 = -\infty$ and $\alpha_M = \infty$. The latent normal model is

$$\begin{aligned} Y_{i,1} &= \beta_{0,1} + e_{i,1} \\ \Pr(Y_{i,2} = m) &= \Pr(\alpha_{m-1} < Z_{i,2} < \alpha_m);\ Z_{i,2} = e_{i,2}, \quad m \in 1, \ldots, M \\ \begin{pmatrix} e_{i,1} \\ e_{i,2} \end{pmatrix} &\sim N_2\left[\mathbf{0}, \boldsymbol{\Omega} = \begin{pmatrix} \sigma_1^2 & \sigma_{1,2} \\ \sigma_{1,2} & 1 \end{pmatrix}\right]. \end{aligned} \tag{4.13}$$

An MCMC algorithm for (4.13) has to update the following parameters: $\mathbf{Z}_2, \boldsymbol{\alpha}, \boldsymbol{\beta}, \boldsymbol{\Omega}$, given $(\mathbf{Y}_1, \mathbf{Y}_2)$, where $\boldsymbol{\alpha} = (\alpha_1, \ldots, \alpha_{M-1})^T$. We set up the Gibbs sampler as follows:

1. update $(\mathbf{Z}_2, \boldsymbol{\alpha})$ given $(\boldsymbol{\beta}, \boldsymbol{\Omega}, \mathbf{Y}_1, \mathbf{Y}_2)$;
2. update $(\boldsymbol{\beta}, \boldsymbol{\Omega})$ given $(\mathbf{Y}_1, \mathbf{Y}_2, \mathbf{Z}_2, \boldsymbol{\alpha})$. This is simpler, because given $\mathbf{Y}_1, \mathbf{Z}_2$, we do not need $\mathbf{Y}_2, \boldsymbol{\alpha}$.

Just as before, we draw from $f(\boldsymbol{\beta}, \boldsymbol{\Omega}|\mathbf{Y}_1, \mathbf{Z}_2)$ by noting $f(\boldsymbol{\beta}, \boldsymbol{\Omega}|\mathbf{Y}_1, \mathbf{Z}_2) = f(\boldsymbol{\beta}|\boldsymbol{\Omega}, \mathbf{Y}_1, \mathbf{Z}_2) f(\boldsymbol{\Omega}|\mathbf{Y}_1, \mathbf{Z}_2)$. We can use exactly the same approach for updating $(\mathbf{Z}_2, \boldsymbol{\alpha})$, since

$$f(\mathbf{Z}_2, \boldsymbol{\alpha}|\boldsymbol{\beta}, \boldsymbol{\Omega}, \mathbf{Y}_1, \mathbf{Y}_2) = f(\mathbf{Z}_2|\boldsymbol{\alpha}, \boldsymbol{\beta}, \boldsymbol{\Omega}, \mathbf{Y}_1, \mathbf{Y}_2) f(\boldsymbol{\alpha}|\boldsymbol{\beta}, \boldsymbol{\Omega}, \mathbf{Y}_1, \mathbf{Y}_2).$$

This gives the following MCMC sampler. Choose initial values $\mathbf{Z}_2^0, \boldsymbol{\alpha}^0, \boldsymbol{\beta}^0, \boldsymbol{\Omega}^0$. As usual let α_0 denote $-\infty$ and α_M denote ∞. Then at update step $r = 1, 2, \ldots$

1. conditional on $\boldsymbol{\beta}^{r-1}, \boldsymbol{\Omega}^{r-1}, \mathbf{Y}_1, \mathbf{Y}_2$ draw $\boldsymbol{\alpha}^r$, as described below;
2. conditional on $\boldsymbol{\alpha}^r, \boldsymbol{\beta}^{r-1}, \boldsymbol{\Omega}^{r-1}, \mathbf{Y}_1, \mathbf{Y}_2$, draw $\mathbf{Z}_2^r$ as follows. For each $i \in 1, \ldots, n$:

   (a) draw a proposed
   $$\tilde{Z}_{i,2} \sim N\{(Y_{i,1} - \beta_{0,1}^{r-1})(\boldsymbol{\Omega}_{1,1}^{r-1})^{-1}\boldsymbol{\Omega}_{1,2}^{r-1}, 1 - \boldsymbol{\Omega}_{2,1}^{r-1}(\boldsymbol{\Omega}_{1,1}^{r-1})^{-1}\boldsymbol{\Omega}_{1,2}^{r-1}\}; \tag{4.14}$$

   (b) recall $Y_{i,2}$ is ordinal so that $Y_{i,2} = m$, for some $m \in (1, \ldots, M)$. We thus accept $\tilde{Z}_{i,2}$ if $\alpha_{m-1} < \tilde{Z}_{i,2} \leq \alpha_m$;

   (c) if $\tilde{Z}_{i,2}$ is accepted, set $Z_{i,2}^r = \tilde{Z}_{i,2}$, else return to step 2(a).

3. conditional on $(\mathbf{Y}_1, \mathbf{Z}_2^r)$ update the elements of $\boldsymbol{\Omega}^{r-1}$ to obtain $\boldsymbol{\Omega}^r$, as described on p. 97.
4. recalling $\beta_{0,2}$ is constrained to be zero, draw $\beta_{0,1}^r$ from the conditional normal distribution
$$N\{\bar{\mathbf{Y}}_1 + \bar{\mathbf{Z}}_2^r(\boldsymbol{\Omega}_{2,2}^r)^{-1}\boldsymbol{\Omega}_{2,1}^r, n^{-1}(\boldsymbol{\Omega}_{1,1}^r - \boldsymbol{\Omega}_{1,2}^r(\boldsymbol{\Omega}_{2,2}^r)^{-1}\boldsymbol{\Omega}_{2,1}^r)\}.$$

Note the above has priors $\propto 1$ for all parameters except $\boldsymbol{\Omega}$.

As before, we can avoid the rejection step 2(b), as follows. For $Y_{i,2} = m$, use (4.14) to calculate $p_{i,U} = \Pr(Z \le \alpha_m)$ and $p_{i,L} = \Pr(Z \le \alpha_{m-1})$. Then, draw a uniform random number from the interval $[p_{i,L}, p_{i,U}]$, say u_i and set $Z^r_{2,i} = \Phi_Z^{-1}(u_i)$, where $\Phi_Z^{-1}(.)$ is the inverse cumulative normal distribution corresponding to (4.14).

Updating $\boldsymbol{\alpha}$

We amend the likelihood (4.12) to include information from $\mathbf{Y}_1$ through the conditional normal distribution derived from (4.13). Specifically, recalling that $\alpha_0 = -\infty$ and $\alpha_M = \infty$,

$$\Pr(Y_{i,2} = m) = \pi_{c,m,i} = \int_{\alpha_{m-1}}^{\alpha_m} \frac{1}{\sqrt{2\pi\sigma_c^2}} e^{-0.5(s-\mu_c)^2/\sigma_c^2}\, ds, \quad m \in (1, \ldots, M), \tag{4.15}$$

where at the beginning of update iteration r,

$$\mu_c = (Y_{i,1} - \beta^{r-1}_{0,1})(\boldsymbol{\Omega}^{r-1}_{1,1})^{-1}\boldsymbol{\Omega}^{r-1}_{1,2},$$
$$\sigma_c^2 = 1 - \boldsymbol{\Omega}^{r-1}_{2,1}(\boldsymbol{\Omega}^{r-1}_{1,1})^{-1}\boldsymbol{\Omega}^{r-1}_{1,2}.$$

At values $(\alpha_1, \ldots, \alpha_M)$, we can then calculate

$$L_c(\alpha_1, \ldots, \alpha_M) = \prod_{i=1}^{n}\prod_{m=1}^{M} \pi_{c,m,i}^{1[Y_i=m]}. \tag{4.16}$$

We then take (4.16) in place of (4.12) and update each element of $\boldsymbol{\alpha}$ using the Metropolis-Hastings steps described following (4.12) on p. 100.

Imputing missing data

We draw missing values after we have drawn $\boldsymbol{\alpha}^r$ and $\mathbf{Z}^r_2$, but before updating $\boldsymbol{\beta}, \boldsymbol{\Omega}$. For a missing ordinal observation, $Y_{i,2}$ say, at update r we draw $Z^r_{i,2}$ from the conditional normal distribution (4.14), find the value of m such that $\alpha_{m-1} \le Z^r_{i,2} \le \alpha_m$ and impute $Y_{i,2} = m$.

For a missing continuous observation, we draw $Y^r_{i,1}$ from the conditional normal given $Z^r_{i,1}$:

$$N\{\beta^{r-1}_{0,1} + Z^r_{i,2}(\boldsymbol{\Omega}^{r-1}_{2,2})^{-1}\boldsymbol{\Omega}^{r-1}_{2,1}, \boldsymbol{\Omega}^{r-1}_{1,1} - \boldsymbol{\Omega}^{r-1}_{1,2}(\boldsymbol{\Omega}^{r-1}_{2,2})^{-1}\boldsymbol{\Omega}^{r-1}_{2,1}\}.$$

Restriction of the latent normal model

The latent normal model only allows the mean of the continuous variables to differ between groups described by the binary or ordinal variables, and not the variance. This is the consequence of the underlying normality assumption: binary and ordinal variables are assumed to derive from an underlying continuous variable which has a joint multivariate normal distribution with the continuous variables. In most cases we believe this restriction is reasonable. If it is not, we might consider introducing covariates into the covariance matrix, as discussed in Browne (2006).

4.4 General location model

This approach to a joint imputation model for continuous and categorical data is described in Schafer (1997), Chapter 9. It uses the general location model due to Olkin and Tate (1961). This separates the data into continuous and categorical variables, and then for each cell of the contingency table defined by the categorical variables, fits a separate multivariate normal model to the continuous variables. Since it is appropriate for categorical, not just binary, variables we discuss it in Section 5.4.

4.5 Full conditional specification

With binary data, full conditional specification proceeds as described in Section 3.3, but for binary variables, linear regression is replaced by logistic regression. As described before, it is preferable to first order the variables $\mathbf{Y}_1, \ldots, \mathbf{Y}_p$, so that the missingness pattern is as close to monotone as possible. To initiate the algorithm, fill in the missing values of each variable, typically by drawing with replacement from the observed values of that variable. Then for each $j = 1, \ldots, p$ in turn

1. using logistic regression for binary $\mathbf{Y}_j$ and linear regression for continuous $\mathbf{Y}_j$, regress *the observed part* of $\mathbf{Y}_j$ on all remaining $\mathbf{Y}$ variables, whose missing values are set at their current imputed values;

2. use the appropriate regression imputation algorithm (Section 3.1 for continous data; Section 4.1 for binary data), impute the missing values of $\mathbf{Y}_j$.

As described on p. 86, we cycle through steps (a)-(b) for all p variables n_{burn} times, until we believe the algorithm has converged to the stationary distribution. We then keep the current imputed values to form the first imputed dataset. After $n_{between}$ further cycles, chosen with a view to ensuring the imputed values are stochastically independent, the current values are kept to form the second imputed dataset. The algorithm is then updated a further $n_{between}$ cycles between drawing each subsequent imputed dataset.

4.5.1 Justification

In Section 3.3.1, we cited Hughes *et al.* (2012a), who show that for multivariate normal data the FCS algorithm can be made equivalent to the corresponding joint modelling approach. One requirement for this result is that the parameter space of each conditional distribution is separate from the corresponding marginal distribution, so that parameters of the latter do not constrain, or provide any information about, the former.

We now explore this condition in the setting considered in this chapter. Suppose we have two variables, Y_1 continous and Y_2 binary, drawn from the following distribution (which is a general location model):

$$\begin{aligned} f(Y_2) &\sim \text{Bernoulli}(\pi) \\ f(Y_1|Y_2=0) &\sim N(\mu_0, \sigma^2) \\ f(Y_1|Y_2=1) &\sim N(\mu_1, \sigma^2), \text{ so that} \\ f(Y_1|Y_2) &\sim N(\mu_0 + Y_2(\mu_1 - \mu_0), \sigma^2). \end{aligned} \tag{4.17}$$

Typically, full conditional specification would use logistic regression for Y_2 on Y_1, and linear regression for Y_1 on Y_2.

Now consider the corresponding marginal distribution of Y_1 and the conditional of $Y_2|Y_1$:

$$\begin{aligned} f(Y_1) &\sim (1-\pi) \times N(\mu_0, \sigma^2) + \pi \times N(\mu_1, \sigma^2) \\ f(Y_2|Y_1=1) &\sim \frac{\pi \times N(Y_1; \mu_1, \sigma^2)}{\pi \times N(Y_1; \mu_1, \sigma^2) + (1-\pi) \times N(Y_1; \mu_0, \sigma^2)}, \end{aligned} \tag{4.18}$$

where (4.18) corresponds to a logistic regression model $\text{logit}(\pi) = \alpha_0 + \alpha_1 Y_1$ with $\alpha_0 = \log\{\pi/(1-\pi)\} + (\mu_0^2 - \mu_1^2)/2\sigma$ and $\alpha_1 = (\mu_1 - \mu_0)/\sigma$.

Here the marginal distribution of Y_1 contains information about all the parameters of the conditional. For example, if μ_0 and μ_1 are separated by more than 4σ there is a lot of information about $\pi, \mu_0, \mu_1, \sigma^2$ in the marginal $f(Y_1)$ distribution. This violates the condition of Hughes *et al.* (2012a) for FCS to be equivalent to a joint MCMC sampler for (4.17).

In practice this means an *end effect* can occur, where the distribution of the imputed data will vary slightly depending on whether the last step before imputing was regressing $\mathbf{Y}_1$ on $\mathbf{Y}_2$ or vice-versa. Hughes *et al.* (2012a) report a simulation which confirms this effect occurs, although it appears unlikely to be important in many applications.

4.6 Issues with over-fitting

More practically relevant is the potential for explicit or implicit over-fitting of models with a number of correlated binary variables. Consider the following example, which was also discussed by Carpenter and Kenward (2008), Chapter 5.

Example 4.1 Dental pain data

Three hundred and sixty-six patients who had moderate or severe post-surgical pain following extraction of their third molar were randomised to receive a single dose of one of five increasing doses of test drug A, or active control C, or a placebo. The response was degree of pain relief, measured on an ordinal scale from 0 (none) to 4 (complete). This was measured before the extraction, and 18 times in the 24 hours following extraction. In the latter part of the trial, many subjects withdrew, particularly in the low dose and placebo arms.

Here, we focus on pain relief 6 hours after randomisation. To illustrate imputation of binary data, we dichotomise the pain relief score to 0 if the original scale was 0, 1, 2 and 1 if the original scale was 3, 4. Thus a response of 1 means some, or complete, pain relief.

Patients reported their degree of pain 0.25, 0.5, 0.75, 1, 1.5, 2, 3, 4, 5 and 6 hours after randomisation. For these analyses we ignore subsequent measurements (which were increasingly missing). Five out of 366 patients had interim missing values and are excluded from this analysis. All patients were observed up to 1.5 hours. Subsequently, Table 4.1 shows the withdrawal pattern.

At 6 hours, 179 out of 212 patients remaining had a response of 1. Further, patients often kept the same response for several visits. Indeed, 162 had the same response until withdrawal (152 always 0), and of the remainder 80% made only one transition.

Let $Y_{i,j}$ denote the binary response on subject $i = 1, \ldots, 361$ at $j = 2, \ldots, 6$ hours after the operation. As the missingness pattern is monotone, we use sequential imputation with logistic regression (Section 4.1) when imputing $\mathbf{Y}_j$. Further, preliminary investigation shows there is not enough information in the data to allow a general dependence on past time points. Instead, we impute using a simpler model. Let $\delta_{i,k} = 1$ if subject i is randomised to intervention group k, $k \in (1, \ldots, 7)$. At each time $j = 2, \ldots, 6$, hours, the imputation model is

$$\text{logit}\{\Pr(\mathrm{Y}_{i,j} = 1)\} = \sum_{k=1}^{7} \alpha_{j,k}\delta_{i,k} + \sum_{k=1}^{7} \beta_{j,k}\delta_{i,k}\mathrm{Y}_{i,(j-1)}, \tag{4.19}$$

Table 4.1 Withdrawal pattern for dental data, for observations up to 6 hours after extraction. Unseen observations are denoted '·'. Five patients with interim missing data are excluded.

No. of patients	Hours after tooth extraction				
	2	3	4	5	6
212	✓	✓	✓	✓	✓
11	✓	✓	✓	✓	·
8	✓	✓	✓	·	·
10	✓	✓	·	·	·
33	✓	·	·	·	·
87	·	·	·	·	·
361 patients in total					

Table 4.2 Results of multiple imputation for estimation of the treatment effects 6 hours after tooth extraction, without and with correction for perfect prediction. All parameter estimates are log-odds ratios vs the placebo (i.e., not adjusted for baseline).

Parameter	Complete records		Multiple imputation, with 50 imputations			
	n = 212		Without correction		With correction	
	Estimate	(s.e)	Estimate	(s.e)	Estimate	(s.e)
A, 450 mcg	−0.43	(0.92)	−1.03	(1.72)	−0.33	(0.92)
A, 900 mcg	0.43	(0.94)	−0.41	(2.05)	0.43	(0.92)
A, 1350 mcg	0.54	(0.94)	−0.27	(1.93)	0.60	(0.98)
A, 1800 mcg	1.46	(1.08)	0.46	(2.12)	0.99	(1.06)
A, 2250 mcg	1.23	(1.00)	0.80	(2.19)	1.42	(0.99)
C, 400 mcg	0.05	(0.89)	−0.53	(2.20)	0.35	(0.86)
Placebo, log(odds)	1.25		1.53		0.62	

in other words, for each treatment group, a different linear dependence on the previous observation on the logistic scale.

After imputing the missing data 6 hours after tooth extraction, we fit a logistic regression to estimate the treatment effects. Table 4.2 compares the results of a complete records analysis, and the usual sequential multiple imputation with $K = 50$ imputations. Looking first at the complete records analysis, there is little to choose between the treatments; the comparisons with significant p-values are between drug A at either 2250 mcg or 1800 mcg and drug A at 450 mcg, both with $p = 0.03$. The degree of pain relief increases with each increase in dose of A with the exception of the highest dose when there is a suggestion it falls back.

Turning to the usual sequential MI results in columns 4–5, we see quite substantial changes in the estimated log-odds ratio against placebo, which no longer show any trend with dose. We also see an unexpected increase in the standard errors, suggesting MI is losing quite a lot of information. No comparisons are now significant.

These results are surprising, and turn out to be due to the problem of *perfect prediction*, which we discuss below. □

The problem of perfect prediction may arise when fitting any model to discrete data. With binary data, it occurs if the strata formed by the covariates create cells in which all the responses are either 1 or 0. In this case the maximum likelihood estimate of the probability is either 1 or 0 and under logit or probit links the corresponding parameter estimates on the linear predictor scale tend to $\pm\infty$; the associated standard errors also become very large. Unfortunately, not all software packages will issue a warning when perfect prediction occurs.

This has implications for MI because these unstable parameter estimates and very large standard errors are used in the normal distribution from which, for each imputation, the parameters used to generate the imputed data are drawn (Section 4.5). This means that the parameters used to generate the imputed data give rise to imputation probabilities in the cell that are very different from those observed (i.e., 0 or 1). This in turn means that the models fitted to the resulting imputed data will have erratic parameter estimates and markedly inflated standard errors. This explains the results in columns 4–5 of Table 4.2.

This issue clearly affects the monotone imputation algorithm and the full conditional specification approach. It will also affect the joint latent normal approach, since if the probability in a cell is 1 or 0, the corresponding latent normal will diverge to $\pm\infty$.

White *et al.* (2010) have explored this issue further in the context of monotone imputation and FCS. They propose the following computationally convenient data-augmentation solution, and justify this approach by linking it to more general penalised regression procedures (Firth, 1993). Their algorithm is as follows. Suppose, in either the monotone imputation or the FCS algorithm, we are currently attempting logistic regression of observed binary $\mathbf{Y}_1$ on the remaining $\mathbf{Y}_2, \ldots, \mathbf{Y}_p$, and perfect prediction is detected.

1. For each $j = 2, \ldots, p$, calculate the sample mean and variance, respectively $\bar{Y}_j$, S_j^2.
2. For each of $j = 2, \ldots, p$ in turn, append four records to the data:
$$Y_1 = 1,\ Y_j = \bar{Y}_j - S_j,\ \text{ and for all } j' \neq j, Y_{j'} = \bar{Y}_{j'},$$
$$Y_1 = 1,\ Y_j = \bar{Y}_j + S_j,\ \text{ and for all } j' \neq j, Y_{j'} = \bar{Y}_{j'},$$
$$Y_1 = 0,\ Y_j = \bar{Y}_j - S_j,\ \text{ and for all } j' \neq j, Y_{j'} = \bar{Y}_{j'},$$
$$Y_1 = 0,\ Y_j = \bar{Y}_j + S_j,\ \text{ and for all } j' \neq j, Y_{j'} = \bar{Y}_{j'},$$
making a total of $4(p-1)$ additional records. Give each new record weight $w = p/4(p-1) \approx 1/4$ (all original observations have weight 1).

The weights are chosen to sum to p, the number of parameters in the imputation model for $\mathbf{Y}_1$ (including the constant).

The augmented data is then used to estimate the logistic regression and impute the missing values of $\mathbf{Y}_1$, as described in Section 4.5. The $4(p-1)$ additional records are then deleted, and the algorithm moves on to the next variable. The same approach is used in step 2 for each covariate Y_j, whether it is discrete or continous. If the jth covariate is discrete, simply round to the nearest valid value. In general, this means that results are not invariant to the choice of reference category for variables with more than 2 categories. However, this is unlikely to be a problem in most applications.

This procedure readily extends to more general logistic regression when the response has m levels, augmenting step 2 above to add two new records for each of the m levels, giving $2m(p-1)$ new records in all, each with weight $w = p/\{2(p-1)m\} \approx 1/2m$.

White *et al.* (2010) report a simulation study with 500 observations and three variables: two binary and one continuous (the outcome in the substantive model). Probabilities are chosen so perfect prediction occurs in each simulated dataset. They compare ignoring perfect prediction with three methods that attempt to account for it: the above algorithm, using a Bayesian bootstrap (Rubin and Schenker, 1986) and using a penalised likelihood (Firth, 1993). All three methods that address perfect prediction have negligible bias, coverage within 1% of the nominal level and power within 2% of each other. However, ignoring perfect prediction and using standard FCS leads to marked bias and massive inflation of the standard error.

The above proposal does not apply naturally to the joint modelling setting. Instead, under the latent normal model for binary data, the simplest approach is to bound acceptable draws for the latent $Z_{i,j}$'s. A natural choice for the bounds is $\Phi^{-1}\{1/n\}$, $\Phi^{-1}\{(n-1)/n\}$. Draws outside these bounds are rejected, and this corresponds to a uniform prior of $[1/n, (n-1)/n]$ on the associated probabilities $\pi_{i,j}$. Alternative priors on can readily be incorporated if desired via rejection sampling, considered in more detail on p. 141. Briefly, if we wish to put a prior $f(\pi)$ on fitted probabilities, then we (i) propose $Z_{i,j}$ in the usual way, (ii) calculate the corresponding $\pi_{i,j}$, but (iii) impose an additional acceptance criterion, accepting $Z_{i,j}$ with probability $f(\pi_{i,j})/M$, where $M = \max_\pi f(\pi)$. For example, a natural choice for $f(\pi)$ is the Beta(1,1) distribution, the conjugate distribution for binomial data. If there are 0 out of n events this gives a posterior with mean probability $1/(n+2)$; conversely if there are n out of n events, this gives a posterior with mean probability $n/(n+2)$.

For the ordinal regression model, priors to address over-fitting need to be included in the Metropolis-Hastings update step for the cut points, $\boldsymbol{\alpha}$.

Example 4.1 Dental data *(ctd)*

Returning to the dental pain example, Table 4.2 columns 6–7, show the results of sequential regression imputation addressing perfect prediction using the proposal of White *et al.* (2010) described above. The results clearly show those obtained ignoring perfect prediction are wrong.

After addressing perfect prediction, all standard errors bar one are slightly smaller than the complete records analysis, as we would expect given the additional information from the patients who drop out early which is included in the imputation analysis. In addition, the log-odds ratios now increase steadily with each increasing dose of drug A, which is much more plausible.

In the complete records analysis, the contrasts of the 450 mcg dose of A with both the 1800 mcg and 2250 mcg doses were significant with $p = 0.03$. After imputation under MAR addressing perfect prediction, the contrast between the 450 mcg and 1800 mcg dose is less significant, $p = 0.09$, while that between the 450 mcg and 2250 mcg dose gains marginal significance, $p = 0.02$.

In fact, patients' pain profiles are characterised by relatively few changes between 0 and 1 (or vice-versa) over time. A more appropriate imputation approach should take this into account, possibly in a non-parametric way as discussed in Chapter 8. □

4.7 Pros and cons of the various approaches

In practice, when using MI with a mix of binary and continuous data, unnoticed perfect prediction is the most likely pitfall. While some software attempts to detect perfect prediction, hence triggering the data augmentation algorithm above, this detection is not failsafe. The usual maxim of careful exploratory data analysis before imputation therefore applies. Specifically in this setting, whether embarking on conditional or joint imputation, it may be useful to fit the conditional models using the complete records in a preliminary step, to assess the chance of perfect prediction occurring in the imputation process. With FCS imputation, perfect prediction may arise in the imputation process, even though not present in the complete records, due to imputed values of the covariates.

As the dental pain data also illustrate, with binary data we may need to structure the FCS regression imputation models by carefully choosing the covariates we include. In the joint modelling framework, this corresponds to setting terms in the precision matrix, $\mathbf{\Omega}^{-1}$, to zero. For instance, in the dental pain example, suppose we impute separately in each treatment group, with $\mathbf{Y}_{j-1}$ only as a predictor for $\mathbf{Y}_j$, $j = 2, \ldots, 5$. The corresponding (symmetric) precision matrix has the following elements constrained:

$$\mathbf{\Omega}^{-1} = \begin{pmatrix} \gamma_{1,1} & \gamma_{1,2} & 0 & 0 & 0 \\ \gamma_{1,2} & \gamma_{2,2} & \gamma_{2,3} & 0 & 0 \\ 0 & \gamma_{2,3} & \gamma_{3,3} & \gamma_{3,4} & 0 \\ 0 & 0 & \gamma_{3,4} & \gamma_{4,4} & \gamma_{4,5} \\ 0 & 0 & 0 & \gamma_{4,5} & \gamma_{5,5} \end{pmatrix},$$

where $\gamma_{i,j}$ is the (i, j) element of $\mathbf{\Omega}^{-1}$ which is not simply the inverse of the (i, j) element of $\mathbf{\Omega}$.

While, as discussed in Section 4.5.1 above, with discrete data the joint modelling approach has a stronger theoretical foundation, both in terms of a well-defined joint distribution and a valid MCMC sampler for imputing from this, in practice we have not found these issues important. As the MCMC sampler for the joint model involves loops, if programmed in a high level language it will be slower than FCS, since the regression models used in the latter exploit efficient low-level code for their matrix calculations.

Lee and Carlin (2010) report a simulation study comparing FCS with joint multivariate normal imputation using adaptive rounding for discrete data. Their simulation study sampled datasets of 1000 individuals from a synthetic population of close to 1 million; the model of interest was linear regression of a continuous variable on six covariates: one continuous, one binary, three ordinal and one categorical. The ordinal variables had 5 levels, and the categorical variable two levels. The continuous variables were skew, and best results were obtained when they were log-transformed before imputation and back transformed after imputation. A variety missing at random data mechanisms were explored; the most extensive had missing data on the continous, two of the ordinal and the binary covariates. All mechanisms resulted in about 33% of values missing for each variable. Using adaptive rounding, they found no evidence that joint multivariate normal imputation performs less well than FCS; indeed for a couple of parameters they report slightly better coverage than with FCS.

Similarly Demirtas *et al.* (2008) conclude joint multivariate normal imputation performs well even if multivariate normality does not hold; likewise Bernaards *et al.* (2007) (discussed above) report broadly good performance. Nevertheless, it is clear that for sparse data this approach must break down and that, in general, multivariate normal imputations cannot be compatible with the distribution of the observed data (Yu *et al.*, 2007, van Buuren, 2007).

Drawing this together, research shows that in analyses where (i) the proportion of partially observed cases is less than $\approx 1/3$, and (ii) fitted probabilities from complete record regression models of partially observed binary variables on the other variables lie inside $(0.1, 0.9)$ joint normal imputation and using adaptive rounding is going to be indistinguishable from FCS.

Indeed, the results may be practically indistinguishable more broadly, because in practice much of the information MI recovers is from the observed data on the additional, partially observed units, it includes. A further advantage of joint normal imputation is that in large datasets (say with over 50 variables) it is more robust for semi-automatic use; in such cases FCS often requires specification of reduced sets of covariates in the conditional models (Lee and Carlin, 2010). Joint latent normal modelling is also attractive for larger datasets as this naturally extends the multivariate normal approach to handle binary data. However, in smaller-scale situations FCS may have the edge. We note that we have not considered partially observed categorical data here – this is the subject of the next chapter.

As usual, there is no substitute for careful examination of the data before imputation, especially when there are a number of correlated binary variables with probabilities close to 0 or 1.

4.8 Software

For sequential imputation of monotone missing data, with a mix of binary and continuous variables, the linear and logistic model fitting software in most statistical packages can be used. Analysts need to be careful to create *proper* imputations, by sampling anew from the distribution of the regression coefficients before drawing each imputed dataset. Overfitting can be avoided by checking the results of each regression model are sensible before starting the imputation process.

For the joint multivariate normal approach, the same options discussed in Chapter 3 are available. Some packages include automatic rounding; however, for adaptive rounding users will typically need to write their own post-imputation data step. An advantage of the multivariate normal approach is that it is more robust to perfect prediction errors. However, problems may arise if the variables are highly correlated, as the covariance matrix $\mathbf{\Omega}$ may be close to singular. This can often be successfully stabilised using a ridge parameter, as discussed in Chapter 8.

Turning to full conditional specification, all the packages mentioned in Chapter 3 can be used. Automatic detection and adjusting for perfect prediction, using the approach described in Section 4.6, is implemented in Stata. Analysts should note that the detection of perfect prediction is not guaranteed.

The latent normal approach is available with `REALCOM-impute`. In this software, we can either treat all binary variables explicitly, or treat those where probabilities are not close to 0 or 1 using the normal distribution, with adaptive rounding, reserving explicit latent normal modelling for the remainder.

4.9 Discussion

In this chapter we have described how cross-sectional data, with a mix of binary and continuous variables, may be imputed. Of the various approaches, we will see that the attraction of the latent normal approach is that it allows a unified treatment of different data types and multilevel structure through the latent multivariate normal distribution. However, like the joint multivariate normal and FCS approach, the latent normal approach does not capture any higher order associations in the binary data; it assumes that the binary observations arise from dichotomisation of a genuine (if unseen) normal variable. Thus, the imputed data will not contain the higher order associations. If these are desired, then the general location model approach is needed, since this can allow a general model for the binary data (e.g. Bahadur, 1961, Bowman and George, 1995). However, unless inference concerning higher order moments is the target of interest, the additional work to model such moments is of no practical value.

5

Multiple imputation of unordered categorical data

Thus far we have considered the imputation of a mix of cross-sectional continuous and ordinal data. We have described and contrasted the different approaches that have been proposed in the literature, and considered issues that are likely to arise in practice and how they might be addressed.

In this chapter we consider unordered categorical data, and imputing this alongside ordered and continuous data. Again a number of approaches have been proposed in the literature, which we describe and contrast.

In Section 5.2 we describe how the multivariate normal approach may be used with categorical data. In Section 5.3 we outline how the latent normal approach can be extended to include categorical data, while in Section 5.4 we describe the general location model, which has the richest potential structure. We discuss the FCS approach in this setting in Section 5.5, concluding with a discussion in Section 5.8.

5.1 Monotone missing data

Continuing with sequential imputation for data with a monotone missingness pattern from Section 4.1, recall that we have p variables and suppose that as we work through $j = 2, \ldots, p$, $\mathbf{Y}_j$ is the first unordered categorical variable. In essence, we replace logistic regression with multinomial logistic regression. Specifically,

1. For unordered categorical variable j, suppose $i = 1, \ldots, n_j$ units have $Y_{i,j}$ observed. Using data from these n_j units, as before let $\mathbf{1}$ be a vector of n_j 1's and form $\mathbf{W} = (\mathbf{1}, \mathbf{Y}_1, \ldots, \mathbf{Y}_{j-1})$ so that $\mathbf{W}$ is the $n_j \times j$ regression model with rows $\mathbf{W}_i$, $i \in 1, \ldots, n_j$.

Multiple Imputation and its Application, First Edition. James R. Carpenter and Michael G. Kenward.

2. Choose $m = 1$ as the base category. Let $\pi_{i,j,m} = \Pr(Y_{i,j} = m)$, $m = 1, \ldots, M$. Fit the model

$$\log\left(\frac{\pi_{i,j,m}}{\pi_{i,j,1}}\right) = \mathbf{W}_i \boldsymbol{\beta}_{j,m} \tag{5.1}$$

obtaining the maximum likelihood estimates $(\boldsymbol{\beta}_{j,2}, \ldots, \boldsymbol{\beta}_{j,M})$ with covariance matrix $\widehat{\boldsymbol{\Sigma}}$.

3. Then

(a) draw $(\tilde{\boldsymbol{\beta}}_{j,2}, \ldots, \tilde{\boldsymbol{\beta}}_{j,M})$ from

$$N\{(\hat{\boldsymbol{\beta}}_{j,2}, \ldots, \hat{\boldsymbol{\beta}}_{j,M})^T, \hat{\boldsymbol{\Sigma}})\}$$

(b) for each unobserved $Y_{i,j}$ calculate, for $m = 2, \ldots, M$

$$\tilde{\eta}_{i,j,m} = (1, Y_{i,1}, \ldots, Y_{i,j-1})\tilde{\boldsymbol{\beta}}_{j,m}. \tag{5.2}$$

Then draw $Y_{i,j}$ from the multinomial distribution with probabilities

$$\frac{1}{1 + \sum_{m=2}^{M} \exp(\tilde{\eta}_{i,j,m})}(1, e^{\tilde{\eta}_{i,j,2}}, \ldots, e^{\tilde{\eta}_{i,j,M}})$$

so that all the missing values of $\mathbf{Y}_j$ are imputed. We note that for $j = 3, \ldots, p$ there will be some units with $Y_{i,j}$ missing and with one or more of $Y_{i,2}, \ldots, Y_{i,j-1}$ missing, and imputed at previous steps. These previously imputed values are included in (5.2) when imputing $Y_{i,j}$.

Going forward to the next variable in the sequence to be imputed, we will need to include the categorical variable $\mathbf{Y}_j$ as a covariate. This will typically mean including $(M - 1)$ dummy variables corresponding to the levels of $\mathbf{Y}_j$.

To impute a dataset with a monotone missingness pattern and a mix of unordered categorical, binary and continuous data, we therefore begin by putting the variables in order to make a monotone missing pattern, with the fully observed variables first. Then we impute each partially observed variable in turn, conditional on previous variables, using steps 1–2 from p. 78 if the variable is continuous, steps 1–2 from p. 90 if the variable is binary, and steps 1–3 above if it is unordered categorical.

The whole sequence is repeated to generate successive imputed datasets.

Perfect prediction, where one or more of the multinomial probabilities $\pi_{i,j,m}$ are estimated to be zero, occurs with increasing frequency as the number of categories and number of categorical variables increases. In Section 4.6 we discuss the implication of perfect prediction for imputation, and a data-augmentation approach – which can be used with categorical data – for addressing it in sequential imputation. To reduce problems with perfect prediction, it is usually good practice to reduce, as far as sensible in the context, the number of categories being imputed.

5.2 Multivariate normal imputation for categorical data

As with binary data, the joint multivariate normal model may be applied to categorical data. To illustrate, suppose we have two variables, $\mathbf{Y}_1$ continuous and $\mathbf{Y}_2$ categorical with M levels. The approach here, proposed among others by Allison (2002), is to create $M - 1$ dummy variables, indexing the categories. We re-order the categories if necessary so the most frequently occurring category is $m = 1$ and for $m = 2, \ldots, M$ define dummy variables as:

$$Z_{i,2,m} = \begin{cases} 1 & \text{if } Y_{i,2} = m, \\ 0 & \text{otherwise} \end{cases} \tag{5.3}$$

We then perform multivariate normal imputation, as described in Section 3.2, including $\mathbf{Y}_1, \mathbf{Z}_{2,2}, \ldots, \mathbf{Z}_{2,M}$.

After creating the imputed datasets, we derive imputed values of the categorical variable $\mathbf{Y}_2$ from $\mathbf{Z}_{2,2}, \ldots, \mathbf{Z}_{2,M}$ as follows:

$$\begin{aligned} Y_{i,2} &= 0 \text{ if all } Z_{i,2,2}, \ldots, Z_{i,2,M} < 0.5 \\ Y_{i,2} &= m \text{ if } Z_{i,2,m} > \text{ all } Z_{i,2,m'}, m' \neq m. \end{aligned} \tag{5.4}$$

There is no benefit in applying adaptive rounding (Section 4.2) before deriving the categorical variables (5.4), as this may distort the ordering (Figure 4.1). Notice that the model allows (linearised) chance of being in each category to be a different linear funtion of $\mathbf{Y}_1$, and indeed of all the other catgory indicators. Thus, if used with a number of categorical variables, each with two or more categories, over-parameterisation is likely to become an issue. A natural proposal is to fix the covariance of category indicators within the same categorical variable to be zero; e.g. in the example above $\text{Cov}(\mathbf{Z}_{2,m}, \mathbf{Z}_{2,m'}) = 0$, for all $m \neq m'$. As far as we are aware, this approach has not been extensively explored in the literature. Nevertheless, experience with binary data, discussed in Section 4.7, suggests it is likely to perform acceptably in many practical settings.

5.3 Maximum indicant model

A natural development of this approach is the maximum indicant model of Aitchison and Bennett (1970). The attraction of this approach is that it links naturally with the latent normal approach described for binary and ordinal data in Section 4.3.

To introduce this, suppose we have a single unordered categorical variable Y_i, $i \in 1, \ldots, n$ taking values $m = 1, 2, 3$. We set up three independent latent normal variables:

$$V_{i,1} = \alpha_1 + \nu_{i,1}$$
$$V_{i,2} = \alpha_2 + \nu_{i,2}$$
$$V_{i,3} = \alpha_3 + \nu_{i,3}$$
$$\begin{pmatrix} V_{i,1} \\ V_{i,2} \\ V_{i,3} \end{pmatrix} \sim N_3\left[\mathbf{0}, \begin{pmatrix} 0.5 & 0 & 0 \\ 0 & 0.5 & 0 \\ 0 & 0 & 0.5 \end{pmatrix}\right]. \qquad (5.5)$$

We term the V's indicants. The maximum indicant model has

$$Y_i = m \text{ if and only if } V_{i,m} > V_{i,m'} \text{ for all } m' \neq m.$$

Thus if $Y_i = 2$ $V_{i,2}$ must be the maximum indicant, with $V_{i,2} > V_{i,1}$ and $V_{i,2} > V_{i,3}$.

In practice, model (5.5) is not fitted directly; instead the following derivation is used. Define

$$Z_{i,1} = V_{i,1} - V_{i,3}$$
$$Z_{i,2} = V_{i,2} - V_{i,3}$$

Then

$$Z_{i,1} = \alpha_1 - \alpha_3 + e_{i,1}$$
$$Z_{i,2} = \alpha_2 - \alpha_3 + e_{i,2}$$
$$\begin{pmatrix} Z_{i,1} \\ Z_{i,2} \end{pmatrix} \sim N_2\left\{\mathbf{0}, \begin{pmatrix} 1 & 0.5 \\ 0.5 & 1 \end{pmatrix}\right\}. \qquad (5.6)$$

Under this model,

$$Y_i = 1 \iff V_{i,1} > V_{i,2} \text{ and } V_{i,1} > V_{i,3}$$
$$\iff Z_{i,1} - Z_{i,2} > 0 \text{ and } Z_{i,1} > 0.$$

Similarly $Y_i = 2$ if and only if $Z_{i,2} > Z_{i,1}$ and $Z_{i,2} > 0$. Lastly,

$$Y_i = 3 \iff V_{i,3} > V_{i,1} \text{ and } V_{i,2} > V_{i,1}$$
$$\iff Z_{i,1} < 0 \text{ and } Z_{i,2} < 0.$$

As (5.6) has one too many mean parameters, we define $\beta_{0,1} = \alpha_1 - \alpha_3$, and $\beta_{0,2} = \alpha_1 - \alpha_3$. In our context it is convenient to further simplify (5.6) by setting the correlations to be zero.

In the case of M categories, the categorical variable Y_i, $i \in 1, \ldots n$, takes unordered categorical values $1, \ldots, M$. For each Y_i, define $(M-1)$ independent latent normal variables, $Z_{i,m} \sim N(\beta_{0,m}, 1)$ with

$$Y_i = m \iff \left\{ \begin{matrix} Z_{i,m} > Z_{i,m'}, \text{ for } m' \neq m \\ \text{and } Z_{i,m} > 0 \end{matrix} \right\}, m = 1, 2, \ldots, (M-1)$$

$$Y_i = M \iff Z_{i,m} < 0 \text{ all } m = 1, \ldots, (M-1). \tag{5.7}$$

We therefore have $M-1$ parameters, $\beta_{0,m}$, defining the $M-1$ probabilities. These sum to 1, as there are exactly $(M-1)$ possibilities in (5.7). Given values $\beta_1, \ldots, \beta_m$, the probability of each possibility, and hence each category, can be calculated from the normal distributions of $Z_{i,1}, \ldots, Z_{M-1}$.

For example, suppose we have 3 categories, and $\beta_{0,1} = \beta_{0,2} = 0$. Since Z_1 and Z_2 are independent, $\pi_3 = \Pr(Z_1 < 0 \,\&\, Z_2 < 0) = 0.25$. Further, as the chance of Z_1 being both greater than zero and greater than Z_2 is the same as the chance of Z_2 being both greater than Z_1 and greater than zero, we must have $\pi_1 = \Pr(Z_1 > Z_2 \,\&\, Z_1 > 0) = \pi_2 = \Pr(Z_2 > Z_1 \,\&\, Z_2 > 0) = 0.375$.

Unfortunately, in general calculation of the probabilities π_m implied by (5.7) requires numerical integration, typically by Gaussian quadrature, albeit only in one dimension because of the independence of the latent normals. However, when – as detailed below – we have a multivariate response model, with continuous variables alongside categorical ones, then conditioning on the continuous variables induces dependency among the latent $Z_{i,m}$, further complicating calculation of the probabilities. In practice, it often easiest to estimate them using Monte-Carl methods.

We now describe MCMC algorithm to estimate the parameters, before going on to consider the multivariate response setting. Initialise $\beta^0_{0,m} = 0$, $m = 1, \ldots, (M-1)$. At step $r = 1, 2, \ldots$

1. for individual $i = 1, \ldots, n$

   (a) draw

   $$\tilde{\mathbf{Z}}_i \sim N_{M-1}\left[(\beta^{r-1}_{0,1}, \beta^{r-1}_{0,2}, \ldots, \beta^{r-1}_{0,M-1})^T, \boldsymbol{I}_{M-1}\right]$$

   (b) if $Y_i = m$, $m = 1, \ldots, (M-1)$

   $$\text{accept } \tilde{\mathbf{Z}}_i \iff \begin{cases} \tilde{Z}_{i,m} > \tilde{Z}_{i,m'} \text{ for all } m' \neq m \\ \text{and } \tilde{Z}_{i,m} > 0 \end{cases}$$

   else if $Y_i = M$,

   $$\text{accept } \tilde{\mathbf{Z}}_i \iff \tilde{Z}_{i,m} < 0, \text{ for all } m = 1, \ldots, M-1;$$

   (c) if $\tilde{\mathbf{Z}}_i$ is accepted, set $\mathbf{Z}^r_i = \tilde{\mathbf{Z}}_i$, otherwise return to (a).

2. Calculate $\bar{Z}^r_m = \sum^n_{i=1} Z^r_{i,m}/n$, $m = 1, \ldots, (M-1)$. Draw

$$(\beta^r_1, \beta^r_2, \ldots, \beta^r_{M-1})^T \sim N_{M-1}\left\{(\bar{Z}^r_1, \bar{Z}^r_2, \ldots \bar{Z}^r_{M-1})^T, \boldsymbol{I}_{M-1}/n\right\}.$$

For a unit with missing response, at update step r, we simply draw a latent normal in step 1, and then impute the missing response using the rule (5.7).

Along the same lines discussed when considering rejection sampling for ordinal data on p. 102, we can avoid the rejection sampling in step 1 above, which may speed up the computations.

Suppose first that $Y_i = m$, $m = 1, \ldots, (M-1)$. Let $\mathbf{Z}_{i,-m}$ denote the latent $\mathbf{Z}_i$ excluding the mth, i.e., $(Z_{i,1}, \ldots, Z_{i,(m-1)}, Z_{i,(m+1)}, \ldots Z_{i,(M-1)})$, with mean vector, at the current iteration of the MCMC sampler, $\boldsymbol{\beta}_{0,-m}$. Then:

1. draw
$$\tilde{\mathbf{Z}}_{i,-m} \sim N_{M-2}(\boldsymbol{\beta}_{0,-m}, \boldsymbol{I}_{M-2}),$$
and find $\tilde{Z}_{max}$, the largest element of $\tilde{\mathbf{Z}}_{i,-m}$
   - if $\tilde{Z}_{max} < 0$ then calculate $\Pr(Z_m < 0) = u$;
   - otherwise calculate $\Pr(Z_m < \tilde{Z}_{max}) = u$;
2. draw $\tilde{u} \sim$ uniform$[u, 1]$ and draw $\tilde{Z}_{i,m} = \Phi^{-1}(\tilde{u}) + \beta_{0,m}$;
3. set $\mathbf{Z}_i = \left(\tilde{Z}_{i,1}, \ldots, \tilde{Z}_{i,(m-1)}, \tilde{Z}_{i,m}, \tilde{Z}_{i,(m+1)}, \ldots, \tilde{Z}_{i,(M-1)}\right)$.

If $Y_i = M$, then

1. for $m = 1, \ldots, (M-1)$, calculate $u_m = \Pr(Z_m < 0)$, draw $\tilde{u}_m \sim$ uniform $[0, u_m]$, $\tilde{Z}_m = \Phi^{-1}(\tilde{u}_m) + \beta_m$, and
2. set $\mathbf{Z}_i = \left(\tilde{Z}_{i,1}, \ldots, \tilde{Z}_{i,(M-1)}\right)$.

5.3.1 Continuous and categorical variable

Now suppose we have two variables: continuous $\mathbf{Y}_1$ and 3-level unordered categorical $\mathbf{Y}_2$. We consider a 3-level categorical variable below to keep the notation simple; the extension to M levels is direct. The joint model is:

$$Y_{i,1} = \beta_{0,1} + e_{i,1}$$
$$\Pr(Y_{i,2} = 1) = \Pr(Z_{i,2,1} > Z_{i,2,2} \text{ and } Z_{i,2,1} > 0) \text{ where } Z_{i,2,1} = \beta_{0,2,1} + e_{i,2,1}$$
$$\Pr(Y_{i,2} = 2) = \Pr(Z_{i,2,2} > Z_{i,2,1} \text{ and } Z_{i,2,2} > 0) \text{ where } Z_{i,2,2} = \beta_{0,2,2} + e_{i,2,2}$$
$$\Pr(Y_{i,2} = 3) = \Pr(Z_{i,2,1} < 0 \text{ and } Z_{i,2,2} < 0)$$
$$\begin{pmatrix} e_{i,1} \\ e_{i,2,1} \\ e_{i,2,2} \end{pmatrix} = N_3 \left[\mathbf{0}, \boldsymbol{\Omega} = \begin{pmatrix} \sigma_1^2 & \sigma_{1,2,1} & \sigma_{1,2,2} \\ \sigma_{1,2,1} & 1 & 0 \\ \sigma_{1,2,2} & 0 & 1 \end{pmatrix} \right]. \tag{5.8}$$

Notice that, as before, the latent normal variables are marginally uncorrelated, with constrained variance. This means there are two parameters, $\beta_{0,2,1}, \beta_{0,2,2}$ defining the marginal probabilities that $\pi_{2,1} = \Pr(Y_{i,2} = 1)$, $\pi_{2,2} = \Pr(Y_{i,2} = 2)$

with $\pi_{2,3} = 1 - \pi_{2,1} - \pi_{2,3}$. Thus we have one parameter for each of the two 'free' probabilities, and the model is not over-parameterised.

The MCMC algorithm for model (5.8) is as follows. Choose initial values $\boldsymbol{\beta}^0$, $\boldsymbol{\Omega}^0$. At update step $r = 1, 2, \ldots$

1. For $i = 1, \ldots, n$

   (a) draw $\tilde{\mathbf{Z}}_i = (\tilde{Z}^r_{i,2,1}, \tilde{Z}^r_{i,2,2})^T$ from the conditional bivariate normal,

$$N\left\{\begin{pmatrix}\beta^{r-1}_{0,2,1}\\ \beta^{r-1}_{0,2,2}\end{pmatrix} + (Y_{i,1} - \beta^{r-1}_{0,1})(\boldsymbol{\Omega}^{r-1}_{1,1})^{-1}\begin{pmatrix}\boldsymbol{\Omega}^{r-1}_{1,2}\\ \boldsymbol{\Omega}^{r-1}_{1,3}\end{pmatrix},\right.$$

$$\left. \boldsymbol{I}_2 - (\boldsymbol{\Omega}^{r-1}_{1,2}, \boldsymbol{\Omega}^{r-1}_{1,3})^T(\boldsymbol{\Omega}^{r-1}_{1,1})^{-1}(\boldsymbol{\Omega}^{r-1}_{1,2}, \boldsymbol{\Omega}^{r-1}_{1,3})\right\} \tag{5.9}$$

   (b) if $Y_{i,2} = m$, $m = 1, 2$

$$\text{accept } \tilde{\mathbf{Z}}_i \text{ if and only if } \begin{cases}\tilde{Z}_{i,m} > \tilde{Z}_{i,m'} \text{ for all } m \neq m'\\ \text{and } Z_{i,m} > 0\end{cases}$$

   if $Y_i = 3$,

$$\text{accept } \tilde{\mathbf{Z}}_i \text{ if and only if } \tilde{Z}_{i,m} < 0, m = 1, 2.$$

   (c) If $\tilde{\mathbf{Z}}_i$ is accepted, set $\mathbf{Z}^r_i = \tilde{\mathbf{Z}}_i$, else return to 1 (a).

2. Let $\mathbf{Z}_{2,m} = (Z_{1,2,m}, Z_{2,2,m}, \ldots, Z_{n,2,m})^T$, $m = 1, 2$. Given $\mathbf{Y}_1, \mathbf{Z}^r_{2,1}, \mathbf{Z}^r_{2,2}$ update $\boldsymbol{\Omega}^{r-1}$ elementwise, as described in Chapter 4, p. 96, subject to the constraints in (5.8). This gives $\boldsymbol{\Omega}^r$.

3. Calculate $\bar{Y}_1 = \sum_{i=1}^n Y_{i,1}/n$, and $\bar{Z}^r_{2,m} = \sum_{i=1}^n Z^r_{i,2,m}/n$, $m = 1, 2$. Draw

$$\begin{pmatrix}\beta^r_{0,1}\\ \beta^r_{0,2,1}\\ \beta^r_{0,2,2}\end{pmatrix} \sim N_3\left\{\begin{pmatrix}\bar{Y}_1\\ \bar{Z}^r_{2,1}\\ \bar{Z}^r_{2,2}\end{pmatrix}, \boldsymbol{\Omega}^r/n\right\}.$$

Avoiding rejection sampling

We can again avoid direct rejection sampling in step 1. Suppose first that $Y_{i,2} = 1$. Then, given $Y_{i,2}$, we must have $Z_{i,2,1} > Z_{i,2,2}$ and $Z_{i,2,1} > 0$. We assume we are at update step r, and omit the superscripts identifying the iteration. Paralleling the approach on p. 116:

1. first draw $Z_{i,2,1}$ from the conditional normal given $Y_{i,1}$, i.e., draw

$$\tilde{Z}_{i,2,1} \sim N\{\boldsymbol{\beta}_{0,2,1} + (Y_{i,1} - \beta_{0,1})(\boldsymbol{\Omega}_{1,1})^{-1}\boldsymbol{\Omega}_{1,2}, 1 - \boldsymbol{\Omega}_{2,1}(\boldsymbol{\Omega}_{1,1})^{-1}\boldsymbol{\Omega}_{1,2}\}$$

$$\tilde{Z}_{i,2,1} > 0$$

2. set $V = \max(0, \tilde{Z}_{i,2,1})$. Then, using the conditional normal density of $Z_{i,2,2}|Z_{i,2,1}, Y_{i,1}$, calculate $p_{i,L} = \Pr(Z_{i,2,2} < V) = \Phi\{(V - \mu_c)/\sigma_c\}$ where

$$\mu_c = \beta_{0,2,2} + (Y_{i,1} - \beta_{0,1}^{r-1}, \tilde{Z}_{i,2,1} - \beta_{0,2,1}) \begin{pmatrix} \mathbf{\Omega}_{1,1} & \mathbf{\Omega}_{1,2} \\ \mathbf{\Omega}_{2,1} & \mathbf{\Omega}_{2,2} \end{pmatrix}^{-1} \begin{pmatrix} \mathbf{\Omega}_{1,3} \\ \mathbf{\Omega}_{2,3} \end{pmatrix}$$

and

$$\sigma_c^2 = 1 - (\mathbf{\Omega}_{1,3}, \mathbf{\Omega}_{2,3}) \begin{pmatrix} \mathbf{\Omega}_{1,1} & \mathbf{\Omega}_{1,2} \\ \mathbf{\Omega}_{2,1} & \mathbf{\Omega}_{2,2} \end{pmatrix}^{-1} \begin{pmatrix} \mathbf{\Omega}_{1,3} \\ \mathbf{\Omega}_{2,3} \end{pmatrix}.$$

3. draw a $\tilde{u} \sim \text{uniform}(p_{i,L}, 1)$, set $\tilde{Z}_{i,2,2} = \Phi^{-1}(\tilde{u})\sigma_c + \mu_c$ and finally set $\mathbf{Z}_{i,2}^r = (\tilde{Z}_{i,2,1}, \tilde{Z}_{i,2,2})^T$.

If $Y_{i,2} = 2$, we use steps 1–3 above but interchange the roles of $Z_{i,2,1}$ and $Z_{i,2,2}$.

If $Y_{i,2} = 3$, then, given $Y_{i,1}$, we require both $Z_{i,2,1} < 0$ and $Z_{i,2,2} < 0$. To achieve this:

1. Calculate $p_{i,L} = Pr(Z_{i,2,1} < 0|Y_{i,1})$ under the conditional normal density of $Z_{i,2,1}|Y_{i,1}$,

$$N\{\boldsymbol{\beta}_{0,2,1} + (Y_{i,1} - \beta_{0,1})(\mathbf{\Omega}_{1,1})^{-1}\mathbf{\Omega}_{1,2}, 1 - \mathbf{\Omega}_{2,1}(\mathbf{\Omega}_{1,1})^{-1}\mathbf{\Omega}_{1,2}\} \quad (5.10)$$

2. Draw $\tilde{u} \sim \text{uniform}(0, p_{i,L})$ and use the inverse of the cumulative normal distribution defined by (5.10) to draw $\tilde{Z}_{i,2,1}$.

3. Using the conditional normal density of $Z_{i,2,2}|Z_{i,2,1}, Y_{i,1}$, calculate $p_{i,L} = \Pr(Z_{i,2,2} < 0) = \Phi\{(-\mu_c)/\sigma_c\}$ where

$$\mu_c = \beta_{0,2,2} + (Y_{i,1} - \beta_{0,1}, \tilde{Z}_{i,2,1} - \beta_{0,2,1}) \begin{pmatrix} \mathbf{\Omega}_{1,1} & \mathbf{\Omega}_{1,2} \\ \mathbf{\Omega}_{2,1} & \mathbf{\Omega}_{2,2} \end{pmatrix}^{-1} \begin{pmatrix} \mathbf{\Omega}_{1,3} \\ \mathbf{\Omega}_{2,3} \end{pmatrix}$$

and

$$\sigma_c^2 = 1 - (\mathbf{\Omega}_{1,3}, \mathbf{\Omega}_{2,3}) \begin{pmatrix} \mathbf{\Omega}_{1,1} & \mathbf{\Omega}_{1,2} \\ \mathbf{\Omega}_{2,1} & \mathbf{\Omega}_{2,2} \end{pmatrix}^{-1} \begin{pmatrix} \mathbf{\Omega}_{1,3} \\ \mathbf{\Omega}_{2,3} \end{pmatrix}.$$

4. draw a $\tilde{u} \sim \text{uniform}(0, p_{i,L})$, set $\tilde{Z}_{i,2,2} = \Phi^{-1}(\tilde{u})\sigma_c + \mu_c$ and finally set $\mathbf{Z}_{i,2}^r = (\tilde{Z}_{i,2,1}, \tilde{Z}_{i,2,2})^T$.

5.3.2 Imputing missing data

Suppose that the categorical variable $Y_{i,2}$ is missing. Then at Step 1(a) of the MCMC algorithm for the joint model on p. 117, we draw $(Z_{i,2,1}^r, Z_{i,2,2}^r)$ from the conditional normal distribution (5.9), and use rule (5.7) to impute $Y_{i,2}$.

Now suppose that $Y_{i,1}$ is missing. Then we draw $(Z_{i,2,1}, Z_{i,2,2})$ from the marginal bivariate normal distribution

$$N_2\left[\begin{pmatrix}\beta_{0,2,1}^{r-1}\\ \beta_{0,2,2}^{r-1}\end{pmatrix}, \boldsymbol{I}_2\right],$$

accepting a draw, denoted $(Z^r_{i,2,1}, Z^r_{i,2,2})$ which satisfies the constraint implied by the observed value $Y_{i,2} = m$.

Given this, we draw $Y^r_{i,1}$ from the conditional normal distribution given $(Z^r_{i,2,1}, Z^r_{i,2,2})$, which has mean

$$\beta_{0,1} + (Z^r_{i,2,1} - \beta^{r-1}_{0,2,1}, Z^r_{i,2,2} - \beta^{r-1}_{0,2,2})\boldsymbol{I}_2\begin{pmatrix}\boldsymbol{\Omega}^{r-1}_{1,2}\\ \boldsymbol{\Omega}^{r-1}_{1,3}\end{pmatrix},$$

and variance

$$\boldsymbol{\Omega}^{r-1}_{1,1} - (\boldsymbol{\Omega}^{r-1}_{1,2}, \boldsymbol{\Omega}^{r-1}_{1,3})\boldsymbol{I}_2(\boldsymbol{\Omega}^{r-1}_{1,2}, \boldsymbol{\Omega}^{r-1}_{1,3})^T.$$

Once we have drawn values for the missing data in step 1, we proceed to update the remaining parameters as before.

Summary

We have set out the MCMC algorithm for a joint model for a continuous and unordered 3-category response using latent normal variables and the maximum indicant model. This extends directly to more than three categories. Through the latent normal structure we can add additional binary or ordinal variables, categorical variables and continuous variables. The latent normal model therefore provides a unified approach to the modelling of different response types. The attraction of this approach is that it extends naturally to the multilevel setting, as we describe in Chapter 9, and other related structures.

5.3.3 More than one categorical variable

We now consider the link between the maximum indicant model above and log-linear models for categorical data. For one M-category variable, $\mathbf{Y}_1$, the log-linear model has $(M - 1)$ parameters which are the log-odds of the multinomial probabilities against the reference category. The corresponding structure in the maximum indicant model (5.7) has $(M - 1)$ independent latent normals, described by $(M - 1)$ mean parameters, all with common variance 1.

Suppose we have two unordered categorical variables, $\mathbf{Y}_1, \mathbf{Y}_2$ with L and M categories respectively. If we model them with the maximum indicant model, then we have $(L - 1)$ parameters (latent normal means) for the marginal distribution of $\mathbf{Y}_1$, $(M - 1)$ parameters (latent normal means) for the marginal distribution of $\mathbf{Y}_2$ and $(L - 1)(M - 1)$ covariance parameters between the latent normal variables. This gives a total of $LM - 1$ parameters, which is the same number for the saturated log linear model for the L by M contingency table defined by $\mathbf{Y}_1$ and $\mathbf{Y}_2$.

Now suppose that we have three categorical variables, $\mathbf{Y}_1, \mathbf{Y}_2, \mathbf{Y}_3$, with respectively L, M and N categories. Fitting them using the maximum indicant model requires $(L-1)+(M-1)+(N-1)$ latent normal mean parameters, plus $(L-1)(M-1)+(L-1)(N-1)+(M-1)(N-1)$ covariance parameters. This is the same number of parameters as for the partial association log-linear model, in which odds ratios relating any two variables are adjusted for levels of a third. As we add more categorical variables, the maximum indicant model continues to correspond to the log-linear model with all the two-way interactions. This will be rich enough for most application settings.

Continuing with three variables, if we wish to parallel the saturated log-linear model, which includes the three way interaction and has $LMN-1$ parameters, then we have to create a new categorical variable with one category corresponding to each cell of the L by M by N contingency table defined by $\mathbf{Y}_1, \mathbf{Y}_2, \mathbf{Y}_3$. We then fit this variable using the maximum indicant model: it has $LMN-1$ categories, so it has $LMN-1$ parameters, just as the saturated log-linear model. We discuss this further in Section 7.2.

5.4 General location model

An alternative model for multivariate normal and categorical data is the general location model of Olkin and Tate (1961). Suppose that we have continuous $(Y_{i,1}, Y_{i,2})$ and binary $(Y_{i,3}, Y_{i,4})$ variables. The binary variables define a contingency table with 4 cells:

	$Y_{i,3}=0$	$Y_{i,3}=1$	total
$Y_{i,4}=0$	n_1	n_2	(n_1+n_2)
$Y_{i,4}=1$	n_3	n_4	(n_3+n_4)
total	(n_1+n_3)	(n_2+n_4)	n

with corresponding probabilities π_g, $g=1,\ldots,4$, $\sum_{g=1}^{4}\pi_g=1$. Given that unit i belongs to cell g,

$$f(Y_{i,1}, Y_{i,2}|Y_{i,3}, Y_{i,4}) \sim N_2(\boldsymbol{\mu}_g, \boldsymbol{\Omega}_g). \tag{5.11}$$

In other words, conditional on unit i belonging to cell g, the continuous variables follow a multivariate normal model with cell-specific mean and covariance matrix.

A key difference with the latent normal model is that (5.11) allows the mean and variance of $(Y_{i,1}, Y_{i,2})$ to differ for each cell g of the contingency table defined by the binary (or in generality categorical) variables. By contrast, the latent normal model has a common covariance matrix. We anticipate few applications in which having a group-specific covariance matrix is important. In the latent normal setting, some flexibility can be introduced by including covariates in the covariance model (Browne, 2006). Model (5.11) with the assumption of a common covariance matrix across groups is the usual linear discriminant analysis model.

Schafer (1999b) has freely available software for fitting and imputing missing data under this model, using a MCMC approach described in Chapters 7–9 of Schafer (1997). Since, in general, the general location model has a saturated log-linear model for the categorical variables and, given this a separate multivariate normal distribution for the continuous variables corresponding to each contingency table cell, both categorical and multivariate normal models usually need to be simplified before it is fitted. While it is strictly congenial with logistic and log-linear models (while the latent normal model is not) it does not extend so naturally to the multilevel setting if we wish to allow a full range of variable types at each level.

5.5 FCS with categorical data

With a mix of continuous, binary and categorical data the FCS approach proceeds as described in Section 4.5, but now using we use multinomial logistic (or multinomial probit) regression for each categorical variable in turn, as described in 5.1, conditioning on all the other variables as covariates. Note that when M-level categorical variables are included as predictors in the regression models that make up the FCS, then they need to be included as M-level categorical variables, in other words using $M - 1$ dummy indicators.

If the missingness pattern is monotone, then appropriately specified FCS will give the same distribution of the imputed data as the sequential regression imputation algorithm, once the former has converged. To see this intuitively, suppose we have ordered the p variables into a monotone missingness pattern. When imputing variables $j > 1$, variables $j' > j$ are always missing, so there is no information 'omitted' from sequential regression imputation that can be recovered by FCS.

Suppose we now have two categorical variables, $\mathbf{Y}_1, \mathbf{Y}_2$ of L and M levels respectively, which define a 2-way contingency table with LM cells. Let $\mu_{l,m}$ be the mean count for each cell. The log-linear model for the contingency table is:

$$\log(\mu_{l,m}) = \lambda + \lambda_l^1 + \lambda_m^2 + \lambda_{l,m}^{12}, \tag{5.12}$$

where (as usual for such models) to avoid over-parameterisation, $\lambda_1^1 = \lambda_1^2 = \lambda_{1.}^{12} = \lambda_{.1}^{12} = 0$, $l = 1, \ldots, L; m = 1, \ldots, M$. The parameters λ_l^1 are the log-odds of $\mathbf{Y}_1$ taking category l to $\mathbf{Y}_1$ taking category 1, when $\mathbf{Y}_2$ is 1. The parameters $\lambda_{l,m}^{12}$ are the $(L - 1)(M - 1)$ odds ratios in the contingency table.

Multinomial logistic regression of $\mathbf{Y}_1$ on $\mathbf{Y}_2$ (including $\mathbf{Y}_2$ as an M level categorical variable) estimates the log-odds λ_l^1 and the log-odds ratios $\lambda_{l,m}^{1,2}$. Likewise, multinomial logistic regression of $\mathbf{Y}_2$ on $\mathbf{Y}_1$ estimates the log-odds λ_m^2 and the log-odds ratios $\lambda_{l,m}^{1,2}$. Therefore the two models are compatible with each other, and any imputed data is congenial with the usual log-linear model for the contingency table. Further, the multinomial logistic regression of $\mathbf{Y}_1$ on $\mathbf{Y}_2$ gives no information on the marginal distribution $\mathbf{Y}_2$ nor places any restriction on it. Using analogous arguments to those for the multivariate normal distribution, Hughes *et al.* (2012a) use this to show that, with appropriate choice of priors, the saturated log-linear model fitted by the Gibbs sampler and the FCS sampler when each multinomial model has the full interaction of the categorical covariates, agree.

If we have three categorical variables, then FCS imputation, where in each multinomial regression the other two variables are included as categorical covariates (but their interaction is not included), corresponds to including all the two-way interactions in the log-linear model. In other words it imputes data that are consistent with the partial association model which estimates odds ratios relating any two factors adjusting for the third. To impute under FCS allowing for heterogeneity in the odds ratios (in other words corresponding to the saturated log-linear model) we need to include the full interaction of the covariates in each of the imputation models. We discuss and illustrate this in Section 7.2.

Now consider the case of a continuous and categorical variable. Here, just as in the case of a continuous and binary variable discussed on p. 103, the conditional mean of the continuous variable given the categorical variable is a linear function of the category indicators. Likewise the conditional distribution of the categorical variable given the continuous variable is linear on the logistic scale. However, as before, because the marginal distribution of the continuous variable does provide information about the parameters of the conditional distribution of the categorical variable given the continuous variable, FCS is not equivalent to a MCMC sampler for the joint model. Simulation studies reported by Hughes *et al.* (2012a) suggest any discrepancy is unlikely to be important in applications.

Example 5.1 Youth Cohort Study

This study was introduced in Chapter 1, Example 1.2. Here, we expand the substantive model to include the different ethnic groups, so it is a linear regression of GCSE educational score (between 0 and 84) on cohort, sex, parental social grouping (derived from questions answered by the students) and ethnicity.

As discussed in Chapter 1, the principal missing data pattern is missing parental social grouping; there are a few missing values of ethnicity, but because this variable has so many groups, it extremely time consuming to impute these, for no practically relevant gain. We therefore restrict ourselves to the 62578 cases where ethnicity is fully observed. The missingness pattern is shown in Table 5.1.

Table 5.1 Missingness pattern in the 62578 YCS records in which ethnicity is observed. Cohort and sex are fully observed.

Pattern	Variable	
Frequency	GCSE score	Parental social grouping
54872	✓	✓
6737	✓	·
673	·	✓
296	·	·

For multiple imputation we use the latent normal model; virtually identical results are obtained with FCS. For student i, let $Y_{i,1}$ denote GCSE score and $Y_{i,2}$ be the three level categorical variable identifying parental social grouping. The imputation model is:

$$Y_{i,1} = \boldsymbol{\beta}_1^T \mathbf{X}_i + e_{i,1}$$

$$\Pr(Y_{i,2} = 1) = \Pr(Z_{i,2,1} > Z_{i,2,2} \text{ and } Z_{i,2,1} > 0) \text{ where } Z_{i,2,1} = \boldsymbol{\beta}_2^T \mathbf{X}_i + e_{i,2,1}$$

$$\Pr(Y_{i,2} = 2) = \Pr(Z_{i,2,2} > Z_{i,2,1} \text{ and } Z_{i,2,2} > 0) \text{ where } Z_{i,2,2} = \boldsymbol{\beta}_3^T \mathbf{X}_i + e_{i,2,2}$$

$$\Pr(Y_{i,2} = 3) = \Pr(Z_{i,2,1} < 0 \text{ and } Z_{i,2,2} < 0)$$

$$\begin{pmatrix} e_{i,1} \\ e_{i,2,1} \\ e_{i,2,2} \end{pmatrix} = N_3 \left[\mathbf{0}, \boldsymbol{\Omega} = \begin{pmatrix} \sigma_1^2 & \sigma_{1,2,1} & \sigma_{1,2,2} \\ \sigma_{1,2,1} & 1 & 0 \\ \sigma_{1,2,2} & 0 & 1 \end{pmatrix} \right]. \qquad (5.13)$$

Rather than put the dummy variables derived from the categorical variables identifying cohort, sex and ethnic group as additional categorical responses in the imputation model, we include them as covariates in the matrix $\mathbf{X}$, which has 12 columns for, respectively, the constant, the 4 cohort contrasts, sex, and the 6 ethnic group contrasts. Thus far, we have not described the extension of the MCMC sampler for imputation models with covariates such as (5.13). This exploits the latent normal structure, and is described in Section 6.2. While for fully observed continuous variables it is computationally simpler and quicker to include them additional responses, rather than covariates, this is not the case for categorical variables, because of the rejection sampling required for the associated latent normal structure. We fitted (5.13) using the `REALCOM-impute` software, with a burn in of 1000 updates, and 10 imputations with 1000 further updates between each imputation.

The results are shown in Table 5.2. The left column shows the complete records analysis and the right column the results of MI under the assumption of MAR using the latent normal imputation model (5.13). Since, as discussed in Chapter 1, the key predictors of missing parental social group are GCSE score and ethnicity, parameter estimates in the model of interest are most likely to change for ethnicity, although other parameters may be more precisely estimated. Table 5.2 shows this is exactly what we find. Of particular note, the estimated coefficients for Black, Pakistani, and Bangladeshi ethnicity move further from the null, and the Bangladeshi estimate moves from nonsignificance in the complete records analysis to being statistically significant at the 0.1% level. We return to this example later in the book, when we carry out sensitivity analysis to the MAR assumption via MI in Chapter 10, and explore how to incorporate the survey weights that are provided with this study in Chapter 11. □

5.6 Perfect prediction issues with categorical data

In Section 4.6 we considered the practical issues raised by perfect prediction with binary data. The same issues arise with categorical data; in fact they are more

Table 5.2 Complete records analysis of the Youth Cohort Study data, and analysis using multiple imputation. Results are based on ten imputed datasets.

Variable	Complete records $n = 54872$	Multiple imputation $n = 62578$
Cohort90	reference	
Cohort93	5.66 (0.20)	5.44 (0.20)
Cohort95	9.42 (0.22)	9.21 (0.20)
Cohort97	8.09 (0.21)	8.03 (0.20)
Cohort99	12.70 (0.22)	12.91 (0.21)
Boys	−3.44 (0.13)	−3.35 (0.13)
Managerial	reference	
Intermediate	−7.42 (0.15)	−7.75 (0.16)
Working	−13.74 (0.17)	−14.32 (0.17)
White	reference	
Black	−5.61 (0.57)	−7.16 (0.51)
Indian	3.58 (0.44)	2.97 (0.42)
Pakistani	−2.03 (0.58)	−3.63 (0.47)
Bangladeshi	0.27 (1.04)	−3.20 (0.74)
Other asian	5.52 (0.68)	4.49 (0.63)
Other	−0.25 (0.70)	−1.32 (0.66)
Constant	39.66 (0.19)	39.09 (0.18)

likely to arise, as there are more categories among which small probabilities may occur.

From a Bayesian perspective, if data are binary taking the conjugate Beta(1,1) prior addresses the issue, bounding probabilities away from 0 and 1. With discrete data, the analogue is the Dirichlet prior, with all parameters set equal to 1. While this can be formally included as a prior for all probabilities in the Bayesian joint model (as described in the context of the general location model in Chapter 7 of Schafer (1997)), this is awkward for the maximum indicant model, at least if it is being fitted using the latent normal approach described here. A simple practically equivalent alternative is to restrict the latent normal variables the interval $[C, D]$, where $C = -3$ and $D = 4$ seems appropriate for most applications. Note the asymmetry of the interval, because (apart from the top category) category probabilities are defined by the probability that the associated latent normal is both positive and greater than all the other latent normals. As part of the update process, a Monte-Carlo estimate of either the marginal or conditional unit specific category probabilities can readily be estimated as a check on whether perfect prediction is close to occurring.

Under the FCS approach, provided perfect prediction is identified by the software, it is a simple matter to automatically apply the approximate data augmentation approach described on p. 104.

While we expect the performance of both adjustments above to be satisfactory, even with a relatively large number of categories, we are not aware of simulation studies which have investigated this, apart from in the binary case.

5.7 Software

There is a range of software packages for imputation with categorical data. Shafer's standalone CAT package uses a joint log-linear model, while the MIX package extends this to a mix of categorical and continuous data using the general location model; see Schafer (1999a). These have been ported to R. As discussed in Section 3.5, FCS is available in Stata and R. Lastly, the maximum indicant approach is available in REALCOM-impute.

5.8 Discussion

In this chapter we have outlined the main approaches in the literature for parametric MI with categorical data. We have seen that all approaches are consistent with a log-linear model with two-way interactions, and all may be extended to be consistent with the saturated log-linear model. The latent normal model extends the approach taken with binary data; the drawback is the relative difficulty of estimating the underlying category probabilities. This, though, is not of primary concern for imputation. When considering multilevel MI in Chapter 9, we will see the latent normal formulation is a key advantage, since it allows modelling and imputation of all types of the data at any level.

By contrast, the general location model, though potentially more general (because it allows for different variances of continuous variables in groups defined by categorical variables) does not extend so naturally to a multilevel structure. Some of this flexibility can be included in the latent normal model through including covariates in the variance model (Browne, 2006).

Lastly, the FCS approach for categorical variables (including all the interactions in each regression imputation model) is equivalent to a joint saturated log-linear model. However, with a mix of variable types this equivalence no longer formally holds, although this is unlikely to be a concern in practice.

So far, we have considered MI for a mix of continuous, ordinal and categorical variables. Our imputation models have all allowed for linear relationships between the variables on the linear predictor (latent normal) scale, and are therefore (at least very close to) congenial with substantive models for cross-sectional data that seek to estimate these effects.

However, frequently we will be interested in nonlinear relationships and interactions between variables. In such cases, the approaches described so far will be inadequate; the imputed data will not have the nonlinear relationships or interactions present. Further, frequently data are multilevel. In the next chapters we therefore consider nonlinear relationships (Chapter 6), interactions (Chapter 7), and survival data (Chapter 8) before going on to full multilevel MI in Chapter 9.

6

Nonlinear relationships

Up to this point we have been concerned with MI for data sets where the substantive scientific model is a regression of one variable on a set of covariates, without nonlinear transformations of, or interactions between, these covariates. In many applications, though, we will be interested in regressing the response on a nonlinear function of the covariates, and exploring the strength of possible interactions. In this chapter we consider nonlinear relationships, and in Chapter 7 the related issue of interactions. The goal in both chapters is the same: to multiply impute data congenially, or at least approximately congenially, when the substantive model includes a linear function of transformed covariates and/or interactions between these covariates.

Nonlinear relationships can either take the form of a linear function of transformed values of the covariates (e.g. typically a polynomial, or fractional polynomial (Royston and Sauerbrei, 2008)), or a nonlinear function of the covariates. In this chapter, our focus is on the former, although the approaches described can be extended to include the latter.

The structure of this chapter is as follows. Following a motivating example, in Section 6.1 we describe the so-called 'passive', or equivalently 'impute then transform' approach, and highlight its shortcomings. In Section 6.2 we describe preferable approaches when the covariates involved in the nonlinear relationship are fully observed. In Section 6.3 we explore the more difficult, but inevitably not uncommon, setting where variables involved in nonlinear relationships themselves have missing values. We review the two principal proposals which have been made in this context: 'Predictive Mean Matching' (PMM) in Section 6.3.1 and 'Just Another Variable' in Section 6.3.2, showing that both are generally biased and inefficient. Then, in Section 6.3.3 we extend the latent normal imputation model to handle nonlinear relationships, and Section 6.3.7 we describe how a similar approach can be adopted within the FCS framework. We conclude with a discussion in Section 6.4.

Multiple Imputation and its Application, First Edition. James R. Carpenter and Michael G. Kenward.

Example 6.1 Nerual degeneration (Bartlett, 2011)

The Alzheimer's Disease Neuroimaging Initiative was launched in 2003 by the National Institute on Aging, the National Institute of Biomedical Imaging and Bioengineering, the Food and Drug Administration, pharmaceutical companies and nonprofit organisations (see http://www.adni-info.org, and the acknowledgements on p. xiii). Using data from cognitively normal individuals in this study, Schott *et al.* (2010) explored the relationship between whole brain atrophy in the first year of follow-up and levels of amyloid $\beta_{1\text{-}42}$ peptides (A$\beta_{1\text{-}42}$), which are measured from cerebrospinal fluid extracted using a lumbar puncture.

Among these cognitively normal individuals, they found evidence of a nonlinear relationship between levels of A$\beta_{1\text{-}42}$ and greater brain atrophy. However, because of the invasive nature of lumbar puncture, A$\beta_{1\text{-}42}$ was only available for around 50% of the sample. Thus the analysis of Schott *et al.* (2010) was based on 105 out of the 199 cognitively normal individuals who had complete records. While data are plausibly MCAR, so that a complete records analysis is likely unbiased, MI nevertheless has the potential to recover information, not least through including auxiliary variables in the imputation model.

Let $Y_{i,1}$ denote the brain atrophy on individual i, in ml/year, and $Y_{i,2}$ denote A$\beta_{1\text{-}42}$ levels in pg/ml. Our substantive model is

$$Y_{i,1} = \beta_0 + \beta_1 Y_{i,2} + \beta_2 Y_{i,2}^2 + e_i, \quad e_i \overset{i.i.d.}{\sim} N(0, \sigma^2). \tag{6.1}$$

Figure 6.1 shows evidence of a nonlinear relationship in the complete records. We are concerned with appropriate imputation strategies for the missing A$\beta_{1\text{-}42}$ values. □

6.1 Passive imputation

One approach to imputing data when the substantive model involves nonlinear transformations of the variables is simply to use the same imputation model that would be adopted if the substantive model did not involve such transformations, and then with each imputed dataset transform the imputed data as required prior to fitting the substantive model.

This method is often referred to as 'passive' imputation, or 'impute then transform' (Von Hippel, 2009), as the imputation model takes no account of the nonlinear relationship between variables in the substantive model. It can be readily applied when the substantive model includes interactions as well. Intuitively, it is clear that data imputed using this procedure does not reflect the nonlinear relationship in the substantive model. However, its simplicity makes it attractive.

Example 6.1 Neural degeneration *(ctd)*

We now apply passive imputation for model (6.1). In addition to the brain atrophy and A$\beta_{1\text{-}42}$ variables, we take as an auxiliary variable a genetic marker ApoE4. This is strongly predictive of A$\beta_{1\text{-}42}$ in the complete records. Under

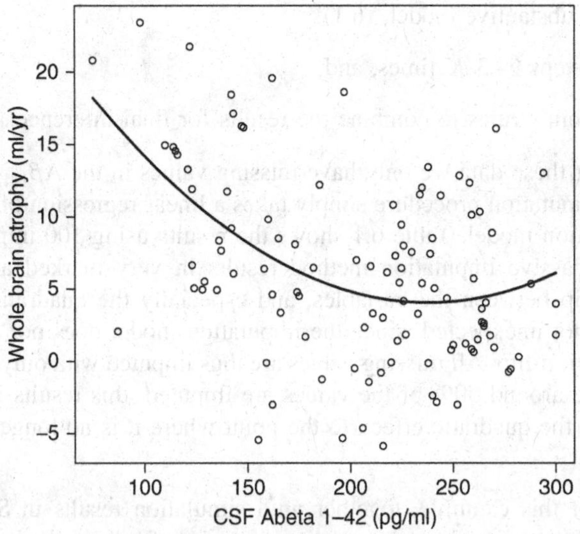

Figure 6.1 ADNI data: plot of whole brain atrophy against $A\beta_{1-42}$ levels in 105 healthy controls with complete records. The curve is from fitting (6.1) to the complete records.

the passive approach, we impute in the same way as if there were no quadratic relationship between the variables. Let $Y_{i,3}$ be a binary variable corresponding to the genetic marker ApoE4. For a general missingness pattern, the latent normal imputation model is:

$$Y_{i,1} = \beta_{0,1} + e_{i,1}$$
$$Y_{i,2} = \beta_{0,2} + e_{i,2}$$
$$\Pr(Y_{i,3} = 1) = \Pr(Z_{i,3} > 0);\; Z_{i,3} = \beta_{0,3} + e_{i,3}$$
$$\begin{pmatrix} e_{i,1} \\ e_{i,2} \\ e_{i,3} \end{pmatrix} \sim N(\mathbf{0}, \boldsymbol{\Omega}), \quad \text{with the constraint } \boldsymbol{\Omega}_{3,3} = 1. \qquad (6.2)$$

It may be computationally more convenient to re-formulate (6.2) to condition on the fully observed variables, particularly categorical variables. For fully observed continuous and binary variables, the conditional distribution for imputing the partially observed variables will be practically equivalent, whether they are included as a response or as covariates.

The analogous FCS approach has: a linear regression of Y_1 on Y_2, Y_3; a linear regression of Y_2 on Y_1, Y_3 and a logistic regression of Y_3 on Y_1, Y_2.

The passive approach proceeds as follows:

1. fit (6.2) using MCMC;
2. draw an imputed data set and calculate any variable transformations required;

3. fit the substantive model, (6.1);
4. repeat steps 2–3 K times, and
5. use Rubin's rules to combine the results for final inference.

In fact, for these data we only have missing values in the A$\beta_{1\text{-}42}$ variable, so the passive imputation procedure simply takes a linear regression of Y_2 on Y_1, Y_3 as the imputation model. Table 6.1 shows the results using 100 imputations. We see that the passive imputation method results in very marked attenuation of the relationship between the variables, and especially the quadratic component (β_2). This is not unexpected, since the imputation model does not allow for the nonlinear relationship. All missing values are thus imputed with only a linear relationship; since around 50% of the values are imputed, this results in substantial attenuation of the quadratic effect, to the point where it is no longer statistically significant. □

In the light of this example, together with simulation results in Seaman *et al.* (2012a) we do not consider the passive approach further; given the practical alternatives discussed below, we do not advocate its use.

6.2 No missing data in nonlinear relationships

Suppose we have three continuous variables, and substantive model

$$Y_{i,1} = \beta_0 + \beta_1 Y_{i,2} + \beta_2 Y_{i,3} + \beta_3 Y_{i,3}^2 + e_i, \quad e_i \overset{i.i.d.}{\sim} N(0, \sigma^2). \tag{6.3}$$

Recall from Chapter 1 that, in the absence of auxiliary variables, individuals with $Y_{i,1}$ missing contribute no information to the analysis. Thus, suppose that $\mathbf{Y}_2$ is partially observed, but that the other two variables are fully observed.

If $(Y_{i,1}, Y_{i,2})$ are approximately bivariate normal given $Y_{i,3}$, with conditional mean a linear function of $Y_{i,3}$, $Y_{i,3}^2$, then

$$Y_{i,2} = \gamma_0 + \gamma_1 Y_{i,1} + \gamma_2 Y_{i,3} + \gamma_3 Y_{i,3}^2 + \tilde{e}_i, \quad \tilde{e}_i \overset{i.i.d.}{\sim} N(0, \tilde{\sigma}^2) \tag{6.4}$$

is a congenial imputation model. The key is that we need the nonlinear effect of $Y_{i,3}$ in (6.4). If $(Y_{i,1}, Y_{i,2})$ are not plausibly bivariate normal, it will probably be more appropriate to use the approach of Section 6.3.3.

Table 6.1 Parameter estimates (standard errors) from fitting (6.1) to the 105 complete records and after MI using the passive approach.

Parameter	Complete records	Passive imputation
β_0	34.2 (7.0)	20.7 (6.5)
β_1	−0.254 (0.075)	−0.106 (0.067)
$\beta_2(\times 10^4)$	5.33 (1.91)	1.61 (1.65)

Now suppose we have four continuous variables and substantive model

$$Y_{i,1} = \beta_0 + \beta_1 Y_{i,2} + \beta_2 Y_{i,3} + \beta_3 Y_{i,4} + \beta_4 Y_{i,4}^2 + e_i, \quad e_i \overset{i.i.d.}{\sim} N(0, \sigma^2), \tag{6.5}$$

now with $Y_{i,2}, Y_{i,3}$ partially observed.

If $(Y_{i,1}, Y_{i,2}, Y_{i,3})$ are approximately trivariate normal given a linear function of $Y_{i,4}, Y_{i,4}^2$, then $(Y_{i,2}, Y_{i,3})$ are bivariate normal with conditional mean a linear function of $Y_{i,1}, Y_{i,4}, Y_{i,4}^2$, and a congenial imputation model is

$$\begin{pmatrix} Y_{i,2} \\ Y_{i,3} \end{pmatrix} \sim \begin{pmatrix} \beta_{0,2} + \beta_{1,2} Y_{i,1} + \beta_{2,2} Y_{i,4} + \beta_{3,2} Y_{i,4}^2 + e_{i,2} \\ \beta_{0,3} + \beta_{1,3} Y_{i,1} + \beta_{2,3} Y_{i,4} + \beta_{3,3} Y_{i,4}^2 + e_{i,3} \end{pmatrix}$$

$$\begin{pmatrix} e_{i,2} \\ e_{i,3} \end{pmatrix} \sim N_2(\mathbf{0}, \mathbf{\Omega}). \tag{6.6}$$

Summarising, when a quadratic, and in general nonlinear, relationship involving a fully observed variable is important in the substantive model, this nonlinear relationship must be included in the linear predictor for each partially observed variable in the imputation model, whether a joint or FCS approach is adopted. It follows that the approach in Section 3.2, where all variables (partially observed or not) are treated as responses in a multivariate normal model, is not appropriate for this setting.

Since, hitherto, the joint imputation model has just had the mean of each response on the right-hand side, we now give the additional Gibbs sampler step for a model with covariates. In order to do this succinctly, we introduce and illustrate the Kronecker product notation.

Define the Kronecker product of two matrices, A (dimension I by J, elements $a_{i,j}$) and B (dimension K by L) by $C = A \bigotimes B$, of dimension IK by JL where

$$C = \begin{pmatrix} a_{1,1}B & a_{1,2}B & \cdots & a_{1,J}B \\ a_{2,1}B & a_{2,2}B & \cdots & a_{2,J}B \\ \vdots & \vdots & \ddots & \vdots \\ a_{I,1}B & a_{I,2}B & \cdots & a_{I,J}B \end{pmatrix}$$

As an illustration, suppose we write $W_i = (Y_{i,1}, Y_{i,4}, Y_{i,4}^2)$; these are then the covariates in the two response models in the joint imputation model (6.6), with covariates $\boldsymbol{\beta}_2 = (\beta_{0,2}, \beta_{1,2}, \beta_{2,2})^T$ and $\boldsymbol{\beta}_3 = (\beta_{0,3}, \beta_{1,3}, \beta_{2,3})^T$. Let $\boldsymbol{\beta} = (\boldsymbol{\beta}_2^T, \boldsymbol{\beta}_3^T)^T$ (dimension 6×1) and $\mathbf{Z}_i = \boldsymbol{I}_2 \bigotimes W_i$ (dimension 2×6), that is,

$$\mathbf{Z}_i = \begin{pmatrix} Y_{i,1} & Y_{i,4} & Y_{i,4}^2 & 0 & 0 & 0 \\ 0 & 0 & 0 & Y_{i,1} & Y_{i,4} & Y_{i,4}^2 \end{pmatrix}.$$

Let $\mathbf{Y}_i = (Y_{i,2}, Y_{i,3})^T$. Then (6.6) can be written more concisely as

$$\mathbf{Y}_i = \mathbf{Z}_i \boldsymbol{\beta} + \mathbf{e}_i, \quad \mathbf{e}_i \sim N(\mathbf{0}, \mathbf{\Omega}), \tag{6.7}$$

$i = 1, \ldots, n$.

In fact, (6.7) represents the generic imputation model for partially observed continuous variables, where the substantive model includes a nonlinear relationship with variables that are fully observed and the conditional distribution of the partially observed variables given the fully observed variables is multivariate normal.

We now consider the Gibbs sampler for sampling from the posterior distribution of the parameters $\boldsymbol{\beta}$, $\boldsymbol{\Omega}$, in (6.7). We initialise $\boldsymbol{\beta} = \mathbf{0}$, $\boldsymbol{\Omega} = \boldsymbol{I}$. Then at update step $r = 2, 3, \ldots$

1. Given the current draw of $\boldsymbol{\Omega}$, assume an improper prior for $\boldsymbol{\beta}$ and draw the next $\boldsymbol{\beta}$ from the multivariate normal distribution

$$N\left[\left\{\sum_{i=1}^{n} \mathbf{Z}_i^T \boldsymbol{\Omega}^{-1} \mathbf{Z}_i\right\}^{-1} \sum_{i=1}^{n} \{\mathbf{Z}_i^T \boldsymbol{\Omega}^{-1} \mathbf{Y}_i\}, \left\{\sum_{i=1}^{n} \mathbf{Z}_i^T \boldsymbol{\Omega}^{-1} \mathbf{Z}_i\right\}^{-1}\right]. \quad (6.8)$$

2. Given the current draw of $\boldsymbol{\beta}$, choose a $\mathrm{W}(n_p, S_p)$ prior for $\boldsymbol{\Omega}^{-1}$. Calculate the current residuals, $\mathbf{e}_i$. Then draw $\boldsymbol{\Omega}^{-1}$ from $\mathrm{W}(n + n_p, S_u)$, where

$$S_u = \left\{\sum_{i=1}^{n} \mathbf{e}_i \mathbf{e}_i^T + S_p^{-1}\right\}^{-1}.$$

3. For units with missing $\mathbf{Y}_i$, given current draws of $\boldsymbol{\beta}, \boldsymbol{\Omega}$, draw

$$\mathbf{Y}_i \sim N(\mathbf{Z}_i \boldsymbol{\beta}, \boldsymbol{\Omega});$$

should one of the responses be observed, we draw from the conditional normal distribution given the other response, as described in Section 3.2.

We can include categorical variables in the above approach too. If they are fully observed, we include dummy indicators for each level (bar the reference) as covariates in the imputation model (6.7). If they are partially observed, we include them as responses, as described in Section 5.3. This assumes that the joint distribution of the partially observed responses and the latent normals for the categorical variable are multivariate normal given the variable with the quadratic effect, and any other fully observed variables, which will often be reasonable.

With categorical responses, the latent normal structure means that the Gibbs step for updating $\boldsymbol{\beta}$ is the same as above. For $\boldsymbol{\Omega}$, because binary and categorical variables impose constraints on the corresponding elements of $\boldsymbol{\Omega}$, we have to update $\boldsymbol{\Omega}$ elementwise, as described in Chapter 5. Likewise, ordinal responses can be handled as described in Chapter 4.

In general, we recommend including fully observed variables as covariates in the imputation model. If they are discrete, this is also computationally simpler, because element-wise updating of $\boldsymbol{\Omega}$ is more awkward, and may be slower, than drawing direct from the Wishart distribution as in step 2 above.

The above development has focused on simply including 'X^2' in the model. However, the extension to any linear function of fully observed variables, for example fractional polynomials (Royston and Sauerbrei, 2008) is immediate. When we discuss the full multilevel imputation model in Chapter 9, we will extend the imputation model to allow random coefficients. This then allows us to exploit the approach described by Verbyla *et al.* (1999); see also Welham (2010), in which cubic splines can be fitted by specifying a specific design matrix for the random effects.

6.3 Missing data in nonlinear relationships

We now consider the case where the variable involved in the nonlinear relationship is itself partially observed. We will see that this complicates the imputation. Thus, if only a small proportion of units are missing data on variables involved in the nonlinear relationship, it will usually be best simply to omit these units and adopt the approach above.

In situations where this is not the case, though, we will need to impute consistently with the partially observed nonlinear variable. We begin by considering an approach called *predictive mean matching* and a more recent proposal by Von Hippel (2009), which we term *just another variable*.

6.3.1 Predictive Mean Matching (PMM)

Suppose we have two variables, both partially observed, and the substantive model is

$$Y_{i,1} = \beta_0 + \beta_1 Y_{i,2} + \beta_2 Y_{i,2}^2 + e_i, \quad e_i \overset{i.i.d.}{\sim} N(0, \sigma^2), \tag{6.9}$$

with $\mathbf{Y}_2$ marginally normally distributed.

The imputation model remains unchanged under predictive mean matching. Thus, our joint imputation model might be bivariate normal for $(\mathbf{Y}_1, \mathbf{Y}_2)$, while under FCS we would have the linear regression of $\mathbf{Y}_1$ on $\mathbf{Y}_2$ and vice-versa. The difference comes at the point of imputation. For each missing value, at the current iteration of the sampler fitting the imputation model, we find the predicted mean. Then we impute by choosing a value at random from a 'donor pool' of neighbours nearest to that predicted mean. In many implementations, we simply impute the value closest to the predicted mean.

For example, suppose we are imputing $Y_{i,1}$ and at the current iteration the conditional mean of $Y_{i,1}$ given all the other variables is 1.3. If the ordered observed values of $\mathbf{Y}_1$ are $\{\ldots, 0.5, 0.8, 1, 1.2, 1.5, \ldots\}$ and we choose the closest value, then 1.2 would be imputed. Predictive mean matching thus has the potential advantage that imputed values are always within the range of the observed data. In cases, such as this, where the imputation model is substantially mis-specified then it may alleviate the worst effects (though this is not guaranteed). If the imputation model is congenial, or close to, it is best not to use this approach (Lee and Carlin, 2010). Seaman *et al.* (2012a) and Bartlett *et al.* (2012) explore its performance in detail in the context of nonlinear relationships using simulation, and do not recommend it.

6.3.2 Just Another Variable (JAV)

To introduce this approach, suppose we have two continuous variables, $\mathbf{Y}_1$, $\mathbf{Y}_2$, our substantive model is again (6.9), and $\mathbf{Y}_2$ is partially observed but $\mathbf{Y}_1$ fully observed.

The JAV approach proposes imputing Y_2 and $Z = Y_2^2$ treating them as if they were unrelated variables; hence the name 'just another variable.' Thus the joint imputation model is

$$\begin{aligned}
Y_{i,2} &= \beta_{0,2} + \beta_{1,2} Y_{i,1} + e_{i,2} \\
Z_{i,3} &= \beta_{0,3} + \beta_{1,3} Y_{i,1} + e_{i,3} \\
(e_{i,2}, e_{i,3})^T &\overset{i.i.d.}{\sim} \mathrm{N}_2(\mathbf{0}, \mathbf{\Omega}).
\end{aligned}$$

Alternatively, using FCS we cycle between two linear regression imputation models:

$$\begin{aligned}
Y_{i,2} &= \gamma_{0,1} + \gamma_{1,1} Y_{i,1} + \gamma_{2,1} Z_{i,2} + e_{i,1}, \quad e_{i,1} \overset{i.i.d.}{\sim} N(0, \sigma_1^2) \\
Z_{i,2} &= \gamma_{0,2} + \gamma_{1,2} Y_{i,1} + \gamma_{2,2} Y_{i,2} + e_{i,2}; \quad e_{i,2} \overset{i.i.d.}{\sim} N(0, \sigma_2^2).
\end{aligned} \tag{6.10}$$

Comparing (6.9) and (6.10) we see that the method can at best be approximate; first because Y_2 and its square are deterministically related and this is ignored; second because it is not possible that both Y_2 and Z can be normally distributed given Y_1.

Seaman *et al.* (2012a) criticize this approach. They show it only gives valid point estimates for linear regression models when data are MCAR, and note that, even in this setting, the validity of Rubin's combination rules for the variance of an imputation estimator is not guaranteed. The intuition is as follows.

If data are MCAR, then the complete records give consistent estimators of population quantities. Specifically, marginal statistics such as means and cross products estimated from the complete records are consistent for their population values. This means that using the complete records gives consistent estimators of the sums of squares and cross products from which the parameter estimators in (6.10) are derived. This in turn can be shown to imply that, assuming data are MCAR, using the imputed data from (6.10) results in consistent estimators of sums of squares and cross products, from which the parameter estimators in (6.9) are derived. Hence the parameter estimators of (6.9) are themselves consistent.

Of course, if data are MCAR, then there is no need to use JAV to obtain consistent estimators: a complete records analysis will suffice. The advantage of JAV under MCAR is therefore the potential for recovering more information, as reflected in smaller standard errors, which are as usual derived using Rubin's combination rules. Unfortunately, Rubin's rules for the variance of a multiple imputation estimator assume a correctly specified imputation model (see Chapter 2). Since (6.10) cannot be correctly specified, the variance estimator is not guaranteed to work with JAV, even assuming data are MCAR. The practical implication of this latter point should not be overstated, however, since Rubin's rules typically work acceptably well, if slightly conservatively, in such settings.

If data are MAR, however, JAV generally gives biased, inconsistent, parameter estimators. This is because complete records give biased, inconsistent estimators of the marginal moments required to estimate the parameters in (6.10). In turn this means that using imputed data from (6.10) gives inconsistent estimators of the parameters (6.9).

Seaman *et al.* (2012a) describe a series of simulation studies comparing passive imputation, Predictive Mean Matching and JAV. They initially consider linear regression, with 200 observations of a fully observed response on a partially observed covariate and its square under MCAR and MAR. The marginal distribution of the covariate is first normal, then lognormal, and the regression R^2 is 0.1, 0.5 and 0.8.

In line with theory, the bias of JAV is small or negligible when data are MCAR. Under MAR, bias is generally present. Focusing on the quadratic parameter, when the marginal distribution of the covariate is normal, bias can decrease or increase with R^2, depending on the nature of the quadratic relationship. If the covariate is log-normal, bias is larger, and increases with increasing R^2. With logistic regression, under MCAR, the performance of JAV is markedly worse, with nontrivial bias (median absolute 23% bias across scenarios with marginal normal covariate; median absolute 66% bias across scenarios with marginal log-normal covariate). Bias is worse again under MAR; and now in 5/6 scenarios it is worse than the passive option, described at the start of this chapter. Coverage can be very poor when bias is substantial.

The markedly varied and often disappointing performance of JAV, especially in logistic regression, means we cannot recommend this approach in general. Instead, below we describe a modelling approach, which is a natural extension of the joint normal framework we have described, and which can also be approximated using a FCS approach. We will see that when data are MCAR, JAV – though consistent – will be inefficient relative to our approach, because JAV is in essence a moment-based estimator.

6.3.3 Joint modelling approach

We begin by considering the case of two continuous variables, Y_1, Y_2, in detail, before outlining a general algorithm in Section 6.3.4. Suppose the substantive model is (6.9), and $\mathbf{Y}_2$ has values MAR (given $\mathbf{Y}_1$).

So far with MI, our imputation models have taken the partially observed variable(s) as the response(s), conditioning on fully observed variables where appropriate. However, because the joint distribution of Y_1, Y_2 that is congenial with (6.9) does not follow a known probability distribution (cf Section 2.9) we instead specify the joint distribution of (Y_1, Y_2) as

$$f_{1,2}(Y_1, Y_2) = f_{1|2}(Y_1|Y_2) f_2(Y_2). \tag{6.11}$$

If we chose $f_{1|2}(Y_1|Y_2)$ as (6.9) then, regardless of the choice of $f_2(Y_2)$, we ensure the imputation model is congenial with (6.9). It remains to choose $f_2(Y_2)$. The simplest choice is a univariate $N(\tilde{\mu}, \tilde{\sigma}^2)$ distribution, which we adopt below. If this is not appropriate, we may consider a transformation to a latent normal scale, $h(Y_2) = Z$, so that Z is more nearly normally distributed. Then, the usual change of variables formula gives

$$f_2(Y_2) = \frac{|h'(Y_2)|}{\tilde{\sigma}} \phi\left(\frac{h(Y_2) - \tilde{\mu}}{\tilde{\sigma}}\right), \tag{6.12}$$

where $\phi(.)$ is the standard normal density. Alternatives such as the log-normal or gamma distribution may be considered for f_2. When f_2 is not the standard normal step 3 below may itself need to be adapted appropriately.

The starting point for the MCMC algorithm to fit the model is the approach outlined so far, assuming Y_2 is fully observed. To this we add two further steps: one to draw missing $Y_{i,2}$ and the other to update the parameters of $f_2(Y_2) = f_2(Y_2; \tilde{\beta}, \tilde{\sigma}^2)$.

As usual, choose starting values for the parameters $(\boldsymbol{\beta}, \sigma^2)$, $(\tilde{\beta}, \tilde{\sigma}^2)$ and the missing $\mathbf{Y}_1, \mathbf{Y}_2$. Then update the MCMC sampler by iterating steps 1–3:

1. Given the current draws for missing $(\mathbf{Y}_1, \mathbf{Y}_2)$, and the observed data, update the parameters of $f_{1|2}$, $\boldsymbol{\beta}$, σ^2, as described in Section 6.2.

2. Given the current draw for $(\boldsymbol{\beta}, \sigma^2)$, $(\tilde{\beta}, \tilde{\sigma}^2)$, and the observed data, update each missing $Y_{i,2}$ as described below.

3. Given $\mathbf{Y}_2$, (the observed part and the current draws for the missing observations), update the parameters, $(\tilde{\beta}, \tilde{\sigma}^2)$.

As we have chosen $f_2(Y_2)$ to be a normal distribution, we update $(\tilde{\beta}, \tilde{\sigma}^2)$ using the same algorithm used for step 1.

We next discuss two approaches for step 2: the first based on a Metropolis-Hasting step, and the other using rejection sampling. At the end of Section 6.3.4, we discuss pros and cons of the two approaches.

Metropolis-Hastings for drawing Y_2

Under the Metropolis-Hastings approach, we need a proposal distribution for $Y_{i,2}$; a natural choice is $Y^{\star}_{i,2} \sim N(Y_{i,2}, \tau^2)$, where $Y^{\star}_{i,2}$ is the proposed new value,

$Y_{i,2}$ the current value and τ^2 a fraction – for example, a half – of the marginal variance of the observed $\mathbf{Y}_2$. Then, given the current draw of $(\boldsymbol{\beta}, \sigma^2)$, $(\tilde{\beta}, \tilde{\sigma}^2)$, for each i with $Y_{i,2}$ is missing in turn, we:

1. propose a new value $Y_{i,2}^{\star}$ drawn from $N(Y_{i,2}, \tau^2)$. Note this is a symmetric proposal, so the Hastings ratio (see Appendix A) is 1.

2. calculate $L(Y_{i,2}^{\star})$ and $L(Y_{i,2})$ where

$$L(x) = f_{1|2}(Y_1|x; \boldsymbol{\beta}, \sigma^2) f_2(x; \tilde{\beta}, \tilde{\sigma}^2) \tag{6.13}$$

Because the substantive model (6.9) is a linear regression we have

$$f_{1|2}(Y_1|x; \boldsymbol{\beta}, \sigma^2) = \frac{1}{\sqrt{2\pi\sigma^2}} \exp\left\{-\frac{1}{2\sigma^2}(Y_{i,1} - \beta_0 - \beta_1 x - \beta_2 x^2)^2\right\} \tag{6.14}$$

and

$$f_2(x; \tilde{\beta}, \tilde{\sigma}^2) = \frac{1}{\sqrt{2\pi\tilde{\sigma}^2}} \exp\left\{-\frac{1}{2\tilde{\sigma}^2}(x - \tilde{\beta})^2\right\}. \tag{6.15}$$

3. accept the proposal with probability

$$\min\left\{1, \frac{L(Y_{i,2}^{\star})}{L(Y_{i,2})}\right\}; \tag{6.16}$$

and if accepted set $Y_{i,2} = Y_{i,2}^{\star}$.

Rejection approach for drawing Y_2

An alternative to the Metropolis-Hastings sampler is rejection sampling (Bartlett *et al.*, 2012). If we can get a good bound, denoted K below, this may prove more computationally efficient. It also has the attraction that, unlike the Metropolis-Hastings step above, each accepted draw is from the desired distribution.

As above, we draw each missing $Y_{i,2}$ value in turn conditional on all the other parameters. If we draw this from density g, suppose that

$$\max_{Y_{i,2}} \left(\frac{f_{2|1}(Y_{i,2}|Y_{i,1})}{g(Y_{i,2})} \right) \leq K. \tag{6.17}$$

Then, if we accept the proposed value with probability

$$\frac{f_{2|1}(Y_{i,2}|Y_{i,1})}{g(Y_{i,2}) \times K}, \tag{6.18}$$

it is a valid draw from $f_{2|1}(Y_{i,2}|Y_{i,1})$, i.e. the distribution of the missing given observed data (see, e.g. (Ripley, 1987, p. 60)). This also makes sense intuitively: if we were able to sample direct from $f_{2|1}(Y_{i,2}|Y_{i,1})$ and so chose $g = f_{2|1}(Y_{i,2}|Y_{i,1})$, then $K = 1$ and we would always accept.

In the model at hand, suppose we let $g = f_2(Y_{i,2}; \tilde{\beta}, \tilde{\sigma}^2)$ be a univariate normal distribution. Then

$$\begin{aligned} \frac{f_{2|1}(Y_{i,2}|Y_{i,1})}{g(Y_{i,2})} &= \frac{f_{1,2}(Y_{i,1}, Y_{i,2})}{f_1(Y_{i,1})f_2(Y_{i,2})} \\ &= \frac{f_{1|2}(Y_{i,1}|Y_{i,2})}{f_1(Y_{i,1})} \\ &\leq \frac{1}{\sqrt{2\pi\sigma^2}} \times \frac{1}{f_1(Y_{i,1})} \\ &= K, \text{ say,} \end{aligned} \tag{6.19}$$

where the inequality follows because $f_{1|2}(Y_{i,1}|Y_{i,2})$ is the density of model (6.3), which being a normal density has maximum value $1/\sqrt{2\pi\sigma^2}$.

Thus, if we draw a proposed $Y^{\star}_{i,2}$ from f_2 then we accept with probability (6.18), which by substitution is

$$\frac{f_{2|1}(Y^{\star}_{i,2}|Y_{i,1})}{g(Y^{\star}_{i,2}) \times K} = \exp\left\{-\frac{1}{2\sigma^2}(Y_{i,1} - \beta_0 - \beta_1 Y^{\star}_{i,2} - \beta_2 Y^{\star 2}_{i,2})^2\right\}. \tag{6.20}$$

Example 6.2 Simulation study

Bartlett (2011) performed a simulation study for $n = 1000$ units, in which the substantive model is (6.9), i.e.

$$Y_{i,1} = \beta_0 + \beta_1 Y_{i,2} + \beta_2 Y^2_{i,2} + e_i, \quad e_i \sim N(0, \sigma^2), \quad i \in (1, \ldots, n)$$

and marginally, $Y_{i,2} \overset{i.i.d.}{\sim} N(0, 1)$. Values of $Y_{i,2}$ were made either made MCAR with probability 0.5, or missing at random under the mechanism

$$\text{logit}\,\{\Pr(\text{observe } Y_{i,2})\} = 0.37 - 0.41 Y_{i,1}.$$

The rejection sampling approach above was compared with passive imputation (Example 6.1), and JAV (Section 6.3.2). Table 6.2 shows the results. We see that even under MCAR, passive imputation performs poorly; this approach should be avoided. JAV is unbiased under MCAR, but less efficient than rejection sampling. Under MAR, only rejection sampling performs adequately. □

6.3.4 Extension to more general models and missing data patterns

The approach above extends naturally to more complicated settings such as the following, again assuming for the time being that all variables are continuous:

$$\begin{aligned} Y_{i,1} &= \beta_0 + \beta_1 Y_{i,2} + \beta_2 Y_{i,3} + \beta_3 Y^2_{i,3} + \beta_4 Y_{i,4} + \beta_5 Y^2_{i,4} + e_i \\ e_i &\overset{i.i.d.}{\sim} N(0, \sigma^2), \quad i \in (1, \ldots n). \end{aligned} \tag{6.21}$$

Table 6.2 Average point estimates and associated empirical standard deviations from 1000 replicates of model with quadratic effect and missing covariate, comparing passive imputation, JAV and rejection sampling.

Parameter value	Complete records	Multiple imputation using Passive	JAV	Rejection
Data MCAR				
$\beta_0 = 0$	−0.003 (0.094)	0.435 (0.080)	−0.012 (0.082)	−0.002 (0.080)
$\beta_1 = 1$	1.002 (0.079)	0.977 (0.102)	1.012 (0.082)	1.002 (0.079)
$\beta_2 = 1$	1.003 (0.056)	0.561 (0.044)	1.014 (0.059)	1.003 (0.053)
Data MAR				
$\beta_0 = 0$	−0.461 (0.092)	0.649 (0.089)	−0.076 (0.111)	0.000 (0.085)
$\beta_1 = 1$	0.900 (0.096)	0.944 (0.140)	1.267 (0.132)	0.993 (0.099)
$\beta_2 = 1$	0.907 (0.079)	0.527 (0.056)	1.271 (0.103)	1.005 (0.069)

We now suppose data are MAR, but with a general missing pattern. We could generalise the approach of the previous subsection directly to (6.21), which would require specification of, say $f(Y_1|Y_2, Y_3, Y_4)$ (i.e. (6.21)) alongside $f(Y_2|Y_3, Y_4)$ and $f(Y_3, Y_4)$. However, if we assume that (Y_1, Y_2) given (Y_3, Y_3^2, Y_4, Y_4^2) are bivariate normal and that (Y_3, Y_4) are bivariate normal (assumptions we discuss relaxing at the end of this subsection), we can write the imputation model as:

$$\begin{aligned} Y_{i,1} &= \beta_{0,1} + \beta_{1,1}Y_{i,3} + \beta_{2,1}Y_{i,3}^2 + \beta_{3,1}Y_{i,4} + \beta_{4,1}Y_{i,4}^2 + e_{i,1} \\ Y_{i,2} &= \beta_{0,2} + \beta_{1,2}Y_{i,3} + \beta_{2,2}Y_{i,3}^2 + \beta_{3,2}Y_{i,4} + \beta_{4,2}Y_{i,4}^2 + e_{i,2} \\ \begin{pmatrix} e_{i,1} \\ e_{i,2} \end{pmatrix} &\sim N_2(\mathbf{0}, \boldsymbol{\Omega}), \end{aligned} \tag{6.22}$$

which we denote by $f_{1,2|3,4}(Y_1, Y_2|Y_3, Y_4; \boldsymbol{\beta}, \boldsymbol{\Omega})$.

The MCMC procedure for fitting this model follows the same essential steps as that described on page 136, but we now need to impute any missing (Y_3, Y_4) following step 1. Denote the bivariate normal distribution of (Y_3, Y_4) by $f_{3,4}(Y_3, Y_4; \tilde{\boldsymbol{\beta}}, \tilde{\boldsymbol{\Omega}})$. Choose starting values for all parameters and missing data. Then update the MCMC sampler by iterating steps 1–3 below:

1. Given the current draws for missing data, and the observed data, update the parameters $(\boldsymbol{\beta}, \boldsymbol{\Omega})$ of $f_{1,2|3,4}$ as described in Section 6.2.
   (a) Impute missing values of $(Y_{i,1}, Y_{i,2})$ by drawing them from (6.22) (or the appropriate conditional) at the current parameter values.
2. Given the current draw for $(\boldsymbol{\beta}, \boldsymbol{\Omega})$, $(\tilde{\boldsymbol{\beta}}, \tilde{\boldsymbol{\Omega}})$, and observed and current imputed values for $(\mathbf{Y}_1, \mathbf{Y}_2)$, draw missing $(Y_{i,3}, Y_{i,4})$ as described below.
3. Given the observed and current imputed values for $(\mathbf{Y}_3, \mathbf{Y}_4)$ update the parameters, $\tilde{\boldsymbol{\beta}}$, $\tilde{\boldsymbol{\Omega}}$ of $f_{3,4}(Y_3, Y_4; \tilde{\boldsymbol{\beta}}, \tilde{\boldsymbol{\Omega}})$, again as described in Section 6.2.

As before, we now consider first Metropolis-Hastings sampling, and then rejection sampling, for step 2.

6.3.5 Metropolis-Hastings sampling

We work in turn through units (indexed by i) where one, or both, of $(Y_{i,3}, Y_{i,4})$ is missing. Either, or both, could be missing: we indicate how the procedure adapts as we go through.

1. Propose new values $(Y^\star_{i,3}, Y^\star_{i,4})$ by drawing from the bivariate normal distribution whose mean is the current values $(Y_{i,3}, Y_{i,4})$ and whose variance is $\tau\hat{\Sigma}$, where $\hat{\Sigma}$ is the sample variance of the observed $(\mathbf{Y}_3, \mathbf{Y}_4)$ and the value of τ can be adapted during the burn-in of the sampler to achieve an acceptance rate of around 50%; alternatively $\tau = 0.5$ may be a reasonable choice. Note this is a symmetric proposal, so the Hastings ratio (see Appendix A) is 1.

   (a) If one of $Y_{i,3}$ or $Y_{i,4}$ is observed, draw a proposal for the other from the marginal normal corresponding to the bivariate proposal in the previous paragraph (if we wish to use the conditional normal, we need to include the Hastings ratio as it will no longer be 1). Again, write $(Y^\star_{i,3}, Y^\star_{i,4})$ for what is now the pair of observed and drawn values.

2. Calculate $L(Y^\star_{i,3}, Y^\star_{i,4})$ and $L(Y_{i,3}, Y_{i,4})$ where $\mathbf{x} = (x_1, x_2)^T$ and

$$L(\mathbf{x}) = f_{1,2|3,4}(Y_1, Y_2|\mathbf{x}; \boldsymbol{\beta}, \boldsymbol{\Omega}) f_{3,4}(\mathbf{x}; \tilde{\boldsymbol{\beta}}, \tilde{\boldsymbol{\Omega}}) \tag{6.23}$$

   Since the imputation model (6.22) is a multivariate normal density, here with $p = 2$ response variables,

$$f_{1,2|3,4}(Y_1, Y_2|\mathbf{x}; \boldsymbol{\beta}, \boldsymbol{\Omega}) = \frac{1}{(2\pi)^{p/2}|\boldsymbol{\Omega}|^{1/2}} \exp\left\{-\frac{1}{2}(\mathbf{Y}_i - \boldsymbol{\mu}_i)^T \boldsymbol{\Omega}^{-1}(\mathbf{Y}_i - \boldsymbol{\mu}_i)\right\}, \tag{6.24}$$

   where $\mathbf{Y}_i = (Y_{i,1}, Y_{i,2}),^T$

$$\boldsymbol{\mu}_i = \begin{pmatrix} \beta_{0,1} + \beta_{1,1}x_1 + \beta_{2,1}x_1^2 + \beta_{3,1}x_2 + \beta_{4,1}x_2^2 \\ \beta_{0,2} + \beta_{1,2}x_1 + \beta_{2,2}x_1^2 + \beta_{3,2}x_2 + \beta_{4,2}x_2^2 \end{pmatrix},$$

   and $f_{3,4}(\mathbf{x}; \tilde{\boldsymbol{\beta}}, \tilde{\boldsymbol{\Omega}})$ is the bivariate normal density evaluated at $\mathbf{x} = (x_1, x_2)^T$.

3. Accept the proposal with probability

$$\min\left\{1, \frac{L(Y^\star_{i,3}, Y^\star_{i,4})}{L(Y_{i,3}, Y_{i,4})}\right\}; \tag{6.25}$$

   and if accepted set $Y_{i,3} = Y^\star_{i,3}$, $Y_{i,4} = Y^\star_{i,4}$.

6.3.6 Rejection sampling

As above, an alternative for drawing missing $(Y_{i,3}, Y_{i,4})$ is rejection sampling. Suppose first that both $(Y_{i,3}, Y_{i,4})$ are missing. We now need to find K such that

$$\max_{Y_{i,3},Y_{i,4}} \left(\frac{f_{3,4|1,2}(Y_{i,3}, Y_{i,4}|Y_{i,1}, Y_{i,2})}{g(Y_{i,3}, Y_{i,4})} \right) < K, \tag{6.26}$$

where g is the proposal density. Suppose we choose $g = f_{3,4}(Y_3, Y_4; \tilde{\boldsymbol{\beta}}, \tilde{\boldsymbol{\Omega}})$ as the bivariate normal density. Following (6.19),

$$\begin{aligned}
\frac{f_{3,4|1,2}(Y_{i,3}, Y_{i,4}|Y_{i,1}, Y_{i,2})}{g} &= \frac{f_{3,4|1,2}(Y_{i,3}, Y_{i,4}|Y_{i,1}, Y_{i,2})}{f_{3,4}(Y_{i,3}, Y_{i,4}; \tilde{\boldsymbol{\beta}}, \tilde{\boldsymbol{\Omega}})} \\
&= \frac{f_{1,2|3,4}(Y_{i,1}, Y_{i,2}|Y_{i,3}, Y_{i,4})}{f_{1,2}(Y_{i,1}, Y_{i,2})} \\
&\leq (2\pi)^{p/2}|\boldsymbol{\Omega}|^{1/2}\frac{1}{f_{1,2}(Y_{i,1}, Y_{i,2})} \\
&= K, \text{ say,}
\end{aligned} \tag{6.27}$$

where p is the dimension of the response in the imputation model (6.22), i.e. $p = 2$ in this case.

Thus if we draw a proposed $(Y^{\star}_{i,3}, Y^{\star}_{i,4})$ from $g = f_{3,4}$, we accept with probability (6.26) which is

$$\frac{f_{3,4|1,2}}{f_{3,4}K} = \exp\left\{-\frac{1}{2}(\mathbf{Y}_i - \boldsymbol{\mu}_i)^T \boldsymbol{\Omega}^{-1}(\mathbf{Y}_i - \boldsymbol{\mu}_i)\right\}, \tag{6.28}$$

where $\mathbf{Y}_i$, $\boldsymbol{\mu}_i$ are defined below (6.24).

Now suppose only $Y_{i,4}$ is missing. We again choose $f_{3,4}(Y_3, Y_4; \tilde{\beta}, \tilde{\Omega})$ as the bivariate normal, and from this calculate the conditional normal $f_{4|3}$. We set $g = f_{4|3}$. Using the same argument leading to (6.26) gives

$$K = (2\pi)^{p/2}|\boldsymbol{\Omega}|^{1/2}\frac{1}{f_{1,2|3}(Y_{i,1}, Y_{i,2}|Y_{i,3})}.$$

The acceptance probability is then given by

$$\frac{f_{4|1,2,3}}{f_{4|3}K} = \exp\left\{-\frac{1}{2}(\mathbf{Y}_i - \boldsymbol{\mu}_i)^T \boldsymbol{\Omega}^{-1}(\mathbf{Y}_i - \boldsymbol{\mu}_i)\right\},$$

in other words the same as (6.28).

Some comments

The situations considered above clearly do not cover the generality of nonlinear relationships that may arise, but exemplify the general approach. Thus, while we have considered quadratic terms, the approach generalises to other nonlinear functions of the covariates in the substantive model. For example, we may have a fractional polynomial relationship involving partially observed covariates. Since, in multivariate imputation models such as (6.22), the responses are multivariate normal conditional on the covariates, nonlinear relationships should be on the RHS.

We have focussed on normally distributed continuous variables. Nonlinear relationships are not meaningful for binary and categorical variables, unless they are part of interactions, which form the subject of Chapter 7. Within the imputation model framework outlined above, we would include them as covariates if they are fully observed and response variables if they were partially observed.

When the marginal distribution of the covariates in (6.22) is not plausibly multivariate normal, we may consider a transformation to a latent normal scale. This could be by introducing a Box-Cox transformation, the parameters of which are updated via a further MCMC step, as sketched by Goldstein *et al.* (2009). It is simpler, and likely to be just as effective, to use the observed values to identify marginal transformations to a latent normal scale. Following (6.12) for variables (Y_3, Y_4) with transformations h_3, h_4, from the usual change of variables formula the density for the covariates is then

$$|h_3'(Y_3)h_4'(Y_4)|\, f(h_3(Y_3), h_4(Y_4); \tilde{\boldsymbol{\beta}}, \tilde{\boldsymbol{\Omega}}),$$

where $f(.,.;\tilde{\boldsymbol{\beta}}, \tilde{\boldsymbol{\Omega}})$ is the bivariate normal density. If we adopt this approach, then in the Metropolis-Hastings step for any missing $(Y_{i,3}, Y_{i,4})$ we should propose new values on the latent normal scale, centred at the current values, as the Hastings ratio then remains 1.

An assumption of imputation model (6.22) is the multivariate normal (or latent multivariate normal for discrete variables) distribution of the responses given the nonlinear function of the covariates, and that this is congenial with the substantive model. For response variables in the imputation model where this is implausible, we cannot simply transform them before imputation and back transform them afterwards, as this breaks the nonlinear relationship we are seeking to preserve in imputation. Instead, such variables may be moved to the RHS of the imputation model and handled as described above.

As we now have a framework for imputing covariate values in the imputation model, we can if desired move all variables, except the response in the original substantive model, to the RHS of the imputation model. In other words we can make the imputation model and the substantive model identical. In this case, because we can sample from the posterior distribution of the parameters, MI is not necessary: we can draw inference from the posterior distribution in the usual way. While, in principle, this can always be done for any substantive model, nevertheless, MI will typically be preferable as:

- we can include auxiliary variables in the imputation model, to increase the plausibility of MAR and improve the prediction of missing values;
- imputation and analysis can be done separately;

- we can impute a relatively large number of variables, and then rapidly explore a variety of models with the resulting imputed data, and
- MI provides a natural route for sensitivity analysis to the MAR assumption, as discussed in Chapter 10.

Indeed, in most cases, handling missing covariates in the imputation model will be cumbersome relative to the approaches described in Chapters 3–5, whether using the joint modelling approach (above) or the FCS approximation (below). Thus, in the absence of nonlinear relationships involving partially observed variables we do not advise it.

6.3.7 FCS approach

The rejection sampling approach can be incorporated into a modified FCS imputation algorithm to handle nonlinearities, and, as we present in Chapter 7, interactions involving nonlinear terms.

Suppose we have three continuous variables, $\mathbf{Y}_1, \mathbf{Y}_2, \mathbf{Y}_3$, a general missingness pattern, we assume MAR and our substantive model is the linear regression

$$Y_{i,1} = \beta_0 + \beta_1 Y_{i,2} + \beta_2 Y_{i,3} + \beta_3 Y_{i,3}^2 + e_i, \quad e_{i,1} \sim N(0, \sigma^2). \tag{6.29}$$

As usual with FCS, we visit, in turn, a conditional model for each partially observed variable given all the others. The difference is (i) that the imputation procedure now needs to know the substantive model and (ii) that we now take account of this information when using a rejection step to impute missing values of covariates in the substantive model. For (6.29) this works as follows. First, choose starting values for missing values of each variable, typically by sampling with replacement from observed values of that variable. Then:

1. Fit model (6.29) to the current observed and imputed data by maximum likelihood, and – as with standard FCS – draw parameter values $\boldsymbol{\beta} = (\beta_0, \ldots, \beta_3), \sigma^2$, from the sampling distribution of the maximum likelihood estimators.
   (a) For each i with missing $Y_{i,1}$, using $\sigma^2, \boldsymbol{\beta}$ drawn in step 1, impute a new value from (6.29).
2. Fit the linear regression of $\mathbf{Y}_2$ on $\mathbf{Y}_3$, with density $f_{2|3}(Y_2|Y_3; \tilde{\boldsymbol{\beta}}, \tilde{\sigma}^2)$, to the current observed and imputed values of these variables using maximum likelihood, and draw parameter values $\tilde{\sigma}^2, \tilde{\boldsymbol{\beta}}$ from the sampling distribution of the maximum likelihood estimators.
   (a) For each i in turn for which $Y_{i,2}$ is missing, draw a proposal, $Y_{i,2}^\star$ from $f_{2|3}(Y_2|Y_{i,3}; \tilde{\boldsymbol{\beta}}, \tilde{\sigma}^2)$, and accept $Y_{i,2}^\star$ with probability

$$\exp\left\{-\frac{1}{2\sigma^2}\left(Y_{i,1} - \beta_0 - \beta_1 Y_{i,2}^\star + \beta_2 Y_{i,3} + \beta_3 Y_{i,3}^2\right)^2\right\} \tag{6.30}$$

If the proposed $Y^{\star}_{i,2}$ is rejected, draw another and repeat until acceptance.

3. Fit the linear regression of $\mathbf{Y}_3$ on $\mathbf{Y}_2$, denoted by $f_{3|2}(Y_3|Y_2; \tilde{\boldsymbol{\alpha}}, \tilde{\tau}^2)$, to the current observed and imputed values of these variables using maximum likelihood, and draw parameter values $\tilde{\tau}^2$, $\tilde{\boldsymbol{\alpha}}$ from the sampling distribution of the maximum likelihood estimators.

   (a) For each i in turn for which $Y_{i,3}$ is missing, draw a proposal $Y^{\star}_{i,3}$ from $f_{3|2}(Y_3|Y_{i,2}; \tilde{\boldsymbol{\alpha}}, \tilde{\tau}^2)$, and accept with probability

$$\exp\left\{-\frac{1}{2\sigma^2}(Y_{i,1} - \beta_0 - \beta_1 Y_{i,2} + \beta_2 Y^{\star}_{i,3} + \beta_3 Y^{\star 2}_{i,3})^2\right\}.$$

   If the proposal for missing $Y_{i,3}$ is rejected, draw another until acceptance.

When the substantive model is a linear regression, e.g. (6.29), the acceptance probability (6.30) is derived in the same way as (6.20). For each additional covariate in the substantive model, (6.29), we simply add another step to the algorithm, analogous to steps 2 and 3.

If the substantive model is logistic regression, for any unit i the maximum value of the probability density function for the substantive model is 1. Following the argument leading to (6.20), the acceptance probability is simply the probability density for the substantive model for unit i. We consider the case when the substantive model is a proportional hazards model in Chapter 8.

If the covariate Y_2 in the substantive model (6.29) is binary, then in step 2 above, the linear regression model of Y_2 on Y_3 is replaced by logistic regression. If the covariate were ordinal, we could use ordinal regression; if it were unordered categorical, a multinomial regression.

As with all FCS imputation procedures, this approach relies on the models – specifically the model for each covariate given all the others – being appropriate. If a continuous covariate does not have a approximately a conditional normal distribution, then if we can find an approximate normalising transformation (say from the observed values) we can regress the transformed covariate on the other covariates, propose a value, back transform, and calculate the acceptance probability as before.

Lastly, in the FCS algorithm, for variables whose distribution, conditional on all the other variables (including nonlinear relationships), is (at least approximately) a known regression, then a standard FCS step can be used. For example,, in (6.29) it may be that Y_2 is (approximately) conditionally normal given Y_1, Y_3, Y_3^2. In this case, step 2 could be replaced by a linear regression.

Bartlett *et al.* (2012) report simulations evaluating FCS with rejection sampling, comparing it with passive imputation and JAV, for model (6.9). They consider MCAR and MAR data, and a marginal normal, log-normal and mixture of normal distributions for the covariate. In line with Table 6.2, FCS with rejection sampling outperforms the other approaches, except for the difficult case

Table 6.3 Parameter estimates (standard errors) from fitting (6.1) using MI with the JAV procedure and using MI incorporating a rejection sampling step.

Parameter	JAV	MI with rejection sampling step
β_0	32.0 (6.3)	31.0 (6.1)
β_1	−0.234 (0.068)	−0.223 (0.064)
$\beta_2(\times 10^4)$	4.91 (1.73)	4.63 (1.60)

when the marginal distribution of the covariate is a mixture of normals (and hence bimodal), where the maximum bias, of 7.5%, is on the linear term (β_1). In this case, a marginal distribution that better reflects the mixture would reduce the bias.

Example 6.1 Neural degeneration *(ctd)*

Continuing with this example, imputing the missing A$\beta_{1\text{-}42}$ values with a rejection sampling step as described above, using ApoE4 as an auxiliary variable, gives the results shown in Table 6.3. For comparison, we include the results of the JAV approach. As missing values are apparently MCAR (the chance of observing them does not vary with brain atrophy or ApoE4), and the substantive model is a linear regression, JAV gives consistent estimators. Thus JAV and rejection sampling give similar results. Note that MI is more efficient, both compared with JAV (though only slightly) and the complete records analysis, as theory predicts. Given the relative lack of power for nonlinear effects, this may be an important benefit in practice. □

6.4 Discussion

In this chapter we have compared various approaches to MI when the substantive model regresses the response on nonlinear transformations of the covariates. In Section 6.1 we showed why the passive approach, in which the imputation model assumes all the relationships are linear, is not appropriate.

When the covariates involved in the nonlinear relationship in the substantive model are fully observed, we showed in Section 6.2 how the approach of earlier chapters could be generalised by including them as covariates in the imputation model. An analogous procedure can be used with FCS: we simply include the nonlinear transformations of the covariates in question in each regression imputation model.

The scenario with missing values among the covariates involved in the nonlinear relationship in the substantive model is more difficult. Thus, if such variables have a small proportion of missing values, discarding these records and using the approach of the previous paragraph – which has the advantage of relative simplicity – will usually be perfectly adequate.

When this is not the case, we have discussed the 'Just Another Variable' approach and also described extending the imputation model to allow missing values in the covariates. This can be done using either a MCMC step or a rejection sampling step. Following Bartlett *et al.* (2012) we have shown how this can be applied with the FCS approach.

Seaman *et al.* (2012a) present the theory behind JAV and report its shortcomings when data are not MCAR. By contrast, the rejection sampling approach is theoretically well founded and gives consistent, fully efficient, inference when the model for the partially observed covariates is correct. In practice, as discussed in Section 6.3.7, results are robust to modest misspecification; where this is a concern, transformation to a latent normal scale may prove helpful.

As discussed in Subsection 6.3.6 a consequence of extending the imputation model fitting procedures to allow for missing covariates is that the distinction between imputation model and substantive model is blurred. Nevertheless, as discussed in Subsection 6.3.6, MI remains attractive. Indeed, handling missing covariates in the imputation model will be cumbersome relative to the approaches described in Chapters 3–5. Thus, when there are no nonlinear relationships involving partially observed variables we do not advise it.

In this chapter we have only considered relationships which are linear in functions of the covariates. However, the MCMC or rejection sampling approaches outlined above can be extended to handle nonlinear functions of the covariates in the substantive model.

7

Interactions

In this chapter we discuss building appropriate MI models when the substantive model contains interactions between covariates. We begin, in Section 7.1, with the case when the variables involved in the interaction are fully observed. Then, in Section 7.2 we consider interactions involving partially observed categorical variables. This leads to interactions involving continuous and categorical variables in Section 7.3. We conclude in Example 7.3 with an illustration from the 1958 UK birth cohort study, where our substantive model includes both interactions and a possible nonlinear effect. Note that we do not consider the 'passive' imputation approach in this chapter because of the shortcomings of this approach, discussed in Chapter 6.

7.1 Interaction variables fully observed

Suppose that the substantive model is

$$Y_{i,1} = \beta_0 + \beta_1 Y_{i,2} + \beta_3 Y_{i,3} + \beta_4 Y_{i,2} Y_{i,3} + e_i, \quad e_i \overset{i.i.d.}{\sim} N(0, \sigma^2), \tag{7.1}$$

with Y_1, Y_2 continuous and Y_3 binary.

If Y_3 is fully observed, but Y_1, Y_2 are partially observed, then since (7.1) fits a straight line for each group identified by Y_3, we can impute as follows:

1. Divide the data into two groups by values of binary Y_3.

2. Separately in each group, impute (Y_1, Y_2) using a bivariate normal model or FCS equivalent (Chapter 3), creating K imputed datasets.

3. For $k = 1, \ldots, K$ append the imputed datasets for the two groups, to give K imputed datasets.

This approach, of imputing separately in the groups defined by categorical variables in the interaction, is by far the simplest approach; clearly we can have more than the two groups in the above discussion. The imputation groups may be defined by levels of a single categorical variable, or the interaction of categorical variables. The only requirement is that these variables be fully observed on each unit.

As this approach is straightforward, it will often be appropriate even when a few values of the categorical variables defining the imputation groups are missing. Since it is always permissible for the imputation model to be richer than the substantive model, it is also appropriate when the substantive model does not have all possible interactions with the categorical variable. For example, if we add an additional variable (binary or continuous) Y_4 to (7.1),

$$Y_{i,1} = \beta_0 + \beta_1 Y_{i,2} + \beta_3 Y_{i,3} + \beta_4 Y_{i,2} Y_{i,3} + \beta_5 Y_{i,4} + e_i, \quad e_i \overset{i.i.d.}{\sim} N(0, \sigma^2) \quad (7.2)$$

the model does not have a all possible interactions involving Y_3, since it does not include $Y_3 Y_4$ as a covariate. However, if binary Y_3 is fully observed and the other variables have missing data, the most sensible approach is again to impute separately in the two groups defined by Y_3.

Example 7.1 Asthma study

We return to the asthma study, introduced in Chapter 1 and last considered in Chapter 3. Recall we have two treatment arms (active and placebo), and lung function measured at baseline, and 2, 4, 8 and 12 weeks post-randomisation.

Let $Y_{i,1}, \ldots, Y_{i,5}$ denote the lung function of patient i at baseline, 2, 4, 8 and 12 weeks. Let $T_i = 1$ if patient i is randomised to the active arm, and 0 otherwise. We focus on the estimated treatment effect, adjusted for baseline, at the final 12 week visit, that is

$$Y_{i,5} = \beta_0 + \beta_1 Y_{i,1} + \beta_2 T_i + e_i, \quad e_i \overset{i.i.d.}{\sim} N(0, \sigma^2). \quad (7.3)$$

Baseline is fully observed, but only 37/90 patients in the placebo arm are present at 12 weeks, and only 71/90 in the active arm. The auxiliary variables are the lung function at the intermediate visits.

We could choose the 6-variable normal distribution as our imputation model:

$$(Y_{i,1}, Y_{i,2}, Y_{i,3}, Y_{i,4}, Y_{i,5}, T_i)^T \sim N_6(\boldsymbol{\mu}, \boldsymbol{\Omega}). \quad (7.4)$$

Note that, since binary T_i is fully observed, having it as a covariate or part of the normally distributed response makes no difference.

However, given the difference in dropout patterns by treatment arm, it is likely (and turns out to be the case) that the covariance matrix varies between the treatment arms. In other words, the dependence of the 12-week measurement on earlier measurements is different in the two treatment arms. Our imputation model should reflect this. Thus, we should impute separately in the two treatment groups, using the unstructured multivariate normal model

$$(Y_{i,1}, Y_{i,2}, Y_{i,3}, Y_{i,4}, Y_{i,5})^T \sim N_5(\boldsymbol{\mu}, \boldsymbol{\Omega}). \tag{7.5}$$

This is congenial with a full baseline-time-treatment interaction, which is richer than we require. However, as usual, having a richer imputation model than substantive model does not unduly affect the validity of the resulting inference.

Thus, this is an example where, although the substantive model (7.3) does not have an explicit interaction, because the relationship between the auxiliary variables and response does vary by treatment group, imputing separately in the two groups is sensible.

Table 7.1 shows the results, obtained using 1000 imputations, where the substantive model is (7.3). Under the MAR assumption, imputing with the interaction gives more appropriate imputations within each treatment group; as Figure 7.1 shows, this results in a larger treatment estimate. For a detailed analysis of these data, see Carpenter *et al.* (2013). □

Separate imputation in potentially distinct groups is therefore worth considering, even if the substantive model does not explicitly have an interaction. This approach only runs into difficulty when the numbers in the categories become small, for then we will need to borrow information across categories in order to fit the imputation model; in other words impose some constraints on the interaction model.

The simplest constraint is to have a common covariance matrix across some of the categories, while retaining a different mean structure. Taking the trial illustration above, one might have a common covariance structure across genetic sub-types within a treatment group, while allowing the mean structure to differ. In this case, in the clinical trial illustration, we would impute separately within each group, with genetic subtype indicator as either an additional response, or a covariate, in the imputation model.

Beyond this, one may well wish to consider shrinkage, so that subgroups have a random covariance (or precision) structure, drawn from an inverse Wishart (or Wishart) distribution with common parameters across subgroups. This approach has been explored by Yucel (2011), and we return to it in the context of multilevel multiple imputation in Subsection 9.5.1.

Table 7.1 Asthma data: estimates of 12-week treatment effect on FEV_1 (litres), adjusted for baseline, using complete records and imputing without, and with, a full treatment group interaction.

Analysis	Treatment estimate	Std. Error	p-value
Complete records	0.247	0.100	0.0155
MI, imputation model (7.4)	0.283	0.093	0.0024
MI, imputation model (7.5)	0.335	0.106	0.0015

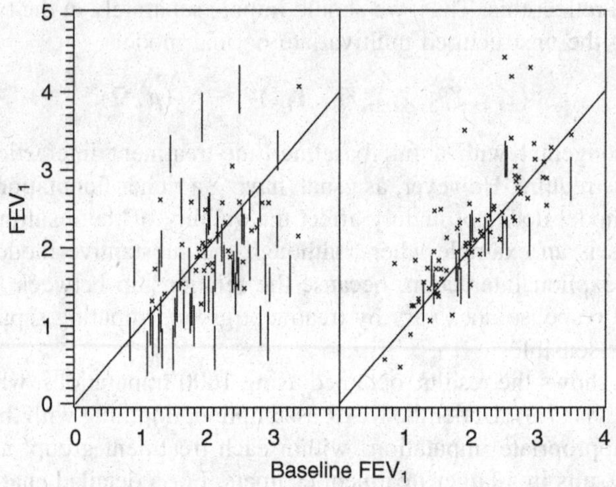

Figure 7.1 Plot of baseline FEV_1 (litres) versus 12 week FEV_1 (litres) by treatment group, under imputation model (7.5). For patients whose 12 week observation is missing, the inter-quartile range from 1000 imputations is shown. Left panel: placebo group, right panel: lowest active treatment group.

To conclude this section, consider again (7.2), now supposing Y_1, Y_4 have missing values, but Y_2, Y_3 are fully observed. In other words we have an interaction between a fully observed continuous and categorical variable. In this setting, paralleling the discussion in Section 6.2, the imputation model has the interaction terms as covariates:

$$Y_{i,1} = \beta_{0,1} + \beta_{1,1}Y_{i,2} + \beta_{2,1}Y_{i,3} + \beta_{3,1}Y_{i,2}Y_{i,3} + e_{i,1}$$
$$Y_{i,4} = \beta_{0,2} + \beta_{1,2}Y_{i,2} + \beta_{2,2}Y_{i,3} + \beta_{3,2}Y_{i,2}Y_{i,3} + e_{i,2}$$
$$\begin{pmatrix} e_{i,1} \\ e_{i,2} \end{pmatrix} \sim N_2(\mathbf{0}, \mathbf{\Omega}).$$

The corresponding FCS algorithm follows in the usual way. The extension to additional interactions involving fully observed variables is direct. In many cases, even if a small proportion of units are missing terms involved in the interaction, this will be sufficient.

Imputing in groups when group indicator has missing values

Consider (7.2), where Y_3 is now categorical, the other variables are continuous and all variables have missing values.

If the context and complete records suggest it is plausible to assume that the probability Y_3 is missing is independent of Y_1 given the other covariates, Y_2, Y_4, then – as explained in Chapter 1 – omitting cases with missing Y_3 does not bias the analysis. So one strategy is to do this, and then impute separately in groups defined by the remaining observed categorical Y_3. This approach can often work quite well, particularly if there are predictive auxiliary variables which can be included in the imputation model (e.g. Carpenter and Plewis, 2011).

However, if a substantial proportion of categorical Y_3 values are missing, this approach excludes a non-negligible proportion of the data and the associated information (which was likely to have been expensive to collect). In this case one of the more complex approaches described below is likely preferable, but the approach of the previous paragraph can still serve as a useful check on the plausibility of the results.

In summary, if either (i) we wish to investigate the possibility of interactions involving fully observed variables in our substantive model, or (ii) we would like to allow a different relationship between variables in the imputation model, in groups defined by a categorical covariate, we can use one of the approaches described above, with a preference for imputing in separate groups.

7.2 Interactions of categorical variables

In this section we consider two scenarios. In the first, the substantive model is a linear regression on two categorical variables and their interaction; in the second, the substantive model is a multinomial regression on two categorical variables and their interaction.

Linear regression

Suppose Y_1 is continuous, Y_2, Y_3 are both unordered categorical taking values $1, \ldots, L$ and $1, \ldots, M$ respectively. As usual let $1[.]$ be an indicator for the event in brackets. Suppose the substantive model is the linear regression

$$Y_{i,1} = \beta_0 + \sum_{l=1}^{L}\sum_{m=1}^{M} \beta_{l,m} 1[Y_{i,2} = l] \times 1[Y_{i,3} = m] + e_i, \quad e_i \overset{i.i.d.}{\sim} N(0, \sigma^2), \tag{7.6}$$

with $\beta_{1,1} = 0$. In other words the covariates defining LM groups, within each of which Y_1 potentially has a different mean.

Suppose there are missing values in all variables. For imputation, the simplest approach is then to define a LM-level unordered categorical variable, Z, taking values

$$Z_i = Y_{i,2} + L(Y_{i,3} - 1)$$

and then impute Y_1, Z either jointly or using FCS (with a linear regression and multinomial regression respectively).

In fact, unless both $Y_{i,2}$ and $Y_{i,3}$ are missing, then Z_i is restricted: for example if $Y_{i,3} = 2$, then $Z \in (L+1, \ldots, 2L)$. This information must be used to reject inadmissible values at each step of the imputation algorithm.

If (as is likely) the substantive model (7.6) contains additional variables, then these are handled in the imputation model in the usual way.

Categorical regression

Suppose we have an I by J by L contingency table defined by unordered categorical variables $Y_{i,1}, Y_{i,2}, Y_{i,3}$, $i \in 1, \ldots, n$, each of which may have missing values, and the substantive model is the multinomial regression of one factor on the other two and their interaction. The imputation model is then the saturated model for the 3-way contingency table.

To apply the joint latent normal approach, we parallel the development above by generating an IJL level categorical variable

$$Z_i = Y_{i,1} + I \times (Y_{i,2} - 1) + IJ \times (Y_{i,3} - 1). \qquad (7.7)$$

which is then treated as an IJL level categorical response model, as described in Chapter 5. However, Z_i is never unrestricted, for at least one of Y_1, Y_2, Y_3 are observed for each i. These restrictions must be incorporated in the imputation model. For example, if $Y_{i,1} = 1$, $Y_{i,3} = 3$, then Z_i can only take values $1 + 3IJ, 1 + I + 3IJ, 1 + 2I + 3IJ, \ldots, 1 + I(J - 1) + 3IJ$. This can most easily be done by rejecting latent normal values which correspond to inadmissible values of of the categorical variable at each update step of the MCMC sampler for fitting the imputation model; this can be viewed as a unit-specific prior on the missing values.

We now consider the FCS approach. We use the notation described in Chapter 5 for modelling contingency tables. Let $\mu_{i,j,l}$ be the mean count in cell i, j, l for $i \in 1, \ldots, I$; $j \in 1, \ldots, J$ and $l \in 1, \ldots, L$. The saturated log-linear model for the contingency table is

$$\log(\mu_{i,j,l}) = \lambda + \lambda_i^1 + \lambda_j^2 + \lambda_l^3 + \lambda_{i,j}^{1,2} + \lambda_{i,l}^{1,3} + \lambda_{j,l}^{2,3} + \lambda_{i,j,l}^{1,2,3}, \qquad (7.8)$$

subject to the usual identifiability constraints: $\lambda_1^1 = \lambda_1^2 = \lambda_1^3 = 0$; whenever $k = 1$ or $j = 1$ or $l = 1$, $\lambda_{i,j}^{1,2}, \lambda_{i,l}^{1,3}, \lambda_{j,l}^{2,3}$ and $\lambda_{i,j,l}^{1,2,3}$ are also constrained to zero.

With no missing data, instead of fitting the saturated log-linear model (7.8), we can fit the multinomial logistic regression of:

1. $\mathbf{Y}_1$ on dummy variables derived from $\mathbf{Y}_2$, $\mathbf{Y}_3$ and their interaction, giving identical estimates and inference for $\lambda_i^1, \lambda_{i,j}^{12}, \lambda_{i,l}^{1,3}$, and $\lambda_{i,j,l}^{123}$;

2. $\mathbf{Y}_2$ on dummy variables derived from $\mathbf{Y}_1$, $\mathbf{Y}_3$ and their interaction, giving identical estimates and inference for $\lambda_j^2, \lambda_{i,j}^{1,2}, \lambda_{j,l}^{2,3}$, and $\lambda_{i,j,l}^{1,2,3}$, and

3. $\mathbf{Y}_3$ on dummy variables derived from $\mathbf{Y}_1$, $\mathbf{Y}_2$ and their interaction, giving identical estimates of $\lambda_l^3, \lambda_{j,l}^{2,3}, \lambda_{i,l}^{1,3}$, and $\lambda_{i,j,l}^{1,2,3}$;

Thus for compatible FCS imputation with the three-way interaction, we need to use three multinomial logistic models with each variable taking it in turn as the response, and the other two *and their interaction* as covariates.

Consider the model in step 1 above. The conditional distribution $\mathbf{Y}_1$ on $\mathbf{Y}_2$, $\mathbf{Y}_3$ does not contain any information on, or in any way constrain, the association in the marginal contingency table defined by $\mathbf{Y}_2$, $\mathbf{Y}_3$. In other words, the analysis in step 1 does not have any information on, or in any way constrain, the parameters λ^2_j, λ^3_l or $\lambda^{2,3}_{j,l}$.

Analogous results hold for the models in step 2 and step 3. Thus the conditions set out for FCS to be equivalent to joint modelling (Hughes *et al.*, 2012a) (see p. 122) will hold for *saturated* log-linear models provided an appropriate prior is chosen (if the models are not saturated, this equivalence does not exactly hold).

To conclude this Section, suppose we have an additional continuous covariate, so that the substantive model is multinomial regression of $\mathbf{Y}_1$ on categorical $\mathbf{Y}_2$, $\mathbf{Y}_3$, their interaction, and continuous $\mathbf{Y}_4$. Under the joint modelling approach described above, $\mathbf{Y}_4$ becomes an additional response variable in the imputation model. Under FCS, $\mathbf{Y}_4$ is included as a covariate in each of the imputation models in steps 1–3, and the imputation model for $\mathbf{Y}_4$ is the regression on categorical $\mathbf{Y}_1$, $\mathbf{Y}_2$, $\mathbf{Y}_3$ (included as dummy variables) and their full interaction.

Example 7.2 Simulation study

The following simulation study is similar to one of a series reported by Tilling *et al.* (2012), who evaluate various FCS imputation strategies when the substantive model contains an interaction involving one or more categorical variables.

Consider three binary variables, $\mathbf{Y}_1$, $\mathbf{Y}_2$, $\mathbf{Y}_3$ whose joint distribution is given by Table 7.2. The corresponding logistic regression of $\mathbf{Y}_1$ on $\mathbf{Y}_2$, $\mathbf{Y}_3$ is

$$\text{logit}\Pr(Y_{i,1} = 1) = 0.5Y_{i,2} + 0.5Y_{i,3} + 0.6Y_{i,2}Y_{i,3}. \tag{7.9}$$

In each simulation, $n = 20000$ observations were drawn from the joint distribution shown in Table 7.2. Each observation, $i = 1, \ldots, 20000$, was then randomly allocated to one of three groups with probability 1/3. Within each group, missing data were generated as follows:

$$\begin{aligned}
&\text{Group 1:}\quad \text{logit}\Pr(\text{observe } Y_{i,1}) = -1.5 + 0.6Y_{i,2} + 1.9Y_{i,3}\\
&\text{Group 2:}\quad \text{logit}\Pr(\text{observe } Y_{i,2}) = -2 + 0.8Y_{i,1} + 1.3Y_{i,3}\\
&\text{Group 3:}\quad \text{logit}\Pr(\text{observe } Y_{i,3}) = -2 + Y_{i,1} + Y_{i,2}
\end{aligned} \tag{7.10}$$

Thus data are MAR with a nonmonotone missingness pattern.

Table 7.2 Joint probability distribution for Y_1, Y_2, Y_3.

		$Y_3 = 0$	$Y_3 = 1$
$Y_1 = 0$	$Y_2 = 0$	0.030	0.095
	$Y_2 = 1$	0.226	0.353
$Y_1 = 1$	$Y_2 = 0$	0.030	0.057
	$Y_2 = 1$	0.137	0.072

The substantive model is (7.9). For each simulated data set, this was fitted before any data were made missing (full data); to the remaining complete records after missingness mechanism (7.10) was applied, and after multiple imputation using FCS with various imputation models. Under FCS, the three conditional models used for imputation are logistic regressions. Five different ways of specifying the covariates in these imputation models were compared:

(i) no interactions in any of the imputation models;

(ii) the imputation model for Y_2 contains the interaction of Y_1, Y_3 and the imputation model for Y_3 contains the interaction of Y_1, Y_2;

(iii) the imputation model for Y_1 contains the interaction of Y_2, Y_3 and the imputation model for Y_2 contains the interaction of Y_1, Y_3;

(iv) the imputation model for Y_2 contains the interaction of Y_1, Y_3 and the imputation model for Y_3 contains the interaction of Y_1, Y_2; and

(v) each imputation model contains its two-way interactions.

Note that (v) corresponds to imputing from a saturated model.

The simulation was replicated 100 times and the results are shown in Table 7.3. Imputing without the interactions gives poorer results than the complete records analysis, even though data are MAR. Imputing with two of the three interactions improves results, but means that the three imputation models in FCS are incompatible with each other, so the sampler cannot converge (though this may be hard to detect in practice). Only when all interactions are included in each imputation model is valid inference obtained.

The results are thus consistent with the exposition above: interactions need to be included in the imputation model if they are to be accurately estimated in the

Table 7.3 Median log-odds ratio (coverage probability) for each of the three coefficients in the substantive model (7.9), estimated from 100 replications.

Analysis	Coefficient of		
	Y_2	Y_3	Y_2Y_3
True values	0.5	0.5	0.6
Full data	0.49	0.49	0.61
Complete records	0.44; 82%	0.40; 76%	0.56; 91%
Imputation (i)	0.56; 83%	0.61; 67%	0.43; 50%
Imputation (ii)	0.53; 96%	0.55; 87%	0.52; 87%
Imputation (iii)	0.53; 96%	0.53; 91%	0.55; 94%
Imputation (iv)	0.53; 96%	0.54; 89%	0.54; 90%
Imputation (v)	0.49; 94%	0.46; 95%;	0.61; 93%

substantive model. Moreover, failure to include them may undermine inference for the main effects. □

7.3 General nonlinear relationships

We now consider the case where the substantive model contains a general nonlinear relationship. For example, consider:

$$Y_{i,1} = \beta_0 + \beta_1 Y_{i,2} + g(\boldsymbol{\beta}, Y_{i,3}, Y_{i,4}) + e_i, \quad e_i \overset{i.i.d.}{\sim} N(0, \sigma^2). \tag{7.11}$$

Here, $\boldsymbol{\beta}$ is a vector of parameters associated with the transformation $g(\,.\,)$, which is linear in the covariates $\boldsymbol{\beta}$. For example, g could be

$$g(\beta_3, \beta_4, \beta_5, Y_3, Y_4) = \beta_3 Y_3 + \beta_4 Y_4 + \beta_5 Y_3 Y_4.$$

We thus have in mind substantive models which are (i) a linear function of one or more untransformed covariates, together with (ii) a linear function (in $\boldsymbol{\beta}$) of a nonlinear function of covariates. The discussion in Subsection 6.3.4 was a particular case of this. Using the methods described in Chapters 4, 5, we can extend to ordinal and categorical variables; here to keep the algebra simple we assume $Y_1, \ldots, Y_4$ are continuous. The approach we describe is thus directly applicable to fractional polynomial type analyses with interactions.

Example 7.3 Adult Educational qualifications in the NCDS

Carpenter and Plewis (2011) explore predictors of no educational qualifications age 23 in the UK 1958 birth cohort study, known as the National Childhood Development Study (NCDS). The substantive model relates the probability of having any educational qualifications at age 23 to four variables measured at birth and in early childhood: birth weight, mothers age, living in social housing and spending a period in care. Taking a probit model (though a logistic could equally be used),

$$\begin{aligned}\Phi^{-1}\ & \Pr\{\text{no qualifications age 23}\}\\ &= \beta_0 + \beta_1 1[\text{in care}] + \beta_2 1[\text{in social housing}] + \beta_3(\text{inverse birth weight})\\ &+\beta_4(\text{mother's age}) + \beta_5(\text{mother's age})^2\\ &+1[\text{in social housing}] \times \{\beta_6(\text{mother's age}) + \beta_7(\text{mother's age})^2\}, \quad (7.12)\end{aligned}$$

where $1[\,.\,]$ is an indicator for the event in brackets.

After allowing for death and emigration (Plewis *et al.*, 2004), the target sample size age 23 was 15 885. Table 7.4 shows the patterns of item nonresponse. There are two key patterns: (2) missing educational qualifications at age 23, and (3) missing the 'In care' and 'Social housing' variables. We are left with only 10279 complete records. If we restrict ourselves to the five variables in (7.12), then MI

Table 7.4 NCDS data: missing value patters for covariates and response in model (7.12).

In care	Social housing	Birth weight	Mo's age	Edu. qual. age 23	No. of records	% (n = 15882)	pattern
✓	✓	✓	✓	✓	10279	65	1
✓	✓	✓	✓	·	2824	18	2
·	·	✓	✓	✓	1153	7.3	3
·	·	✓	✓	·	765	4.8	4
✓	✓	·	✓	✓	349	2.2	5
Other patterns					513	3.2	–

has the potential to recover information for records where educational qualification age 23 is observed (i.e. patterns 3, 5). We would need to include auxiliary variables, measured between birth and age 23, in order to recover information for patterns 2, 4.

Imputation congenial with (7.12) requires handling an interaction and a nonlinearity, and thus serves to motivate the development below, after which we return to this example. □

We now consider joint modelling imputation, and then an FCS approach, congenial with models like (7.11). In both approaches we need to postulate a model for the variables involved in the interaction and apply a separate MCMC or rejection sampling step to impute them.

Joint modelling approach

Consistent with Section 6.2, all partially observed variables not involved in nonlinear relationships and/or interactions are treated as responses. A congenial imputation model for (7.11) is therefore

$$\begin{aligned} Y_{i,1} &= \beta_{0,1} + g(\boldsymbol{\beta}_{1,1}, Y_{i,3}, Y_{i,4}) + e_{i,1} \\ Y_{i,2} &= \beta_{0,2} + g(\boldsymbol{\beta}_{1,2}, Y_{i,3}, Y_{i,4}) + e_{i,2} \\ \begin{pmatrix} e_{i,1} \\ e_{i,2} \end{pmatrix} &\sim N_2(\mathbf{0}, \boldsymbol{\Omega}), \end{aligned} \tag{7.13}$$

assuming the conditional distribution of (Y_1, Y_2) is bivariate normal and g is linear in $\boldsymbol{\beta}$.

To fit and impute from (7.13) we need to specify a model for (Y_3, Y_4). We assume this is $f_{3,4} = N_2(\tilde{\boldsymbol{\beta}}, \tilde{\Omega})$ and refer to the discussion on p. 142 when this assumption is not plausible.

As usual, choose starting values for missing observations, parameters $\boldsymbol{\beta} = (\beta_{01}, \boldsymbol{\beta}_{1,1}^T, \beta_{0,2}, \boldsymbol{\beta}_{1,2}^T)^T$, $\boldsymbol{\Omega}$ of (7.13) and $\tilde{\boldsymbol{\beta}}, \tilde{\boldsymbol{\Omega}}$. Then update the MCMC sampler by iterating steps 1–3:

1. Given observed values of, and current draws for missing, $\mathbf{Y}_1, \ldots, \mathbf{Y}_4$, update the parameters $\boldsymbol{\beta}, \boldsymbol{\Omega}$ of (7.13) as described in Section 6.2. The algorithm described there can be used because we have stipulated $g(.)$ is linear in the covariates.

2. Given the current draw for $(\boldsymbol{\beta}, \boldsymbol{\Omega})$, $(\tilde{\boldsymbol{\beta}}, \tilde{\boldsymbol{\Omega}})$ update missing $(Y_{i,3}, Y_{i,4})$ as described below.

3. Given the observed values of, and current draws for missing, $\mathbf{Y}_3, \mathbf{Y}_4$, update the parameters of $f_{3,4}$, $(\tilde{\boldsymbol{\beta}}, \tilde{\boldsymbol{\Omega}})$. Since $f_{3,4}$ is bivariate normal, we can use the approach of Section 6.2.

As with nonlinear relationships, we can either use a Metropolis-Hastings step or rejection sampling for Step 2. The MCMC algorithm for step 2 closely parallels Subsection 6.3.5 and the rejection sampling approach parallels Subsection 6.3.6. We therefore only briefly describe the former.

Metropolis-Hastings sampling

As before we work in turn through units (indexed by i) where one, or both, of $(Y_{i,3}, Y_{i,4})$ is missing. Either, or both, could be missing: we indicate how the procedure adapts as we go through.

1. Propose new values $(Y^{\star}_{i,3}, Y^{\star}_{i,4})$ by drawing from the bivariate normal distribution whose mean is the current values $(Y_{i,3}, Y_{i,4})$ and whose variance is $\tau\hat{\Sigma}$, where $\hat{\Sigma}$ is the sample variance of the observed $(\mathbf{Y}_3, \mathbf{Y}_4)$ and τ can be adapted during the burn-in of the sampler to achieve an acceptance rate of around 50%; alternatively $\tau = 0.5$ may be a reasonable choice.

   (a) If one of $Y_{i,3}$ or $Y_{i,4}$ is observed, draw a proposal for the other from the marginal normal corresponding to the bivariate proposal in the previous paragraph (if we wish to use the conditional normal, we need to include the Hastings ratio as it will no longer be 1). Again, write $(Y^{\star}_{i,3}, Y^{\star}_{i,4})$ for what is now the pair of observed and drawn values.

2. Calculate $L(Y^{\star}_{i,3}, Y^{\star}_{i,4})$ and $L(Y_{i,3}, Y_{i,4})$ where $\mathbf{x} = (x_1, x_2)^T$ and

$$L(\mathbf{x}) = f_{1,2|3,4}(Y_1, Y_2|\mathbf{x}; \boldsymbol{\beta}, \boldsymbol{\Omega}) f_{3,4}(\mathbf{x}; \tilde{\boldsymbol{\beta}}, \tilde{\boldsymbol{\Omega}}). \tag{7.14}$$

   Since the imputation model (7.13) is a multivariate normal density, here with $p = 2$ response variables,

$$f_{1,2|3,4}(Y_1, Y_2|\mathbf{x}; \boldsymbol{\beta}, \boldsymbol{\Omega}) = \frac{1}{(2\pi)^{p/2}|\boldsymbol{\Omega}|^{1/2}} \exp\left\{-\frac{1}{2}(\mathbf{Y}_i - \boldsymbol{\mu}_i)^T \boldsymbol{\Omega}^{-1}(\mathbf{Y}_i - \boldsymbol{\mu}_i)\right\}, \tag{7.15}$$

where $\mathbf{Y}_i = (Y_{i,1}, Y_{i,2}),^T$

$$\boldsymbol{\mu}_i = \begin{pmatrix} \beta_{0,1} + g(\boldsymbol{\beta}_{1,1}, x_1, x_2) \\ \beta_{0,2} + g(\boldsymbol{\beta}_{1,2}, x_1, x_2) \end{pmatrix},$$

and $f_{3,4}(\mathbf{x}; \tilde{\boldsymbol{\beta}}, \tilde{\boldsymbol{\Omega}})$ is the bivariate normal density evaluated at $\mathbf{x} = (x_1, x_2)^T$.

3. Accept the proposal with probability

$$\min\left\{1, \frac{L(Y^\star_{i,3}, Y^\star_{i,4})}{L(Y_{i,3}, Y_{i,4})}\right\}; \tag{7.16}$$

and if accepted set $Y_{i,3} = Y^\star_{i,3}, Y_{i,4} = Y^\star_{i,4}$.

Provided the distributional assumptions made are reasonable for the data, this algorithm will impute data which will give valid inference for model (7.11). As already mentioned, we need to check that the distribution for the covariates in the in the imputation model (7.13) is broadly appropriate. If it is not, as discussed on p. 142, we can transform Y_3, Y_4 to a latent normal scale.

We now consider the case where $Y_{i,3}$ is binary and $Y_{i,4}$ continuous. The only aspect of the above that changes is the density $f_{3,4}$, which is no longer bivariate normal. We again use the latent normal model:

$$\begin{aligned} \Pr(Y_{i,3} = 1) &= \Pr(Z = \tilde{\beta}_1 + e_{i,1} > 0) \\ Y_{i,4} &= \tilde{\beta}_2 + e_{i,2} \\ \begin{pmatrix} e_{i,1} \\ e_{i,2} \end{pmatrix} &\sim N_2(\mathbf{0}, \tilde{\boldsymbol{\Omega}}), \quad \text{where } \boldsymbol{\Omega}_{1,1} = 1. \end{aligned} \tag{7.17}$$

Let $\tilde{\mu}_{3|4,i} = \tilde{\beta}_1 + (Y_{i,4} - \tilde{\beta}_2)\tilde{\boldsymbol{\Omega}}_{1,2}/\tilde{\boldsymbol{\Omega}}_{2,2}$ and $\tilde{\sigma}^2_{3|4} = 1 - \tilde{\boldsymbol{\Omega}}^2_{1,2}/\tilde{\boldsymbol{\Omega}}_{2,2}$. Then, under (7.17) the conditional distribution of $Z = \tilde{\beta}_1 + e_{i,1}$ given $Y_{i,4}$ is $N(\tilde{\mu}_{3|4,i}, \tilde{\sigma}^2_{3|4})$ so that

$$\Pr(Y_{i,3} = 1|Y_{i,4}) = \Pr(Z > 0|Y_{i,4}) = \Phi(\tilde{\mu}_{3|4,i}/\tilde{\sigma}_{3|4}) = \pi_{3|4,i},$$

say. Then, as the marginal density of $Y_{i,4}$ is $f_4(Y_{i,4}) = N(\tilde{\beta}, \tilde{\Omega}_{2,2})$, we have

$$f_{3,4}(Y_{i,3}, Y_{i,4}) = f_{3|4}(Y_{i,3}|Y_{i,4}) f_4(Y_{i,4}) = \pi^{Y_{i,3}}_{3|4,i}(1 - \pi_{3|4,i})^{1-Y_{i,3}} f_4(Y_{i,4}). \tag{7.18}$$

The MH algorithm now proceeds as follows:

1. Propose new values $(Y^\star_{i,3}, Y^\star_{i,4})$. The simplest approach (because it means the Hastings ratio is 1) is to draw $Z^\star \sim \mathrm{N}(Z, 1)$ and independently $Y^\star_{i,4} \sim \mathrm{N}(Y_{i,4}, \tau^2)$ where τ^2 is a fraction – for example, a half – of the marginal variance of the observed $\mathbf{Y}_3$. If $Z^\star > 0$ we have $Y^\star_{i,3} = 1$, otherwise $Y^\star_{i,3} = 0$.
   (a) If either of $Y_{i,3}$ or $Y_{i,4}$ is observed, draw a proposal for the other from the marginal distribution in step 1 above; Again, write $(Y^\star_{i,3}, Y^\star_{i,4})$ for what is now the pair of observed and drawn values.
2. Using $f_{3,4}$ given by (7.18) in (7.14), calculate $L(Y^\star_{i,3}, Y^\star_{i,4})$ and $L(Y_{i,3}, Y_{i,4})$.

Table 7.5 Average parameter estimates and standard error of mean, from 100 replications of the simulation study (7.20).

Parameter	True value	Average over replications	Std. Error of Mean
β_0	0	0.002	0.004
β_1	0.5	0.497	0.002
β_2	0.5	0.502	0.001
β_3	0.5	0.496	0.002
β_4	0.5	0.503	0.002
σ_u^2	0.1	0.104	0.002
σ_e^2	0.5	0.498	0.001

3. Accept the proposal with probability

$$\min\left\{1, \frac{L(Y^\star_{i,3}, Y^\star_{i,4})}{L(Y_{i,3}, Y_{i,4})}\right\}; \tag{7.19}$$

and if accepted set $Y_{i,3} = Y^\star_{i,3}$, $Y_{i,4} = Y^\star_{i,4}$.

Note that while this approach generalises to unordered categorical variables, in this case estimating the category probabilities will generally need a separate Monte-Carlo step (see p. 116).

Example 7.4 Simulation study: interaction and nonlinear effects

Goldstein *et al.* (2012a) report a number of simulation studies using this algorithm, including the following, based on the structure of the 'tutorial dataset' (Goldstein, 2010, Chapter 3). This is a multilevel dataset, with 4059 pupils (level-1 units) nested within 65 schools (level-2 units). The simulation is multilevel, and readers unfamiliar with this setting may find it helpful to refer to the early part of Chapter 9.

Goldstein *et al.* (2012a) simulated $i = 1, \ldots, 4059$ level-1 units nested within $j = 1, \ldots, 65$ level-2 units, as follows:

$$\begin{aligned}
\begin{pmatrix} Z_{i,j} \\ Y_{i,j,3} \end{pmatrix} &\sim N\left[\begin{matrix}0\\0\end{matrix}, \begin{pmatrix}1 & 0.5\\ 0.5 & 1\end{pmatrix}\right]; \\
\text{and set } Y_{i,j,2} &= \begin{cases} 1 \text{ if } Z_{i,j} > 0, \\ 0 \text{ if } Z_{i,j} < 0, \end{cases} \\
Y_{i,j,1} &= 0.5Y_{i,j,2} + 0.5Y_{i,j,3} + 0.5Y_{i,j,2}Y_{i,j,3} + 0.5Y^2_{i,j,3} + u_j + e_{i,j} \\
u_j &\sim N(0, 0.1) \\
e_{i,j} &\sim N(0, 0.5).
\end{aligned} \tag{7.20}$$

They then made both $Y_{i,j,2}, Y_{i,j,3}$ independently MCAR with probability 0.2, so that around 4% of records had missing values for both, and 32% had one or other missing.

For each replication of the simulation study, they fitted the model

$$\begin{aligned} Y_{i,j,1} &= \beta_0 + \beta_1 Y_{i,j,2} + \beta_2 Y_{i,j,3} + \beta_3 Y_{i,j,2} Y_{i,j,3} + \beta_4 Y_{i,j,3}^2 + u_j + e_{i,j} \\ u_j &\sim N(0, \sigma_u^2) \\ e_{i,j} &\sim N(0, \sigma_e^2) \end{aligned}$$

to the partially observed dataset, using the Monte Carlo algorithm described above for handling missing data in covariates with an interaction and a nonlinear effect – extended to the multilevel setting as described in Chapter 9. For each model fit, they burned in the MCMC sampler for 500 iterations and updated it for 1000 iterations, and estimated the posterior mean for each coefficient.

They replicated the simulation study 100 times, and for each coefficient they then took the 100 posterior means to calculate the Monte Carlo standard error of the mean. The results are shown in Table 7.5. We see that the average of each coefficient's posterior mean is within two standard errors of the mean of the true parameter value. This confirms the utility of this algorithm for both (i) directly fitting models with partially observed covariates which include quadratic and interactions terms and (ii) creating multiply imputed data sets congenial with substantive models which include nonlinear effects and interactions. □

FCS approach

Following the discussion in Section 6.3.7, we show how the modified FCS algorithm can be used with interactions and nonlinear relationships. Consider again the substantive model, where all covariates are assumed continuous:

$$Y_{i,1} = \beta_0 + \beta_1 Y_{i,2} + g(\boldsymbol{\beta}_3, Y_{i,3}, Y_{i,4}) + e_{i,1}, \quad e_{i,1} \overset{i.i.d.}{\sim} N(0, \sigma^2), \tag{7.21}$$

where, as above, g is a linear function, in covariates $\boldsymbol{\beta}$, of possibly nonlinear transformations of $(Y_{i,3}, Y_{i,4})$ and/or their interaction. For example, $g(\boldsymbol{\beta}_3, Y_{i,3}, Y_{i,4}) = \beta_{3,1} Y_{i,3} + \beta_{3,2} Y_{i,4} + \beta_{3,3} Y_{i,4}^2 + \beta_{3,4} Y_{i,3} Y_{i,4}$.

As usual with FCS, we visit, in turn, a conditional model for each partially observed variable given the others. We describe how to proceed with rejection sampling, though an Metropolis-Hastings sampler could be used. Following the procedure in Subsection 6.3.7, we choose a conditional distribution for each of the covariates in (7.21) given all the others, which we denote generically by $f_{\text{cov}=j|\text{cov}\neq j}$ for $j = 2, 3, 4$ in the case of (7.21). We do this is in the usual way for the FCS algorithm, so that if covariate j is a continuous, we choose a linear regression, if it is binary we choose a logistic regression, and so on.

We begin by choosing initial values for missing values of $\mathbf{Y}_1, \ldots, \mathbf{Y}_4$. Then:

1. Fit the substantive model, (7.21) to the current data (i.e. observed and current imputed values). Draw from the sampling distribution of the parameters, and denote these values by $\tilde{\beta}_0, \tilde{\beta}_1, \tilde{\boldsymbol{\beta}}_3, \tilde{\sigma}^2$. Using these values, impute missing values of $\mathbf{Y}_1$ from model (7.21).

2. For Y_2, fit the regression model $f_{\text{cov}=2|\text{cov}\neq 2}$ to the current data. Draw from the sampling distribution of the parameters, and – using this draw – for each missing value

   (a) propose a value $Y^{\star}_{i,2}$ by drawing from $f_{\text{cov}=2|\text{cov}\neq 2}$, and

   (b) accept this value with probability

$$\exp\left\{-\frac{1}{2}(Y_{i,1} - \tilde{\beta}_0 - \tilde{\beta}_1 Y^{\star}_{i,2} - g(\tilde{\boldsymbol{\beta}}_3, Y_{i,3}, Y_{i,4}))^2\right\}, \qquad (7.22)$$

   where (7.22) is derived in Subsection 6.3.7 and $\tilde{\beta}_1, \tilde{\beta}_2, \tilde{\boldsymbol{\beta}}_3$ are drawn in step 1.

3. repeat step 2 for the other covariates, $j = 3, 4$.

The above defines one cycle of the modified FCS algorithm. As usual, we update the process for a number of cycles, then retain the current data set as the first imputed data set, update the algorithm for further set of cycles, retain the current data as the second imputed data set, and so on.

For covariates like Y_2 in (7.21), that are not involved in the nonlinear relationship or interaction, we can replace step 2 with a standard FCS step, that is a regression (here a linear regression) of Y_2 on all the other variables. In general, this is an approximation; however it will generally reduce the computational time which may be important in large datasets.

If the substantive model (7.21) is a logistic regression, then as discussed in on p. 144, the acceptance probability is simply the probability density for the substantive model for unit i. We consider the case of a survival model in Chapter 8.

Comments

In the case that continuous covariates in the substantive model are not normally distributed, we may consider transformations, exactly along the lines discussed on p. 144.

The simulations of Bartlett *et al.* (2012) suggest that non-normality of the covariates has to be quite severe (e.g. bimodality) for practically important bias to arise. Nevertheless, in the case of linear regression, if data are plausibly MCAR, one could apply JAV as a diagnostic: because the justification for JAV is moment based, it is not affected by missspecification of the covariate distribution.

We note that the above approaches, both joint modelling and FCS, extend directly to both the case of additional interactions and nonlinear terms, but also to functions g which – unlike those above – are nonlinear in *both* parameters and covariates, provided we have an algorithm for fitting such a model to complete data.

Example 7.3 Adult Educational qualifications in the NCDS *(ctd)*

Using the above approach, we now impute data congenial with our substantive model (7.12). Let $\mathbf{Y}_2, \ldots, \mathbf{Y}_5$ be respectively the four covariates as they appear on the RHS of (7.12), that is: in care (binary) in social housing (binary) inverse birthweight (continuous), mothers age (continuous). The two continuous variables are well approximated by marginal normal distributions.

We take a joint latent-normal model for these covariates:

$$\begin{aligned}
\Pr(Y_{i,2} = 1) &= \Pr(\tilde{Z}_{i,1} = \tilde{\beta}_1 + e_{i,1} > 0) \\
\Pr(Y_{i,3} = 1) &= \Pr(\tilde{Z}_{i,2} = \tilde{\beta}_2 + e_{i,2} > 0) \\
Y_{i,4} &= \tilde{\beta}_3 + e_{i,3} \\
Y_{i,5} &= \tilde{\beta}_4 + e_{i,4}
\end{aligned}$$

$$(e_{i,1}, e_{i,1}, e_{i,1}, e_{i,1})^T \sim N_4(\mathbf{0}, \tilde{\mathbf{\Omega}}), \tag{7.23}$$

with constraints $\tilde{\mathbf{\Omega}}_{1,1} = \mathbf{\Omega}_{2,2} = 1$.

Considering the three steps on p. 157, we can use the algorithm for updating the latent normal model with covariates to perform step (1) (update parameters $\boldsymbol{\beta}$ of (7.12)); we can perform step (2) (update missing covariates) using proposal distributions given below, and we can again use the algorithm for updating the latent normal model to perform step (3) (update parameters $\tilde{\boldsymbol{\beta}}, \tilde{\mathbf{\Omega}}$ of (7.23)).

To perform step 2, we use independent proposal distributions on the latent normal scale: $\tilde{Z}^{\star}_{i,1} \sim \mathrm{N}(\tilde{Z}_{i,1}, 1)$, $\tilde{Z}^{\star}_{i,2} \sim \mathrm{N}(\tilde{Z}_{i,2}, 1)$, $Y^{\star}_{i,4} \sim \mathrm{N}(Y_{i,4}, \tau_4^2)$, $Y^{\star}_{i,5} \sim \mathrm{N}(Y_{i,4}, \tau_5^2)$. The final step is to generalize the argument below (7.17) to the case of two binary and two continuous variables. To do this, write the probability distribution of (Y_2, Y_3, Y_4, Y_4) given by (7.23) as $f_{2,3,4,5}(Y_2, Y_3, Y_4, Y_4, \tilde{\boldsymbol{\beta}}, \tilde{\mathbf{\Omega}})$. Then write $f_{2,3,4,5} = f_{2|3,4,5} f_{3|4,5} f_{4,5}$. $f_{4,5}(Y_4, Y_5)$ is the marginal normal implied by (7.23). $\Pr(Y_3 = 1|Y_4, Y_5)$ can be derived from the latent normal model following the argument given below (7.17); the same argument then gives $\Pr(Y_2 = 1|Y_3, Y_4, Y_5)$. This completes step 2.

In this analysis we do not include auxiliary variables. In this case, as the substantive model coincides with the imputation model, we do not use multiple imputation; we simply run the MCMC sampler for the substantive model/ imputation model, and summarise the posterior distribution of the parameter chains by the posterior mean and standard deviation. We used a burn in of 500 updates, and drew a sample of 1000 from the posterior. The results are shown in Table 7.6, alongside the analysis of the complete records for comparison.

Table 7.6 Parameter estimates (std. errors) for model (7.12), from complete records (left) and using joint modelling congenial with the interaction and quadratic relationship.

Coefficient:	Complete records (N = 10 279)		Full model	
β_0	−1.6	(0.103)	−1.5	(0.073)
β_1	0.65	(0.096)	0.64	(0.090)
β_2	0.57	(0.037)	0.57	(0.035)
β_3	75	(10.9)	73	(7.8)
β_4	−0.016	(0.0040)	−0.016	(0.0030)
β_5	0.0019	(0.0005)	0.0019	(0.0004)
β_6	0.013	(0.0053)	0.013	(0.0052)
β_7	−0.00065	(0.00067)	−0.00077	(0.00066)

The complete records show evidence of strong association between the variables. Of particular interest is the interaction between mother's age and social housing. Here the reduction in the probability of no qualifications age 23 with increasing mothers age (centred at 28 years) appears to be largely negated when the family was in social housing. However, the effect is borderline significant, with a z-score of 2.43. It is interesting to see the extent to which this effect is maintained when information from all the records is used. Passive imputation would tend to dilute nonlinear and interaction associations, so is not appropriate here. JAV is only appropriate for linear regression under MCAR. Using the approach outlined here for imputing congenial with nonlinear effects and interactions, we include the information from the partially complete records. This results in smaller standard errors for all parameters, but little change in the covariates. In particular, the negation – among those in social housing – of the reduction in the probability of no qualifications age 23 with increasing mother's age at birth, is confirmed.

A natural next step in this analysis would be to include auxiliary variables in the imputation model, particularly those recorded closer to age 23 (whether before or after) which provide information on the missing qualifications. In this setting, the imputation model would not coincide with the substantive model, so it would be natural to use the full multiple imputation approach. □

7.4 Software

Standard MI software is not able to handle general interactions and/or nonlinear relationships except via the 'Just Another Variable' approach.

For categorical data, standard packages which handle categorical variables, either through FCS or through joint modelling (like Schafer's CAT package), should allow saturated log-linear imputation models for categorical data, thus imputing congenial with any interactions among categorical variables in the substantive model.

The approach set out here is implemented in the `REALCOM-impute` software, and a version of the FCS algorithm is available from www.missingdata.org.uk.

7.5 Discussion

Interaction structure is often present in datasets, even if it is not the direct focus of the substantive model. For example, this may take the form of different relationships between variables among those who are harder to follow-up than among those whose follow-up is relatively complete (Seaman *et al.*, 2012). Such interaction structure needs to be reflected in the imputation model.

This chapter completes the development begun in Chapter 6, presenting a general strategy for congenial imputation with substantive models which include nonlinear relationships in the covariates, and interactions which may additionally involve these nonlinear relationships. We have discussed both a full joint modelling approach, and a FCS alternative. The joint modelling approach can be applied directly with multilevel multiple imputation described in Chapter 9.

In practice, the form of the interaction we are considering, together with the missingness pattern in the data, will often mean that simpler approaches, outlined earlier in the chapter, will suffice. In this case, these should be adopted.

The most flexible approach we have described can be summarised as allowing missing values in the covariates of the imputation model. It thus allows the imputation model and the substantive model to be identical. When this is the case, fitting the 'imputation' model gives estimates of the parameters in the substantive model direct, without recourse to generating imputed datasets and proceeding down the usual MI route (see Example 7.3). However, as discussed in more detail in Subsection 6.3.6, imputation will still be useful when we have auxiliary variables in the imputation model (which will typically be the case) and also for sensitivity analysis, considered in detail in Chapter 10.

PART III

ADVANCED TOPICS

8

Survival data, skips and large datasets

Up to this point we have described and illustrated the use of MI for cross-sectional data with a mix of continuous and discrete variables, linear and nonlinear relationships, and interactions. In this chapter we consider some further issues with cross-sectional data, and then in Chapter 9 we explore the use of MI for problems with a hierarchical (multilevel) structure.

We begin in Section 8.1 by discussing the use of MI methods with time-to-event analyses, and follow this in Section 8.2 with a brief discussion nonparametric, or *hot-deck* MI. We then consider in Section 8.3 the problem of imputation with skips, which typically arise in questionnaires. In some settings, it may be useful to break the imputation process into two or more stages, and this is discussed in Section 8.4. The handling of large datasets can introduce a range of practical issues that require special approaches, and some compromises. We consider some of these problems and associated solutions in Section 8.5. Such datasets are often assembled using record linkage, and using MI to tackle uncertainty in record linkage is discussed in Section 8.6. Finally we then consider measurement error and the imputation of imputation of aggregated subscores in Sections 8.7 and 8.8 respectively. We conclude with a brief discussion in Section 8.9.

8.1 Time-to-event data

Time-to-event data, where units or individuals are followed until an event occurs, arise in almost all areas of scientific research. We consider the context of medical research, so unit i corresponds to individual i, who is followed up from entry into a study until either (i) death or (ii) loss to follow-up – which typically occurs

Multiple Imputation and its Application, First Edition. James R. Carpenter and Michael G. Kenward.

because the individual is still alive at the end of the study period. Let T_i be the time at which follow-up of individual i ends, with $D_i = 1$ indicating follow-up ends at death (so that T_i is the survival time) while $D_i = 0$, indicating that individual i is still alive when follow-up ends (so that T_i is the censoring time).

Survival data is thus a special case of missing data, where we know the range in which the missing value must fall: for unit i, if $D_i = 0$ then the event is at some $\tilde{T}_i > T_i$. We can therefore consider the mechanism that gives rise to the censored (i.e. missing) data in the same way as with other kinds of missing data. Specifically, we consider two processes: (i) the time to the event of interest and (ii) the time to censoring. If censoring occurs before the event, so $D = 0$, then the event time is missing; we simply know it occurs after T_i, the time of censoring. Conversely, if censoring occurs after the event, so $D_i = 1$, the censoring time is missing; we simply know it occurs after T_i, the time of the event.

The censoring mechanism therefore can be thought of in the same way as the missingness mechanism. Specifically, we have three kinds of censoring mechanisms, respectively paralleling MCAR, MAR and MNAR:

1. Survival data are said to be censored completely at random (CCAR) when the distribution of time to censorship is completely independent of the survival process under investigation. This typically happens when censoring is caused by the cessation of study follow-up, provided each unit's entry into the study is independent of its survival time.

2. Survival data are said be censored at random (CAR) if *conditional on covariates in the survival model*, such as treatment or exposure group, the censoring process is independent of the survival time.

3. Survival data are said to be censored not at random (CNAR) if, even given covariates, the censoring time is dependent on the survival time.

Mechanisms 1 and 2 are often referred to as 'noninformative' or 'ignorable' while mechanism 3 is often referred to as 'informative'.

In survival analysis, we typically aim to model the association between the time-to-event and covariates. These covariates can be measured at baseline, but may also be measured during the follow-up. Here, we only consider baseline covariates. Nevertheless, the approaches extend in principle to the more complex settings of time-varying covariates, and competing risks.

We consider two settings. In the first, in Subsection 8.1.1, we focus on imputing missing values of covariates in a survival analysis. In the second, in Subsection 8.1.3, we consider imputation of censored survival times. This is appropriate if our substantive model involves a subset of the variables needed for CAR to hold. Although we deal with the two settings separately, this is artificial in practice, and we may well wish to impute censored survival times and covariates together. Imputation of censored survival times leads naturally to exploring sensitivity analysis to the CAR assumption, which we discuss in Subsection 10.3.2.

As usual, MI is not the only method for inference, but it does provide a unified, conceptually accessible and computationally practical approach. For instance, suppose that in a prognostic study, survival times are CAR conditional on both intervention and a number of prognostic variables. Then we can use MI including all these variables, to impute missing survival times. We can then estimate the marginal relationship between survival and only a specific subset of covariates (e.g. the intervention), by fitting the model to each imputed data set in turn and combining the results for inference using Rubin's rules.

8.1.1 Imputing missing covariate values

As above, for individual i, let T_i be the time-to-event, D_i be the status indicator ($D_i = 1$ if the event occurs at T_i and 0 if it occurs subsequently), and suppose we have two covariates $Y_{i,1}$, $Y_{i,2}$.

Recall that for a survival time distribution $f(t)$, $t \geq 0$, with cumulative distribution function $F(t)$, the survival function is $S(t) = \Pr(T > t) = 1 - F(t)$, the hazard is $h(t) = f(t)/S(t)$ and the cumulative hazard is

$$H(t) = \int_0^t h(s)\, ds = -\log\{S(t)\}.$$

The log-likelihood for T_i given baseline covariates $Y_{i,1}$, $Y_{i,2}$ is thus

$$\begin{aligned} D_i \log\{f(T_i|Y_{i,1}, Y_{i,2})\} &+ (1 - D_i)\log\{S(T_i|Y_{i,1}, Y_{i,2})\} \\ &= D_i \log\{h(T_i|Y_{i,1}, Y_{i,2})\} - H(T_i|Y_{i,1}, Y_{i,2}). \end{aligned} \tag{8.1}$$

We now consider the Cox proportional hazards model, which is ubiquitous in survival modelling. Corresponding derivations can be made for parametric models in a similar manner. Under the proportional hazards model, $h(T_i|Y_{i,1}, Y_{i,2}) = h_0(T_i)\exp(\beta_1 Y_{i,1} + \beta_2 Y_{i,2})$, and $H(T_i|Y_{i,1}, Y_{i,2}) = H_0(T_i)\exp(\beta_1 Y_{i,1} + \beta_2 Y_{i,2})$, so (8.1) becomes

$$\begin{aligned} \ell(T_i, D_i, Y_{i,1}, Y_{i,2}, \boldsymbol{\beta}) = D_i[\log\{h_0(T_i)\} &+ \beta_1 Y_{i,1} + \beta_2 Y_{i,2}] \\ &- H_0(T_i)\exp(\beta_1 Y_{i,1} + \beta_2 Y_{i,2}). \end{aligned} \tag{8.2}$$

The second term in (8.2) implies that, excluding a couple of special cases outlined below, the conditional distribution of covariates given survival time will not follow any common distribution. Thus, for a joint imputation model the natural approach is to factor $f(T, Y_1, Y_2) = f(T|Y_1, Y_2) f_{12}(Y_1, Y_2)$. We assume that survival or censorship times are known, and that the censoring time is not required for MAR. Also, assume (Y_1, Y_2) are marginally bivariate normal, so that $f_{12} = N_2(\tilde{\beta}, \tilde{\Omega})$. When this is not the case, we proceed as discussed on p. 142.

As usual, choose initial values for missing values of $(\mathbf{Y}_1, \mathbf{Y}_2)$, $\boldsymbol{\beta} = (\beta_1, \beta_2)$ in model (8.2) and $\tilde{\beta}, \tilde{\Omega}$. Then update the MCMC sampler by iterating steps 1–3:

1. Given observed values, and current draws for missing values, of $\mathbf{Y}_1, \mathbf{Y}_2$, update the parameters $\boldsymbol{\beta}$ of the proportional hazards model (8.2) and update the hazard, $H_0(t)$, as discussed below.

2. Given the current draw for $\boldsymbol{\beta}$, the baseline hazard, and $(\tilde{\boldsymbol{\beta}}, \tilde{\boldsymbol{\Omega}})$, for each $i = 1, \ldots, n$, if one or both of $(Y_{i,1}, Y_{i,2})$ is missing then draw new values as described below.

3. Given the observed values, and current draws for missing values, of $\mathbf{Y}_1, \mathbf{Y}_2$, update the parameters of $f_{12}(\tilde{\boldsymbol{\beta}}, \tilde{\boldsymbol{\Omega}})$. Since f_{12} is bivariate normal, we can use the approach described in Chapter 2 for this.

For step 1, for a full Bayes approach, we need an MCMC algorithm for the Cox proportional hazards model. This is beyond the scope of this book; see for example Clayton (1991). Alternatively, we may approximate this by fitting the Cox model using the usual maximum partial likelihood, drawing $\boldsymbol{\beta}$ from the approximate bivariate normal sampling distribution of the maximum partial likelihood estimators, $N(\hat{\boldsymbol{\beta}}, \hat{\Omega})$ and then extracting a revised estimate of the baseline hazard. However, this is strictly improper, and thus may result in reduced confidence interval coverage, although as all the remaining uncertainty is acknowledged this error is likely to be small.

For step 2, we work in turn through units (indexed by i) where one, or both, of $(Y_{i,1}, Y_{i,2})$ is missing, as follows:

1. Propose new values $(Y^\star_{i,1}, Y^\star_{i,2})$ by drawing from the bivariate normal distribution whose mean is the current values $(Y_{i,1}, Y_{i,2})$ and whose variance is $\tau\hat{\Sigma}$, where $\hat{\Sigma}$ is the sample variance of the observed $(\mathbf{Y}_1, \mathbf{Y}_2)$ and τ can be adapted during the burn-in of the sampler to maximise the acceptance rate; alternatively $\tau = 0.5$ may be a reasonable choice.

   (a) If one of $Y_{i,1}$ or $Y_{i,2}$ is observed, draw a proposal for the other from the marginal normal corresponding to the bivariate proposal in 1. Again, write $(Y^\star_{i,1}, Y^\star_{i,2})$ for what is now the pair of observed and drawn values.

2. Accept the proposed values $(Y^\star_{i,1}, Y^\star_{i,2})$ with probability

$$\min\left\{1, \frac{L(Y^\star_{i,1}, Y^\star_{i,2})}{L(Y_{i,1}, Y_{i,2})}\right\},$$

   where

$$L(x_1, x_2) = \exp\{\ell(T_i, D_i, x_1, x_2; \boldsymbol{\beta}\} f_{12}(x_1, x_2; \tilde{\boldsymbol{\beta}}, \tilde{\boldsymbol{\Omega}}), \qquad (8.3)$$

   and ℓ is given by (8.2).

Since it is derived without approximation from the joint distribution, this algorithm is congenial with the Cox proportional hazards model. Should the substantive model be parametric, we simply replace ℓ in (8.3) by the corresponding parametric log-likelihood. The attractive aspect of this approach is that, as described in Chapters 6–7, we can extend to the case of binary and categorical covariates, together with their interactions and nonlinear transformations.

FCS approximation

We can apply the FCS approach described by Bartlett *et al.* (2012), and described on p. 143 directly in this setting. For this we need to derive the formula for the acceptance probability.

The first step in each cycle of the FCS algorithm is to fit the substantive model – here proportional hazards model – to the observed and current imputed values of the data. This gives maximum partial likelihood estimators $\hat{\beta}$ and associated covariance matrix $\hat{\boldsymbol{\Omega}}$. We then approximate a draw from the Bayesian posterior by (i) drawing $\boldsymbol{\beta}$ from $N(\hat{\boldsymbol{\beta}}, \hat{\boldsymbol{\Omega}})$, and then at the values of $\boldsymbol{\beta}$ extracting the estimate of $H_0(t)$, $h_0(t)$.

Now, consider the FCS step for variable Y_1, conditional on the others. Define the proposal distribution $g(.)$ for Y_1 given Y_2 as described on p. 143, and consider the proposal $Y_{i1}^\star$ for the ith individual missing Y_1. Following the derivation of (6.30), at the current value of $\boldsymbol{\beta}$, this is accepted with probability

$$\frac{S(T_i|Y_1^\star, Y_2; \boldsymbol{\beta})}{\max_{Y_1} S(T_i|Y_1, Y_2; \boldsymbol{\beta})} \tag{8.4}$$

if $D_i = 0$, and

$$\frac{f(T_i|Y_1^\star, Y_2; \boldsymbol{\beta})}{\max_{Y_1} f(T_i|Y_1, Y_2; \boldsymbol{\beta})} \tag{8.5}$$

if $D_i = 1$. For a censored observation, $D_i = 0$, since the maximum of the survivor function is 1, from (8.4) the acceptance probability is

$$S(T_i|Y_{i,1}^\star, Y_{i,2}; \boldsymbol{\beta}). \tag{8.6}$$

For an uncensored individual we have

$$\begin{aligned}\max_{Y_1} f(t) &= \max_{Y_1}[h(t)\exp\{-H(t)\}]\\ &= \max_{Y_1}\left[h_0(t)\exp\{(Y_1\beta_1 + Y_2\beta_2) - H_0(t)\exp(Y_1\beta_1 + Y_2\beta_2)\}\right],\end{aligned} \tag{8.7}$$

which takes its maximum when

$$(Y_1\beta_1 + Y_2\beta_2) - H_0(t)\exp(Y_1\beta_1 + Y_2\beta_2) \tag{8.8}$$

takes its maximum in Y_1. Differentiating with respect to Y_1 and solving shows (8.8) is at a maximum in Y_1 at $\log H_0(t) = -(Y_1\beta_1 + Y_2\beta_2)$. Substituting into (8.7) we see this is bounded by

$$h_0(t)\exp[-\{1 + \log H_0(t)\}].$$

Hence, when $D_i = 1$, we accept $Y^{\star}_{i,1}$ with probability

$$\frac{f(T_i|Y^{\star}_1, Y_2; \boldsymbol{\beta})}{\max_{Y_1} f(T_i|Y_1, Y_2; \boldsymbol{\beta})} = h_0(t)\exp\left[(Y^{\star}_{i,1}\beta_1 + Y_{i,2}\beta_2) - H_0(t)\exp\{Y^{\star}_{i,1}\beta_1 + Y_{i,2}\beta_2\}\right] \times \frac{e^1 H_0(t)}{h_0(t)}$$

$$= H_0(t)\exp\left[1 + (Y^{\star}_{i,1}\beta_1 + Y_{i,2}\beta_2) - H_0(t)\exp\{Y^{\star}_{i,1}\beta_1 + Y_{i,2}\beta_2\}\right].$$

As with the joint modelling approach described above, this approach extends to allow interactions and nonlinear transformations of the covariates. This approach is not difficult to program in specific cases, but currently there is no general software. Instead, one of the approaches discussed below is typically used.

Survival data as transformed normal

The Metropolis-Hastings step / rejection step is needed in the above algorithm because, under the proportional hazards model, the joint distribution of the survival time and the covariates does not take a known form. However, while to interpret the substantive, time-to-event, model we need to model time on the original scale, this is not necessary for the imputation model.

Instead we may transform the survival time to approximate normality and then include the resulting variable in the imputation model as normally distributed. We may use any appropriate order-preserving transformation, fit the imputation model, and then back-transform afterwards. A further attraction of this approach is that we do not have to model the censoring indicator directly. Instead, if unit i is censored at T_i, we put a prior of 0 on $[0, T_i]$ and an improper prior on (T_i, ∞), and set T_i to be missing. This can readily be accommodated in the joint modelling and FCS approaches outlined in the previous chapters.

This approach will work well if (i) we can find a good normalising transformation for the survival time data and (ii) the relationships between the normalised survival time data and the other variables are appropriately modelled. Unfortunately, the second point is harder in general because, if the proportional hazards assumption holds and the log-hazard is linear in the covariates, the log-hazard for transformed survival time will not be linear in the covariates.

Thus, in practice this approach is likely to be satisfactory if survival is approximately log-normal, but could introduce bias otherwise.

This approach is equally applicable to the FCS setting; the transformed survival time is modelled using linear regression conditional on the other covariates. Censored survival times contribute the appropriate cumulative distribution to the log-likelihood. Such models are often referred to as *Tobit* models and can be fitted in most software packages.

8.1.2 Survival data as categorical

One way around the issues raised by transformation of the survival time is to discretise the survival variable into a categorical variable, and include this derived categorical variable in the imputation model. This could be done either as an ordinal variable, or as an unordered categorical variable. The latter is preferable because it does not impose a linear relationship between survival time and the other variables; instead it allows an interaction between them. Thus the hazard is not constrained to vary linearly with time, so a range of survival time distributions can be approximated. This approach has been adopted more generally for modelling survival data in a multilevel setting (Steele *et al.* 2004). Censored survival times are then handled via a prior on the categorical variable. Suppose the derived categorical survival variable has $m = 1, \ldots, M$ categories, and unit i is censored at the time interval corresponding to category m'_i. Then we set unit i's survival time to be missing, but put a prior of 0 on all categories $\leq m'_i$ and an uninformative (uniform) prior across the remaining categories. Imputation of any missing survival times then proceeds in the same way as imputing a missing categorical variable (Chapter 5); imputation of other variables conditional on survival likewise follows the approaches described in Chapters 3–4.

This is a natural approach if the survival data are already grouped, for example to the nearest week, month or year. If the survival data are not grouped, it makes sense to group them over regions of approximately constant hazard. This could be assessed prior to imputation using the nonparametric Nelson-Aalen estimate of the cumulative hazard. However, if the number of categories becomes large relative to the number of observations, it will be computationally demanding, and possibly unstable.

Again, this method can be applied using FCS, using multinomial logistic regression for the categorised survival time, and handling censored observations through an appropriate unit-specific prior.

Using the cumulative hazard

This approach was proposed by White and Royston (2009), from consideration of the conditional distribution of covariates given the survival time, under the proportional hazards model.

Suppose that $\mathbf{Y}_1$ is partially observed, and $\mathbf{Y}_2$ fully observed. Denote the conditional density of $Y_1|Y_2$ by $f(Y_1|Y_2)$. Then we have

$$f(Y_1|T, D, Y_2) = \frac{f(T, D, Y_1, Y_2)}{f(T, D, Y_2)} = \frac{f(T, D|Y_1, Y_2) f(Y_1, Y_2)}{f(T, D, Y_2)}$$

$$= f(T, D|Y_1, Y_2) f(Y_1|Y_2) \left\{ \frac{f(Y_2)}{f(T, D, Y_2)} \right\}. \tag{8.9}$$

Because the last term on the RHS of (8.9) is constant with respect to Y_1, it follows from (8.2) that the the log conditional distribution of Y_1 given Y_2 and survival time is, up to a constant of proportionality,

$$\log\{f(Y_1|T, D, Y_2)\} = \log\{f(Y_1|Y_2)\} + D[\log\{h_0(T)\} + (\beta_1 Y_1 + \beta_2 Y_2)] - H_0(T)\exp(\beta_1 Y_1 + \beta_2 Y_2). \quad (8.10)$$

Suppose first that Y_1 is binary. From (8.10) we have

$$\begin{aligned}\text{logit}\{f(Y_1 = 1|T, D, Y_2)\} &= \text{logit}\{\Pr(Y_1 = 1|Y_2)\} + D\beta_1 - H_0(T)(e^{\beta_1} - 1)e^{\beta_2 Y_2} \\ &\approx \varsigma_0 + \varsigma_1 Y_2 + \varsigma_2 D + \varsigma_3 H_0(T) + \varsigma_4 H_0(T) \times Y_2,\end{aligned} \quad (8.11)$$

for constants $\varsigma_0, \ldots, \varsigma_4$, provided $\text{Var}(Y_2)$ is small. In other words, (8.11) is approximately the logistic regression of Y_1 on $Y_2, D, H_0(T)$ and the interaction of Y_2 and $H_0(T)$. If Y_2 is not present, then the logistic regression result is exact; otherwise it is approximate, and the approximation is poorer the larger the variance of Y_2.

Now suppose that Y_1 is continuous, specifically $Y_1|Y_2 \sim N(\alpha_0 + \alpha_1 Y_2, \sigma^2)$. From (8.10) we have

$$\log f(Y_1|Y_2, T, D) \propto -\frac{(Y_1 - \alpha_0 - \alpha_1 Y_2)^2}{2\sigma^2} + D\beta_1 Y_1 - H_0(T)e^{(\beta_1 Y_1 + \beta_2 Y_2)}. \quad (8.12)$$

The term $\exp(\beta_1 Y_1 + \beta_2 Y_2)$ means that (8.12) is not normal, nor any common distribution. However, it turns out (White and Royston, 2009) that if $\text{Var}(Y_1)$ and $\text{Var}(Y_2)$ are small, then (8.12) is approximately a linear regression on $D, H_0(T), Y_2, H_0(T) \times Y_2$.

The implication is that the conditional distribution of covariates is approximately linear (or linear on the logistic scale for binary variables) if we include the cumulative hazard, and the censoring indicator D_i and the interaction of the cumulative hazard with the covariates. Whether a joint modelling or FCS approach is adopted, this becomes increasingly difficult, and potentially numerically unstable, with increasing numbers of variables in the imputation model. Because all the interactions may well not be important in every dataset, preliminary variable selection based on the complete records may be appropriate.

As discussed above, under the proportional hazards model we extract the estimate of the baseline cumulative hazard. Under parametric models, such as exponential or more generally Weibull, the cumulative hazard has a parametric form. The relevant parameters need to be updated at the appropriate step of the MCMC or FCS algorithm.

Example 8.1 Simulation study

White and Royston (2009) report simulations studies with a single covariate (binary, then continuous) and also two covariates. We briefly review results for the latter here, and refer readers to the paper for full details.

In the two covariate study, survival times were drawn from an exponential distribution with hazard $h(t) = \lambda \exp(\beta_1 Y_1 + \beta_2 Y_2)$ where $\lambda = 0.002$, and (Y_1, Y_2) are bivariate normal, mean zero, variance 1 and correlation ρ. Censoring times were independently drawn with exponential hazard, again with $\lambda = 0.002$, giving about 50% censoring. Only Y_1 was allowed to be missing; MCAR and MAR mechanisms dependent on Y_2 were explored and around 50% of the $\mathbf{Y}_1$ values were missing.

As only one variable had missing data, there was only one imputation model, a linear regression for missing $\mathbf{Y}_1$ values. The following methods were compared.

Imputation from model regressing Y_1 on:

1. $Y_2, D, \log(T)$;
2. Y_2, D, T, (appropriate for the exponential hazard);
3. Y_2, D, T^2, (appropriate for a Weibull hazard with shape parameter $\kappa = 2$);
4. $Y_2, D, \hat{H}(T)$, where $\hat{H}(T)$ is the Nelson-Aalen estimate of $H(T)$;
5. $Y_2, D, \hat{H}(T), Y_2 \times \hat{H}(T)$ ($\hat{H}(T)$ again the Nelson-Aalen estimate), and
6. $Y_2, D, \hat{H}_0(T)$, where $H_0(T)$ is re-estimated only on the first two cycles of the FCS algorithm, by fitting the Cox proportional hazards model to the current observed and imputed data and then extracting the baseline cumulative hazard.

Method 4 approximates the baseline cumulative hazard $H_0(T)$ by $H(T)$, and this may cause bias with larger effects. For method 6, the results showed that re-estimating the baseline hazard at each cycle of the FCS algorithm did not materially change the results.

With data MCAR, focusing first on β_1, bias towards the null is present and increases slowly with increasing β_1, β_2, ρ. Bias is least for method 4 (maximum -5% when $\beta_1 = \beta_2 = \rho = 0.5$), but similar for all methods with maximum of 10% for method 3 when $\beta_1 = \beta_2 = \rho = 0.5$. Including the interaction (method 5) gives no detectable benefit The difference between empirical and imputation standard errors is smallest with method 4, with a maximum of 11% too high when $\beta_1 = \beta_2 = \rho = 0.5$. Power was weaker for method 3, but otherwise comparable.

Still focusing on β_1, under MAR the same pattern is observed; method 4 and 5 give the least bias, of around -10% when $\beta_1 = \beta_2 = \rho = 0.5$. For the standard error, MI estimates are again larger than empirical estimates; but now method 5 is best with a maximum of 12% too high when $\beta_1 = \beta_2 = \rho = 0.5$; method 1 and 4 peak at 15 – 16.% Confidence interval coverage ranged between 94–97%.

Turning to β_2, bias was much smaller, and comparable across all methods, with a maximum of +5% when $\beta_1 = \beta_2 = \rho = 0.5$. Overall, method 4 was better than, or as good as, the other methods in all scenarios. Method 4 also performed well for agreement between MI and empirical standard errors, with a maximum difference of 9%; however, there was less to choose between methods here as the maximum difference across all methods was an overestimation by 11%.

In summary, White and Royston (2009) conclude that method 4, using the Nelson-Aalen estimate of the cumulative hazard, $H(T)$, and the censoring indicator as covariates is the 'best method in general'. □

Although, from a theoretical standpoint, including the censoring indicator and Nelson-Aalen estimate of cumulative hazard falls short of the full joint modelling approach of Subsection 8.1.1, at the time of writing the latter has yet to be investigated with comparable simulation study to that of White and Royston (2009).

If the hazard is approximately constant, then while including T as a covariate may be appropriate, the simulations suggest that for moderate effect sizes, including the Nelson-Aalen estimate of hazard works at least as well, if not slightly better. Likewise if the survival time is approximately log-normal, then using log-survival time, and D, as suggested in Subsection 8.1.1 above will work well; again if effect sizes are moderate, the simulations suggest the Nelson-Aalen estimate will work just as well. Splitting the survival time into intervals and handling as a categorical variable approximates including the interaction between covariates and cumulative hazard (method 5 above); however, in the scenarios considered by White and Royston (2009) including this interaction made little difference.

Finally, note that the discussion has focused on proportional hazards models. For other scenarios, such as accelerated failure time models, the conditional distribution is much more complicated, and a joint modelling approach, as discussed above, may be preferable.

Example 8.2 Cancer registry data

Nur *et al.* (2010) describe the application of MI for missing covariates in relative survival analysis for colorectal cancer patients. The data consist of all adults (15 – 99 years) resident in the North West of England who were registered in the North West Cancer Intelligence Service with malignant, invasive colorectal cancer diagnosed during 1997–2004. A total of 29 563 records were linked to hospital episode statistics on co-morbidity and treatment, and available for analysis.

Unfortunately, a substantial proportion of patients were missing important covariates, specifically stage at diagnosis (40%), morphology (12%) and grade (25%). The proportion of missing values rose with age, deprivation, nonsurgical treatment, and was strongly associated with vital status and survival time. Thus a complete records analysis was reduced to 16 233 cases, 55% of the total.

Data were imputed using FCS and follow-up time was categorized as 0–6 months, 6–12 months, yearly up to 5 years, and >5 years; over each of these periods the hazard is approximately constant. The three FCS imputation models included all the other variables in the substantive model, together with vital status, follow-up time categorised as above, and two interactions: deprivation and follow-up time and age and follow-up time. Stage and grade were imputed with ordinal logistic regression; unordered categorical (multinomial logistic) regression was used for morphology. Ten imputed datasets were created.

A regression model to estimate relative survival was fitted to the complete records and imputed data, where the relative survival $R(t)$ is defined as

$$R(t) = \frac{S_c(t)}{S_r(t)},$$

where $S_c(t)$ is the survivor function for the cancer cases in the registry, and $S_r(t)$ is the survivor function for the general population, taken from life tables stratified by age, sex and calendar period. Specifically, an additive hazards model was used to estimate the excess hazard ratio for patient i,

$$h_i(t) = h_0(t) + \exp(\mathbf{x}_i^T \boldsymbol{\beta}),$$

for a background hazard $h_0(t)$ estimated from life tables, and a patient with covariates $\mathbf{x}_i$. Roughly speaking, the adjusted excess hazard ratio for a factor x estimated by such models, can be thought of as the probability of dying from cancer when one has factor x, divided by the probability when x is absent.

Table 8.1 shows the results. Here, morphology types A–C are, respectively, adenocarcinoma, mucinours and serous and other; site A–C are, respectively colon, rectosigmoid and rectum. These data are clearly not MCAR, and the probability of missing data is associated with the outcome. MAR is therefore a good working approximation, especially given the number of predictors in the model. We see that the analysis of the imputed data recovers information from the partially observed records, resulting in narrower confidence intervals. In addition, the estimated excess hazard ratios with age are markedly higher, the estimated excess hazard ratios with deprivation are slightly higher, while the excess hazard of stages III and IV, while still dominating the model, are markedly reduced. □

8.1.3 Imputing censored survival times

MI is useful if survival times are plausibly censored at random, conditional on all of a number of variables, $Y_1, \ldots, Y_p$, but we wish to estimate either the marginal survival distribution, or a survival regression with fewer covariates. Just as in the standard regression setting, discussed in Chapter 1, fitting the model to the observed data with no covariates (i.e. a marginal summary), or with only a subset of the p covariates, gives invalid results – because we are not conditioning on all the variables required for CAR to hold. In addition, as in the regression setting, we may also have additional variables predictive of survival time, which we might wish to include to improve our prediction of censored survival times, but which we do not wish to include in our substantive model.

Table 8.1 Adjusted excess hazard ratio (EHR) of death in the first year following diagnosis, estimated from complete records and after MI with 10 imputations using FCS (from Nur *et al.*, 2010). Details of categorical variables are in the text.

Covariate	Complete records (16 223 cases)			MI (29 563 cases)		
	EHR	95% CI		EHR	95% CI	
Stage: 1			reference			
2	3.56	2.69	4.72	2.56	2.17	3.02
3	10.20	7.72	13.48	7.02	5.86	8.40
4	26.39	19.60	35.53	16.53	13.80	19.80
Morphology: type A			reference			
B	1.03	0.94	1.13	1.02	0.95	1.10
C	1.17	0.61	2.24	0.99	0.75	1.30
Grade: I			reference			
II	1.18	1.07	1.30	1.22	1.14	1.30
II/IV	2.04	1.82	2.28	1.94	1.77	2.14
Site: A			reference			
B	0.82	0.73	0.91	0.90	0.84	0.97
C	0.76	0.70	0.82	0.88	0.85	0.92
Sex: male			reference			
female	0.93	0.88	0.99	0.95	0.91	0.98
Age group: 15–44			reference			
45–54	1.08	0.77	1.53	1.29	1.04	1.60
55–64	1.40	1.02	1.91	1.75	1.44	2.11
65–74	1.99	1.47	2.69	2.38	1.97	2.88
75–84	2.72	2.01	3.69	3.56	2.95	4.29
85–99	3.97	2.87	5.49	5.41	4.45	6.57
Deprivation: 1 (least)			reference			
2	0.99	0.85	1.15	1.05	0.97	1.14
3	1.12	0.97	1.29	1.16	1.07	1.26
4	1.20	1.05	1.39	1.24	1.14	1.34
5	1.29	1.13	1.47	1.37	1.27	1.47
Charlson index: 0			reference			
1	1.41	1.21	1.65	1.20	1.08	1.34
2	1.46	1.14	1.87	1.31	1.13	1.53
>3	2.06	1.25	3.41	2.45	1.84	3.26

The strategy is to use MI to impute the censored survival times, including in the imputation model all the covariates necessary for CAR as well as those not involved in the CAR mechanism but nevertheless predictive of survival. We proceed as follows:

1. use the model with all p covariates as an imputation model, and impute the censored survival times, creating K 'completed' datasets with no censored observations;
2. fit the substantive model to each imputed datatset; and
3. combine the results for inference using Rubin's rules.

As usual, the imputation model needs to contain the covariates needed for (i) CAR to hold and (ii) that are in the substantive model, compatible with any interactions, or nonlinear relationships, among covariates in the substantive model. We also need to be careful that we apply Rubin's rules to quantities with at least approximately normal sampling distributions.

The algorithms described thus far in this chapter all include steps for updating the coefficients of the survival model, which in turn allow the calculation of an estimate of the survivor function $\hat{S}(t|\boldsymbol{\beta}, Y_1, \ldots, Y_p)$. At each iteration of the algorithm, immediately following this update step impute the censored survival times as follows:

1. for each censored unit i, censored at T_i, calculate

$$p_i = 1 - \hat{S}(T_i, |\boldsymbol{\beta}, Y_{i,1}, \ldots, Y_{i,p});$$

2. draw $u_i \sim \text{uniform}[p_i, 1]$; and
3. impute the censored survival time, say $T_i^\star$, as the solution of $u_i = 1 - \hat{S}(t, |\boldsymbol{\beta}, Y_{i,1}, \ldots, Y_{i,p})$.

This ensures that each imputed survival time is greater than the time at which the unit was censored.

If we wish to do sensitivity analysis with respect to the CAR assumption, we will need to impute censored survival times with a hazard modified from the CAR estimate. We discuss this in Chapter 10, Subsection 10.3.2.

In summary, we have discussed imputing missing covariates, and censored survival times, using a range of strategies, and have sketched their relative merits. The key difficulty is that the distribution of covariates given survival times is not generally linear in either survival time or cumulative hazard. Simulation studies suggest that approximations are acceptable, but may nevertheless lead to coefficients of imputed variables being attenuated.

We now consider nonparametric MI, and then discuss a nonparametric approach to MI for survival data proposed by Hsu *et al.* (2006).

8.2 Nonparametric, or 'hot deck' imputation

So far, we have only discussed parametric imputation models, that is choosing, estimating and imputing from a parametric statistical model for the distribution of the missing data given the observed data. Here, we briefly consider nonparametric imputation, also known as 'hot deck' imputation – we explain the name below.

To describe the approach, suppose we have $Y_1, \ldots, Y_{p'}$ fully observed discrete variables, and $Y_{p'+1}, \ldots, Y_p$ partially observed variables of any type. Then the p' discrete variables form G exclusive subgroups of the data, indexed by $g = 1, \ldots, G$, each with n_g members, where $\sum_{g=1}^{G} n_g = n$, the sample size. We further assume that within each group one or more units have all of the remaining $p - p'$ variables observed. Within each group, we order the observations so that $i = 1, \ldots, n_{go}$ units are fully observed, and $i = n_{go}, \ldots, n_g$ are partially observed.

Nonparametric imputation proceeds independently within each group g as follows:

1. Sample with replacement, n_{go} times, from the fully observed units $i \in (1, \ldots, n_{go})$, each with probability $1/n_{go}$, to form the donor pool, $\{\mathbf{Y}_1^\star, \ldots, \mathbf{Y}_{n_{go}}^\star\}$.

2. For each unit $i = (n_{go} + 1), \ldots, n_g$, with missing data, draw a donor from the donor pool $\{\mathbf{Y}_1^\star, \ldots, \mathbf{Y}_{n_{go}}^\star\}$ with equal probability with replacement. Impute missing values of $\mathbf{Y}_i$ with values from this donor.

These two steps give an imputed group g, with no missing data. Applying the same algorithm for each group $g = 1, \ldots, G$ gives a complete imputed dataset.

Repeating the whole process gives a series of imputed data sets, $k = 1, \ldots, K$. The substantive model is then fitted to each imputed data set in turn, and the results combined for inference using Rubin's rules. This algorithm was proposed by Rubin and Schenker (1986).

The term 'hot-deck' imputation arose when data were stored on punched cards. A deck of cards was 'hot' because it was currently being processed; for a unit with missing data we select a card from the from the current, 'hot deck' and substitute it (i.e. impute from it).

The double resampling in the above algorithm approximates the Bayesian bootstrap (Rubin, 1981). While the standard bootstrap samples with replacement from n observations, say $\mathbf{Y}_1, \ldots, \mathbf{Y}_n$, with probability $1/n$, $i = 1, \ldots, n$, the Bayesian bootstrap:

1. draws and orders $(n - 1)$ uniform[0, 1] variables;

2. calculates $p_1 = u_1$, $p_i = u_i - u_{i-1}$, $p_n = 1 - u_{n-1}$; and

3. resamples the n observations with replacement with probability p_i, $i = 1, \ldots, n$.

Rubin (1981) shows this simulates the posterior distribution of a statistic $\theta = \theta(p_1, \ldots, p_n, \mathbf{Y}_1, \ldots, \mathbf{Y}_n)$ under the improper prior proportional to $\prod_{i=1}^{n} p_i^{-1}$; see also Lo (1986).

The nonparametric imputation algorithm above is therefore a version of the Bayesian bootstrap. Relative to the bootstrap, it reflects uncertainty in estimating the resampling probabilities p_i within each group g, which is required for the application of Rubin's variance formula.

Rubin and Schenker (1986) showed the validity of Rubin's rules in this context for constructing a confidence interval for large n and fixed K. They also showed the consistency of the variance estimator as sample size and number of imputations tend to infinity. However, Kim (2002) considers nonparametric imputation for the sample mean, and shows that the MI variance formula underestimates the variance with the bias of order n^{-2}. In the context of the sample mean, Kim gives a formula for a reduced donor group size to compensate for this. Rao and Wu (1988) discuss related points in the context of survey sampling.

However, nonparametric imputation is attractive in very large datasets, such as a census, where parametric imputation is likely to prove cumbersome. Thus, in practice, the principal concern is not likely to be the validity of Rubin's rules, but instead how to form appropriate the donor groups – in other words deciding on the groups within which units are exchangeable. In our motivating discussion, we avoided this issue by assuming that the fully observed variables were categorical, and using their values to form groups. More generally, one might consider using Malhanobis distance or k^{th} nearest neighbours. An alternative is to use the propensity score (Rosenbaum and Rubin, 1983). Simply speaking, one uses logistic regression to estimate the probability of data being missing, and then forms donor groups from units with similar probabilities. This is discussed more fully in, for example Lavori *et al.* (1995).

The key advantage of nonparametric imputation is that it is compatible with all interactions and complex relationships within the data, and these do not have to be specified. Unfortunately, this advantage will not be realised if the matching itself introduces bias. Assuming that it does not, however, the remaining disadvantage is that it is inefficient relative to parametric imputation. One can look at it in terms of a bias-variance trade off. If we form valid donor pools, then nonparametric imputation will be unbiased, but the parameter estimates will be less precise than a correctly specified parametric imputation model.

In very large datasets, such as census data, there is a lot of information to form donor pools, and precision is not a major concern; thus nonparametric imputation is attractive. Conversely, in smaller studies, such as those considered in this book, parametric imputation is most likely preferable. For an application in imputing health records, including consideration of issues raised by MNAR data, see Siddique and Belin (2008). Andridge and Little (2010) give a good overview, highlighting the diversity of approaches to nonparametric imputation and the lack of consensus on how to obtain inferences from the completed data set.

8.2.1 Nonparametric imputation for survival data

As the proportional hazards model is semi-parametric, with the baseline hazard unspecified, it is natural to consider nonparametric imputation. Hsu, Taylor and Murray consider this in a series of articles (Taylor *et al.*, 2002; Hsu *et al.* 2006, 2007; Hsu and Taylor 2009); we outline their approach. As discussed in Subsection 8.1.3, the aim is to impute censored survival times using auxiliary variables, thus increasing the plausibility of CAR, and then estimate either the marginal survival distribution or the marginal effect of a subset of covariates.

For unit $i = 1, \ldots, n$, we have as before data T_i and D_i, where T_i is the survival time if $D_i = 1$ and T_i is the censoring time if $D_i = 0$. We denote the ith unit's covariates by the p by 1 column vector $\mathbf{Y}_i = (Y_{i,1}, \ldots, Y_{i,p})^T$, so that each unit's data are $(T_i, D_i, \mathbf{Y}_i)$. The algorithm is then as follows:

1. Sample the n units with replacement, and form the corresponding bootstrap dataset
$$\{(T_i, D_i, \mathbf{Y}_i)^{\star}\}_{i=1,\ldots,n}.$$
2. Use the bootstrap data to estimate an appropriate metric defining the distance $d(i, j)$ 'between' unit i and j, as discussed below.
3. For each unit i with censored survival time,
   (a) identify the set of N nearest neighbours using the distance metric;
   (b) using the set of data from the nearest neighbours, calculate the Kaplan-Meier estimate of the survivor function, $\hat{S}_i$; and
   (c) use $\hat{S}_i$ to impute the unseen survival time, $\tilde{T}_i$ for unit i, subject to $\tilde{T}_i \geq T_i$, the censoring time.

Steps 1–3 create a single imputed dataset; we repeat the whole process to obtain K imputed datasets. Repeating step 1 as part of each imputation is important, as discussed on p. 180, to ensure appropriate between-imputation variability for the MI variance estimator. Using the Kaplan-Meier estimate in step 3, the procedure will always impute a survival time from one of the observed survival times among the nearest neighbours, unless the last observation time among the nearest neighbours is censored, in which case occasionally a censored time may be imputed.

The metric is derived as follows:

(i) fit the proportional hazards model to the bootstrap data generated in Step 1, using all the available covariates, giving parameter estimates $\hat{\boldsymbol{\beta}}^{\star}$;

(ii) using $\hat{\beta}^{\star}$, calculate each unit's risk score, that is, their linear predictor, $Z_i = \mathbf{Y}_i^T \hat{\boldsymbol{\beta}}^{\star}$;

(iii) calculate $d_i^S = (Z_i - \bar{Z})/\hat{\sigma}_Z$, where $\bar{Z}$ and $\hat{\sigma}_Z$ are respectively the sample mean and standard deviation of the Z_i's and

(iv) define $d^S(i, j) = (d_i^S - d_j^S)^2$.

Within the current bootstrap dataset, we then construct the donor pool for unit i as the $j = 1, \ldots, N$ 'nearest neighbours' as measured by $d^S(i, j)$. If the covariates have missing values, one option is to generate a single imputed data set using one of the approaches of Subsection 8.1.1 in order to generate a working data set to calculate the distances.

In applications, Hsu *et al.* (2006) show performance can be further improved by, in step (i), additionally fitting a second model with time to censorship, rather than event time, as the outcome. This is simply achieved by defining $C_i = 1 - D_i$, and fitting the proportional hazards model to $(T_i, C_i, \mathbf{Y}_i)$. Then for unit i, we can analogously define d_i^C, and $d^C(i, j)$. We can then choose the N nearest neighbours for unit i in terms of

$$\sqrt{w_S d^S(i, j) + w_C d^C(i, j)}, \tag{8.13}$$

where w_S and w_C are nonnegative weights that sum to 1, and typically $w_S = w_C = 0.5$.

As Hsu *et al.* demonstrate, the advantage of this procedure is that it induces a form of double robustness: if either the model for the time-to-event or the censoring time is correct, then in large samples the survival estimate from this procedure will be have good properties, because conditional on the two risk scores, survival and censoring times will be independent. In smaller samples, bias may occur because, within the neighbourhood, censoring and survival time may not be independent. In moderate sample sizes (n = 300 – 500), their simulation study demonstrates small bias and good coverage if both time-to-event and time-to-censoring models are correct. If not, there is some bias, but this can be alleviated if in (8.13), instead of weighting d^S and d^C equally, we up-weight the model that is correct. The simulation studies suggest that $N = 10$ is a reasonable choice for the number of nearest neighbours.

Hsu *et al.* (2007) describe the application of this approach to interval censored survival data. Here, the model required to determine the distances, and to impute survival times within sets of nearest neighbours, is no longer the proportional hazards/Kaplan-Meier model, but the nonparametric model for the interval censored data (Peto, 1973). Further, with interval censored data they report that using linear interpolation to smooth the estimated survivor function before imputing reduces bias. This is because interpolation compensates for the fact that survivor functions estimated from interval-censored data inevitably have fewer, larger, jumps than the underlying survival curve. Again, a simulation study shows good performance.

In applications, Monte Carlo error is likely to be larger than with parametric imputation methods, so a greater number of imputations may be desirable, say $K = 100$.

8.3 Multiple imputation for skips

Frequently in questionnaires, the answer to a particular question will determine the immediately succeeding questions. For example, if an interviewee reports that he or she is in paid employment, succeeding questions may ask about the nature of the work and remuneration. However, if the interviewee reports he or she is not in paid employment, questions about the nature of the work and remuneration will be *skipped* and possibly a different set of succeeding questions may be asked. Imputation of a large-scale database will inevitably run up against the issue of skips. For recent examples see He *et al.* (2010) and Drechsler (2011).

Imputation for questionnaire, or other data with skips, is potentially more complex than for the cross-sectional data considered so far, because questions that are skipped should not be imputed (or if imputed then discarded), while imputation of missing data on questions that determine skip patterns requires consistent imputation for succeeding skip questions. As usual with imputation, careful consideration of the context is needed to avoid making the imputation model unduly complex on the one hand, and on the other to avoid inappropriate imputation of important associations.

Example 8.3 Youth Cohort Study

GCSE exam results from the YCS illustrate how formulating imputation in terms of skips may be useful, even when the data are not actually presented in terms of skips, but instead as a single variable – here GCSE points score. We may imagine this was derived in answer to a series of questions along the lines of (a) did you obtain any GCSE at grade G or higher? and (b) if yes, in which subjects and with what grades. If the answer to (a) is 'no', (b) is skipped. Each GCSE grade is given a point score, from A/A* = 7 through to G = 1, these are added and and the score is capped at 84. Figure 8.1 shows the histogram of GCSE scores among pupils who had at least one pass at grade G or higher; 2468/64 045 (3.9%) did not obtain any GCSEs.

In the YCS data only a small proportion of GCSE scores are missing. Thus imputing assuming GCSE score has a normal distribution, and then rounding any negative imputed values to zero is going to give similar results to more complex methods, and is likely to be acceptable.

However, more generally if a variable has a distribution with a spike at a particular value, then it is awkward to model and thus impute. Considering the variable as a binary skip indicator plus a response if the skip indicator is 1 is potentially an attractive way around this problem, which connects to the literature on zero inflated, and more general, mixture models.

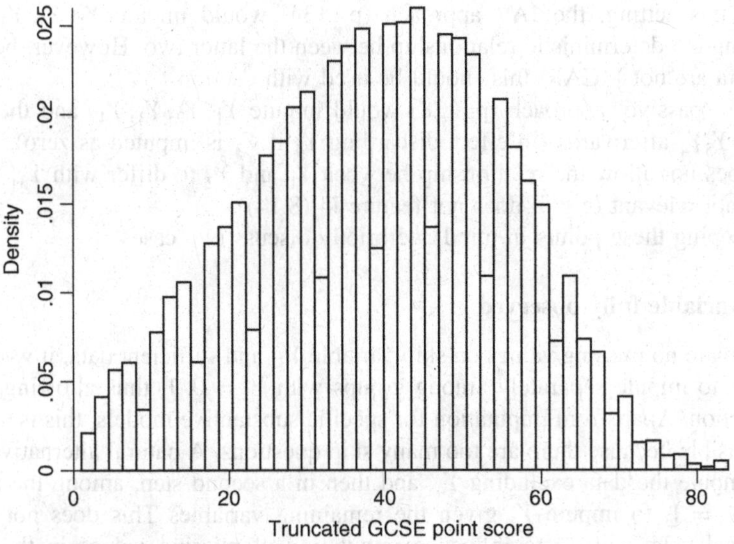

Figure 8.1 Histogram of GCSE points score, for pupils who obtained one or more GCSEs at grade G or above.

Thus, even when skips are not explicit in the variables in the substantive model, the approaches described below may be useful. □

To explore this further, suppose the following linear regression is of interest:

$$Y_{i,1} = \beta_0 + \beta_1 Y_{i,2} + \beta_2 Y_{i,3} + \beta_3 (Y_{i,3} Y_{i,4}) + e_i, \quad e_i \overset{i.i.d.}{\sim} N(0, \sigma^2), \tag{8.14}$$

where Y_1, Y_2, Y_4 are continuous, and Y_3 is a skip indicator for Y_4, so that if the answer to the question coded in Y_3 is 'no', $Y_3 = 0$ and the information in Y_4 is not asked for, because it is not relevant. In the YCS example Y_3 would be whether any GCSE passes were obtained, and Y_4 the points score; examples abound in all application areas. The discussion below is general, so Y_1, Y_2, Y_4 can be variables, or groups of variables, of different types.

Framing the issue through (8.14), we see that skips are a special case of interactions; special because usually we would fit Y_3, Y_4 and $Y_3 Y_4$, but with a skip we do not fit Y_4 because, if $Y_3 = 0$, it is not relevant. Thus the consideration of interactions in Chapter 7 is directly relevant to skips. With a general missingness pattern, this points to the approach described in Section 7.3. However, as we discuss below, this may not always be necessary.

We note that if Y_4 is observed, Y_3 cannot be missing. However, if Y_3 is 1 and Y_4 is missing, it cannot be MCAR. Also note that what we assume about the distribution of Y_4 when $Y_3 = 0$, and in particular how it relates to that of Y_4 when $Y_3 = 1$, is unlikely to have much effect on imputed values for Y_1, Y_2, as no values of Y_4 are 'seen' if $Y_3 = 0$.

In this setting, the JAV approach (p. 134) would impute Y_1, Y_2, Y_3, Y_3Y_4 ignoring the deterministic relationship between the latter two. However, because the data are not MCAR, this should be used with caution.

The 'passive' approach (p. 128) would impute Y_1, Y_2, Y_3, Y_4, and then calculate Y_3Y_4 afterwards (in effect discarding Y_4 if Y_3 is imputed as zero). While this does not allow the relationship between Y_1 and Y_2 to differ with Y_3, this is often not relevant (e.g. it does not feature in (8.14)).

Keeping these points in mind, we briefly discuss two cases.

Skip variable fully observed

If there are no missing values on skip variable Y_3, and sufficient data, it would be natural to impute separately among groups with $Y_3 = 0, 1$, thus allowing a full interaction. Apart from imputation for specific substantive models, this is usually not feasible because there are too many skip questions. A natural alternative is to first impute the data excluding Y_4, and then in a second step, among the subset with $Y_3 = 1$, to impute Y_4 given the remaining variables This does not allow observed values of Y_4 to influence imputation of missing values in the other variables, but in many settings this loss of information may be minimal.

Alternatively, we may simply impute from a joint model:

$$\begin{aligned} Y_{i,1} &= \beta_{0,1} + \beta_{11}Y_{i,3} + e_{i,1} \\ Y_{i,2} &= \beta_{0,2} + \beta_{12}Y_{i,3} + e_{i,2} \\ Y_{i,4} &= \beta_{0,3} + e_{i,3} \\ (e_{i,1}, e_{i,2}, e_{i,3}) &\sim N_3(\mathbf{0}, \boldsymbol{\Omega}). \end{aligned} \tag{8.15}$$

Here we fit the model as usual, and impute as usual, but then discard imputed values for Y_4 when $Y_3 = 0$. Since $Y_{i,4}$ is always missing when $Y_{i,3} = 0$, when imputing any missing $Y_{i,1}, Y_{i,2}$, when $Y_{i,3} = 0$ we have no explicit information in $Y_{i,4}$ to condition on, only implicit information through the normality assumption. If this is a concern, where $Y_{i,3} = 0$, at the imputation step we could explicitly exclude Y_4 from the conditional distribution for drawing any missing $Y_{i,1}, Y_{i,2}$.

Imputation model (8.15) can clearly be approximated using FCS; note that when imputing Y_4, if we include Y_3 alongside the constant, the imputation model is over-parameterised. Instead we proceed as follows:

1. regress Y_1 on Y_2, Y_3, Y_3Y_4 and impute Y_1;
2. regress Y_2 on Y_1, Y_3, Y_3Y_4 and impute Y_2;
3. in the subset $Y_3 = 1$, regress Y_4 on Y_1, Y_2 and impute.

Here, as usual with FCS, each regression is fitted to records with observed response, but with missing values for covariates at their current imputed values.

Missing values in the skip variable

Now suppose we have missing values of Y_3 (any missing Y_3 for which we have observed Y_4 are set equal to 1). We can again adopt the first approach described above; first we impute Y_1, Y_2, Y_3 setting aside Y_4. Then, in a second step, for each imputed data set separately in turn, among those with $Y_3 = 1$ we impute Y_4 given Y_1, Y_2. This is a form of two-stage imputation, which we consider in Section 8.4 below.

Alternatively, we may simply extend (8.15) including binary skip indicator Y_3 as a response through the latent normal structure:

$$\begin{aligned} Y_{i,1} &= \beta_{0,1} + e_{i,1} \\ Y_{i,2} &= \beta_{0,2} + e_{i,2} \\ \Pr(Y_{i,3} = 1) &= \Pr(\beta_{0,3} + e_{i,3} > 0) \\ Y_{i,4} &= \beta_{0,4} + e_{i,4} \\ (e_{i,1}, e_{i,2}, e_{i,3}, e_{i,4})^T &\sim N_4(\mathbf{0}, \mathbf{\Omega}), \quad \text{with } \mathbf{\Omega}_{3,3} = 1. \end{aligned} \tag{8.16}$$

Because when imputing missing Y_3, Y_4 must be missing, we also constrain their dependence, conditional on (Y_1, Y_2), to be zero by setting $\mathbf{\Omega}^{-1}_{34} = \mathbf{\Omega}^{-1}_{43} = 0$. As in the discussion following (8.15), when $Y_{i,3} = 0$ we have no explicit information in $Y_{i,4}$ to condition on, so whether or not we formally condition on it when imputing any missing $Y_{i,1}$, $Y_{i,2}$ is unlikely to have any practical effect.

We can set up an analogous FCS imputation sampler:

1. regress Y_1 on Y_2, Y_3, Y_3Y_4 and impute;
2. regress of Y_2 on Y_1, Y_3, Y_3Y_4 and impute;
3. regress Y_3 on Y_1, Y_2 and impute;
4. among those units with Y_3 (observed or imputed at step 3) equal to 1, regress Y_4 on Y_1, Y_2 and impute.

Here, as usual with FCS, the each regression is fitted to records with observed response, but with missing values for covariates at their current imputed values.

For each unit, where the skip indicator, $Y_{i,3}$ is missing, that unit's variables will vary between imputed datasets: some will include imputed skip variables because $Y_{i,3}$ was imputed to 1, others will not. While, with models like (8.14) this should not cause a problem, models fitted to, say, the subset of each imputed dataset for which $Y_3 = 1$ will have different numbers of observations (sample size) for different imputations. This triggers an error for some software which applies Rubin's rules. This is a computational issue: the substantive model can still be fitted to each imputed data set and Rubin's rules applied to the results.

However, this computational issue illustrates that the analysis of imputed data with skips may give rise to situations where the substantive model is fitted to a subset of the available data. As discussed in Chapter 2, this is a situation in which Rubin's rules will not, in general, hold. The effect is that inferences are likely to be conservative; in most cases the effect is likely of little practical consequence.

Before leaving skips, note that both the joint modelling and the FCS approach extend directly when (i) there are more skip variables than just Y_4 and (ii) there are more skip indicators than just Y_3. For joint modelling, we simply constrain the covariance matrix so that that skip indicators are uncorrelated with the associated skip variables. For FCS, (i) when imputing skip indicators, we do not include corresponding skip variables and (ii) when imputing skip variables, we restrict ourselves to the subset of records defined by the observed and current imputed values of the corresponding skip indicator.

8.4 Two-stage MI

Harel (2003, 2007) discusses the advantages of performing MI in two stages. This approach is most useful when the missing values fall into two qualitatively different types: for example studies with planned and unplanned missing values, or longitudinal studies with intermittent missing values and attrition. Suppose we can partition the variables into three disjoint sets, where the first set, denoted $\mathbf{Y}_O$, contains all the observed values, and the second and third sets, respectively $\mathbf{Y}_{M,A}$, $\mathbf{Y}_{M,B}$ are two distinct sets of missing values.

Two stage MI proceeds as follows:

1. Take $\mathbf{Y}_O$, $\mathbf{Y}_{M,A}$ and choose an appropriate imputation model for the missing data. Impute K_1 datasets, denoted $\mathbf{Y}_{A,1}, \ldots, \mathbf{Y}_{A,K_1}$.

2. In turn, for each of the $k = 1, \ldots, K_1$ imputed datasets from step 1, take $\mathbf{Y}_O, \mathbf{Y}_{A,k}, \mathbf{Y}_{M,B}$, choose an appropriate imputation model and impute the missing values of $\mathbf{Y}_{M,B}$ K_2 times. This gives $K_1 K_2$ datasets, now with no missing observations remaining, denoted $\mathbf{Y}_{k,l}$, $l = 1, \ldots, K_2$.

In the resulting $K_1 K_2$ imputed datasets, $\mathbf{Y}_{k,l}$, for each $k = 1, \ldots, K_1$, $\mathbf{Y}_{k,1}, \ldots \mathbf{Y}_{k,K_2}$ share the same imputed values for $\mathbf{Y}_{M,A}$, i.e. the $l = 1, \ldots, K_2$ imputations can be thought of as 'nested' within the kth first stage imputation.

In this setting, we now have two sets of response indicators: (i) those for the missing observations and (ii) those identifying variables in set A and set B. For imputation to proceed ignoring the missingness indicators, Harel (2003, 2009) and Harel and Schafer (2009) show the following two conditions are sufficient:

(i) missing data in both $\mathbf{Y}_A$, $\mathbf{Y}_B$ are MAR (dependent on $\mathbf{Y}_O$), and

(ii) the process that divides the missing data into the two groups, A and B does not depend on any part of the missing data, given the observed data.

The second condition is practically important: it allows the analyst to partition the data into sets A and B depending on characteristics of the observed data.

Suppose $\hat{\beta}(\mathbf{Y}_{k,l})$ is the quantity of interest, calculated using the $(k,l)^{th}$ imputed dataset, with corresponding estimated variance $\hat{\sigma}^2(\mathbf{Y}_{k,l})$. Under two-stage MI, Shen (2000) shows Rubin's combination rules need to be modified as follows. The MI point estimate is:

$$\hat{\beta}_{TS} = \frac{1}{K_1 K_2} \sum_{k=1}^{K_1} \sum_{l=1}^{K_2} \hat{\beta}(\mathbf{Y}_{k,l}),$$

with variance

$$\widehat{V}_{TS} = \left(1 + \frac{1}{K_1}\right)\widehat{B} + \left(1 - \frac{1}{K_2}\right)\widehat{N} + \widehat{W},$$

(note the minus sign in the multiplier of $\widehat{N}$). In this expression,

$$\widehat{B} = \frac{1}{K_1 - 1} \sum_{k=1}^{K_1} \left\{ \hat{\beta}_{TS} - \frac{1}{K_2} \sum_{l=1}^{K_2} \hat{\beta}(\mathbf{Y}_{k,l}) \right\}^2,$$

$$\widehat{N} = \frac{1}{K_1} \sum_{k=1}^{K_1} \frac{1}{K_2 - 1} \sum_{l=1}^{K_2} \left\{ \hat{\beta}(\mathbf{Y}_{k,l}) - \frac{1}{K_2} \sum_{l=1}^{K_2} \hat{\beta}(\mathbf{Y}_{k,l}) \right\}^2,$$

and

$$\widehat{W} = \frac{1}{K_1 K_2} \sum_{k=1}^{K_1} \sum_{l=1}^{K_2} \hat{\sigma}^2(\mathbf{Y}_{k,l}).$$

To test the hypothesis $\beta = \beta_0$, we refer

$$\frac{\hat{\beta}_{TS} - \beta_0}{\sqrt{\widehat{V}_{TS}}}$$

to a t-distribution with v degrees of freedom, where

$$v^{-1} = \frac{1}{K_1(K_2 - 1)} \left\{ \frac{(1 - K_2^{-1})\widehat{N}}{\widehat{V}_{TS}} \right\}^2 + \frac{1}{K_1 - 1} \left\{ \frac{(1 + K_1^{-1})\widehat{B}}{\widehat{V}_{TS}} \right\}^2.$$

We notice that if $K_2 = 1$ these formulae reduce to Rubin's rules for a scalar, given in Section 2.5, p. 52.

A particular attraction of this approach is it enables us to partition the information lost due to missing data into two parts; that related to part A of the data, and that related to part B. We can derive this as follows. We note that, were all the data observed then all the 'imputed' datasets would be the same, and $\widehat{N}$ and

$\widehat{B}$ would go to zero. Thus the rate of missing information can be estimated as

$$\hat{\lambda} = \frac{\widehat{B} + (1 - K_2^{-1})\widehat{N}}{\widehat{W} + \widehat{B} + (1 - K_2^{-1})\widehat{N}}.$$

Similarly, if $\mathbf{Y}_{M,A}$ had no missing observations, $\hat{\sigma}_B^2$ vanishes, so that the rate of missing information due B given A can be estimated as

$$\hat{\lambda}^{B|A} = \frac{\widehat{N}}{\widehat{W} + \widehat{N}}.$$

Thus $(\hat{\lambda} - \hat{\lambda}^{B|A})/\hat{\lambda}$ represents the proportion of the information lost due to missing values in part B. We can therefore use two-stage MI to highlight the 'part' of the study where we are losing the most information about β. This can be useful if targeted further data collection is an option, or to inform planning for future studies. It also indicates where sensitivity analysis may usefully be focused.

Under standard MI, to accurately estimate missing information substantially more than 5–10 imputations are needed (Schafer, 1997, p. 200). Harel (2007) shows this also holds true for two stage MI. Based on the simulation results he reports, we suggest $K_1 \approx 100$ and K_2 in the range 2–5 is likely to be adequate for most purposes.

If we wish to perform two-stage MI with standard MI software such as FCS, then it may be simplest to proceed as follows:

1. Impute the whole data set, i.e. both $\mathbf{Y}_{M,A}$ and $\mathbf{Y}_{M,B}$ K_1 times using standard FCS software;

2. Set $\mathbf{Y}_{M,B}$ to missing in each of the K_1 imputed data sets, and

3. Given $\mathbf{Y}_O, \mathbf{Y}_{A,k}$, impute $\mathbf{Y}_{M,B}$ K_2 times.

8.5 Large datasets

We now consider issues raised by large datasets. These could be large cross sectional datasets, but they could also be longitudinal with regular observation times. We consider multilevel, or hierarchical, imputation models in Chapter 9. Here our focus is addressing issues raised by imputing a large number of variables simultaneously, rather than those specifically raised by hierarchical/multilevel structure.

We first consider these issues in the context of joint modelling, and then in the context of FCS.

8.5.1 Large datasets and joint modelling

Consider joint multivariate normal modelling first, so that either all the variables are continuous, or they are being treated as continuous for the purpose of imputation. The key difficulty which is likely to arise is an ill-conditioned covariance matrix, whose determinant is close to zero. This can arise when

1. two or more variables are highly correlated, and/or

2. the number of variables is 'large' relative to the number of observations.

The first cause can be dealt with relatively easily; after removing any variables that are structurally dependent on others, we can calculate the sample correlation matrix of the data, taking care to use all available data to estimate each pairwise correlation, and remove variables that have a correlation of above 0.9, say. For the general treatment of such problems see Hansen (1998).

The second potential problem is that with the p-variate normal, there are p mean and $p(p+1)/2$ variance/covariance parameters and issues of both statistical precision and and numerical stability arise in its estimation. A good rule of thumb as far as precision is concerned is that the unstructured covariance matrix will perform well compared with more parsimoniously parameterised alternatives provided $n > 10p$ (see Section 5.6 of Molenberghs and Kenward (2007)). If there are concerns about the numerical stability of the covariance matrix estimator then it is helpful to monitor the convergence to identify potential ill-conditioning. When there are such problems, there are two broad approaches which can be taken:

1. increase the diagonal terms, and/or

2. set some off-diagonal terms of the inverse to zero.

Approach 1 has a long history, and is known as ridge regression (Hoel and Kennard 1970), and see Schafer (1997) p. 155–156 for a discussion in the MI context. For the imputation of quantitative data, recall from p. 82 that the update step for the precision matrix $\mathbf{\Omega}^{-1}$ with prior $\mathrm{W}(\nu, \mathbf{S}_P)$ is

$$f(\mathbf{\Omega}^{-1}|\boldsymbol{\beta}, \mathbf{Y}) \sim \mathrm{W}\left[n+\nu, \left\{\mathbf{S}_P^{-1} + \sum_{i=1}^{n} (\mathbf{Y}_i - \boldsymbol{\beta})(\mathbf{Y}_i - \boldsymbol{\beta})^T\right\}^{-1}\right].$$

Under ridge regression, for a chosen scalar $\lambda > 0$, this becomes

$$f(\mathbf{\Omega}^{-1}|\boldsymbol{\beta}, \mathbf{Y}) \sim \mathrm{W}\left[n+\nu, \left\{\mathbf{S}_P^{-1} + \sum_{i=1}^{n} (\mathbf{Y}_i - \boldsymbol{\beta})(\mathbf{Y}_i - \boldsymbol{\beta})^T + \lambda \boldsymbol{I}_p\right\}^{-1}\right], \tag{8.17}$$

where $\boldsymbol{I}_p$ is the p-dimensional identity matrix. An alternative proposal of Schafer (1997), p. 156, is as follows. Let $\mathbf{S} = \sum_{i=1}^{n} (\mathbf{Y}_i - \boldsymbol{\beta})(\mathbf{Y}_i - \boldsymbol{\beta})^T$ and let $\mathbf{S}^\star$ be a matrix with diagonal elements $\mathbf{S}^\star_{i,i} = \mathbf{S}_{i,i}$, and off diagonal elements $\mathbf{S}^\star_{i,j} = 0$,

$i \neq j$. Then replace (8.17) by

$$f(\mathbf{\Omega}^{-1}|\boldsymbol{\beta}, \mathbf{Y}) \sim \mathrm{W}\left[n+\nu, \left\{\mathbf{S}_P^{-1} + \left(\frac{\lambda}{n+\lambda}\right)\mathbf{S}^\star + \left(\frac{n}{n+\lambda}\right)\mathbf{S}\right\}^{-1}\right].$$

We choose λ large enough so that this empirical prior stabilises the covariance matrix by down-weighting the off-diagonal terms.

In linear regression with covariates, one can show (Hoel and Kennard, 1970) that ridge regression is equivalent to minimising the sum of squared residuals, subject to the constraint that the sum of the squared regression parameters is less than a constant. The greater λ, the smaller the absolute values of β.

In multiple imputation, the usual guidance is to err on the side of complexity in building imputation models, in the expectation that this will recover more information from the data about the distribution of the missing values. Unlike the final model, the imputation model does not aim at a parsimonious description of the data. Consistent with this, it is appropriate to choose λ large enough to allow stable estimates of $\boldsymbol{\beta}$, without imposing marked shrinkage.

Ridge regression is attractive for imputation with a large number of variables, since we only have one shrinkage parameter. In contrast the methods below require specification of which coefficients, or elements of $\boldsymbol{\beta}$, should be estimated and which is set to zero.

Under the joint modelling approach, with a mix of variable types, categorical and ordinal variables impose constraints on the covariance matrix. In this setting, we might impose ridge shrinkage on the part of the covariance matrix for the continuous covariates. In practice, this is most easily done by re-ordering the data so that the q continuous variables come first, and correspond to the top $q \times q$ submatrix of $\mathbf{\Omega}$. Then we add $\lambda\tilde{\boldsymbol{I}}$ to instead of $\lambda\boldsymbol{I}_p$ in (8.17), where $\tilde{\boldsymbol{I}}$ has the first q diagonal elements 1, and the remaining elements 0.

8.5.2 Shrinkage by constraining parameters

The alternative to applying shrinkage to all the parameters, $\boldsymbol{\beta}$, is to explicitly specify which should be set equal to zero. In the FCS approach, for a variable $j \in 1, \ldots, p$, this corresponds to specifying which of the $(p-1)$ covariates should be excluded when imputing $\mathbf{Y}_j$, i.e. excluded from the regression model with dependent variable $\mathbf{Y}_j$.

In joint modelling terms, this corresponds to constraining terms in the inverse covariance matrix to zero. For example, suppose we have $p = 5$ continuous variables and we constrain $\mathbf{\Omega}^{-1}$ so that

$$\mathbf{\Omega}^{-1} = \begin{pmatrix} \omega_{11} & \omega_{12} & \omega_{13} & 0 & 0 \\ \omega_{21} & \omega_{22} & \omega_{23} & \omega_{24} & 0 \\ \omega_{31} & \omega_{32} & \omega_{33} & \omega_{34} & \omega_{35} \\ 0 & \omega_{42} & \omega_{43} & \omega_{44} & \omega_{45} \\ 0 & 0 & \omega_{53} & \omega_{54} & \omega_{55} \end{pmatrix},$$

where as usual the matrix is symmetric so $\omega_{ij} = \omega_{ji}$. When the nonzero terms follow this banded pattern the resulting covariance matrix is said to have an ante-dependence structure, and such matrices play a role in the modelling of nonstationary time-ordered data (Zimmerman and Núnez Antón, 2010).

This is equivalent to the following chained equations specification:

$$Y_{i,1} = \beta_{0,1} + \beta_{2,1}Y_{i,2} + \beta_{3,1}Y_{i,3} + e_{i,1}, \quad e_{i,1} \overset{i.i.d.}{\sim} N(0, \sigma_1^2)$$

$$Y_{i,2} = \beta_{0,2} + \beta_{1,2}Y_{i,1} + \beta_{3,2}Y_{i,3} + \beta_{4,2}Y_{i,4} + e_{i,2}, \quad e_{i,2} \overset{i.i.d.}{\sim} N(0, \sigma_2^2)$$

$$Y_{i,3} = \beta_{0,3} + \beta_{1,3}Y_{i,1} + \beta_{2,3}Y_{i,2} + \beta_{4,3}Y_{i,4} + \beta_{5,3}Y_{i,5} + e_{i,3}, \quad e_{i,3} \overset{i.i.d.}{\sim} N(0, \sigma_3^2)$$

$$Y_{i,4} = \beta_{0,4} + \beta_{2,4}Y_{i,2} + \beta_{3,4}Y_{i,3} + \beta_{5,4}Y_{i,5} + e_{i,4}, \quad e_{i,4} \overset{i.i.d.}{\sim} N(0, \sigma_4^2)$$

$$Y_{i,5} = \beta_{0,5} + \beta_{3,5}Y_{i,3} + \beta_{4,5}Y_{i,4} + e_{i,5}, \quad e_{i,5} \overset{i.i.d.}{\sim} N(0, \sigma_5^2)$$

In applications with FCS, we can either specify which coefficients are set to zero in advance, or we can use variable selection in an initial stage of the algorithm. Neither approaches are wholly satisfactory with large datasets. For example, for imputing a questionnaire with say 100 questions, it is hard to know in advance which coefficients should be set to zero. Conversely, we should be wary of selection based on significance tests.

In longitudinal data, the temporal element can be used to resolve some of these issues. If we have k variables at waves $1, 2, \ldots, t$, (e.g. annual follow up) when imputing wave t we can restrict to data from wave $t-1, t, t+1$. This leads to Nevalainen *et al.* (2009)'s proposal for 'two-fold' MI:

1. at time $t = 1$, use FCS to impute the k variables, using as covariates (but not imputing) the k variables at time $t = 2$;
2. for times $t = 2, \ldots, t-1$:
   use FCS to impute the k variables, using as covariates (but not imputing) the k variables at time $t-1$ and the k variables at time $t+1$; and
3. at time t, use FCS to impute the k variables, using (but not imputing) the k variables from time $t-1$.

FCS at each time t is run for C_w 'within' time cycles, and the whole algorithm is run for C_a 'among' (or 'across') time cycles. The 'window' of time, which is $t \pm 1$ above, can clearly be made wider, and/or only a selection of the k covariates available at any specific time are included in certain imputation models.

Nevalainen *et al.* (2009) report the results of a simulation study with three time points and a mix of variable types, where the algorithm imputes with minimal bias and good coverage; they advise that C_w should be an order of magnitude greater than C_a; for example 10 within cycles and 5 across cycles.

Welch *et al.* (2011) explore the application for imputation of general practice patient record data, as illustrated in Figure 8.2. Here, over the time period of

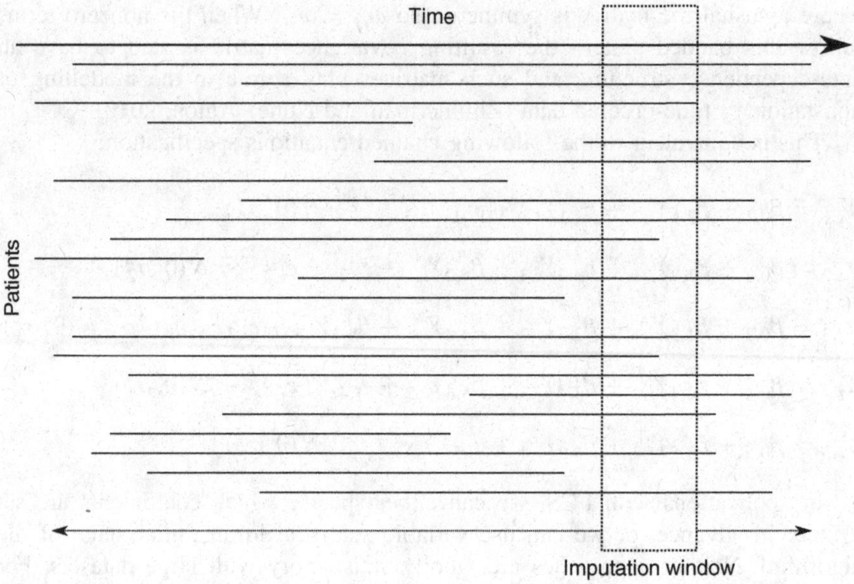

Figure 8.2 Schematic for imputation of longitudinal clinical record data using approach of Nevalainen et al. (2009).

interest, patients may register with the practice, and leave the practice. Certain key health variables, such as smoking and alcohol use, blood pressure and weight, should be measured at registration and subsequently. However, very often some, or even many of them, are missing, particularly for relatively healthy patients. They apply the algorithm above, imputing individuals' clinical measurements using measurements in a surrounding window. This avoids issues with overfitting the imputation model. Strictly following the approach of Nevalainen *et al.* (2009), the imputation window is only run forward through the data set; however it may be advantageous to run it forward and backward through the data. A comprehensive simulation study reported by Welch *et al.* (2011) shows promising performance. It suggests that longitudinal correlations beyond the 'window width' (e.g. if the window with is 1 year, correlations between blood pressure measurements at 2, 3, … years) can be recovered with small bias, but substantially more imputations are required for convergence. In particular, unlike in the three time point setting considered by Nevalainen *et al.* (2009), C_a should now be an order of magnitude greater than C_w: for a 1-year time window: say $C_a = 30$ and $C_w = 10$.

An alternative approach, which to our knowledge has not been explored, is to 'rotate' the window in Figure 8.2. Thus, we model longitudinal measurements for each variable (or group of variables) in turn – say weight, blood pressure, smoking history – conditional on the others; we then cycle round the variables in turn, in the manner of FCS. Each imputation model now needs to be a multilevel imputation model. Such multilevel imputation models are discussed in Chapter 9.

8.5.3 Comparison of the two approaches

Shrinkage using the ridge parameter λ in univariate linear regression can be shown to shrink with respect to the orthonormal basis formed by the principal components. Furthermore, components with the smallest variance are shrunk most. Applying such data-based shrinkage to the multivariate imputation model thus seems preferable to the alternative approach of setting some coefficients to zero, unless time-ordering, or some other natural property of the data, point to likely coefficients. In the absence of this, ridge regression, by its construction, concentrates shrinkage where it will have the least effect on prediction.

We can also use ridge regression to stabilise each of the conditional regressions in FCS. However, this does not correspond directly to the joint modelling case. An attraction of applying shrinkage through the joint model is that it allows a unified approach across response types through the latent normal structure, in a way that does not have a direct analogue in the FCS approach.

8.6 Multiple imputation and record linkage

In many social and health applications, we wish to link individual records across different databases; for example hospital and registry data, or different surveys. Typically, the aim is to add particular variables of interest to the data, for example date and cause of death to hospital records, or information on hospital episodes to general practice research databases.

If we wish to link individuals in a primary and secondary database, we first identify a set of variables, for example surname, date of birth, gender, available in both databases. Ideally, these would give a unique match for all individuals. Unfortunately, this is rarely the case due to errors and omissions in data recording. Individuals in the primary database without a unique match in the secondary database may be discarded from the analysis, or may be assigned their 'most likely' match. Assigning a single 'most likely' match does not reflect the uncertainty in the matching process, though.

An alternative, proposed by Goldstein *et al.* (2012b), is to use *prior informed imputation* (PII). The idea is that, for each individual in the primary database who does not have a unique match, we use the matching weights to calculate a prior distribution for the missing variable. Then, when we impute, we take this as the prior for our variable in the imputation model.

Specifically, suppose we wish to link a categorical variable, with possible values $m = 1, \ldots, M$, from the secondary database. For individual i in the primary database, we suppose we have a set weights $w_{i,j}$ representing the plausibility of a match to individual j in the secondary database, normalised to sum to 1. In the event of a perfect match of i and j' then $w_{i,j'} = 1$ and the remaining weights are zero. For an imperfect match, a number of the weights will be nonzero.

Construction, or estimation, of the $w_{i,j}$ is a specialist area of its own; see for example Clark (2004); Jaro (1995). Essentially, suppose individual i in the primary database and j in the secondary database have a particular pattern p among the matching variables. Then we use individuals where we (i) are sure of a match, to estimate $\Pr(p|\text{match})$, and (ii) are sure that there is no match, to estimate $\Pr(p|\text{no match})$. The traditional record linkage procedure then computes $w_{i,j} \propto \log_2\{\Pr(p|\text{match})/\Pr(p|\text{no match})\}$.

Assuming we have the $w_{i,j}$, and recalling that the variable we wish to link from the secondary database is categorical with M levels, then for individual i we compute the prior probability that the variable takes value m as

$$p_{i,m} = \sum_j w_{i,j}\delta_{j,m} \Big/ \sum_j w_{i,j}, \tag{8.18}$$

where $\delta_{j,m} = 1$ if individual j in the secondary database has a value of m for the categorical variable to be linked, and 0 otherwise.

For each individual i in the primary database, we therefore have a prior for imputing the value from the secondary database. For a perfect match this uniquely identifies one value; for an imperfect match it gives a range of probable values. During imputation we can either

1. impute the missing value, ignoring the prior, using the current estimate of the distribution of the missing given the observed data (i.e. as in standard MI), or

2. impute the linked value by combining (8.18) with an imputation distribution estimated from the rest of the data.

Goldstein *et al.* (2012b) point out that option 1 will work reasonably well for small amounts of unmatched data under the assumption of MAR. They comment that in practice this will often be adequate. They caution, however, against doing this if it is suspected that the probability of a correct match is associated with the values of the variables in the secondary database being linked in. They suggest that in this case option 2 will perform better. They further describe the extension of this approach to handle continuous data, and present a simulation study which gives promising results.

The advantage of this approach is that we can use multiple imputation to unify the handling of missing data and linkage, so that the analysis both increases the number of individuals contributing to the analysis (by including those with an uncertain link) and takes proper account of uncertainty in the linkage process. There is a natural link to measurement error problems, where we can use external data to identify a probability distribution for an individual's underlying value of a variable, given their observed value.

8.7 Measurement error

Here, we briefly review the use of MI in measurement error problems. We first consider the case where there is a 'gold standard' (i.e. error free) measurement available, and then consider the case where no error free measurements are available.

This topic has received some attention in the literature; Ghosh-Dastidar and Schafer (2003) use MI for missing data and measurement error simultaneously and similar strategies are followed by, for example, Yucel and Zaslavsky (2005), Raghunathan (2006) and Cole *et al.* (2006) which we consider further below.

Suppose we have three continuous variables: response Y_1, true exposure, Y_2, and exposure measured with error, Y_3. We take as the substantive model the linear regression

$$Y_{i,1} = \beta_0 + \beta_1 Y_{i,2} + e_i, \quad e_i \overset{i.i.d.}{\sim} N(0, \sigma^2). \tag{8.19}$$

We suppose that in a subset of the data, we have Y_1, Y_2, Y_3 measured, but for the majority of the dataset we have only Y_1, Y_3 measured, so that Y_2 can be regarded as missing.

Often, Y_2 will be missing by design, so the MAR assumption holds (any design variables informing the missingness mechanism would typically need to be included in the imputation model). Here we assume that the error-free measurement Y_2 was recorded on a randomly chosen subset of the full data. We adopt the multivariate normal imputation model, which enables us to accommodate missing values in all variables:

$$\begin{aligned}
Y_{i,1} &= \beta_{0,1} + e_{i,1} \\
Y_{i,2} &= \beta_{0,2} + e_{i,2} \\
Y_{i,3} &= \beta_{0,3} + e_{i,3} \\
(e_{i,1}, e_{i,2}, e_{i,3})^T &\sim N_3(\mathbf{0}, \mathbf{\Omega}).
\end{aligned}$$

We then proceed as in a standard MI analysis, imputing K 'completed' datasets, fitting the substantive model (8.19) to each and combining the results for inference using Rubin's rules. As this is a standard imputation setting, Rubin's rules are valid.

Example 8.4 Simulation study

Cole *et al.* (2006) explore the performance of this approach in a simulation study. Their setting is more complex than that outlined above, because (i) in the substantive model the response, T_i, is a Weibull distributed time-to-event with shape parameter 2, and event indicator D_i and (ii) both $Y_{i,2}$ (the error free exposure measurement) and $Y_{i,3}$, (its measured-with-error counterpart) are binary. Error free exposure, $Y_{i,2}$, is only observed in 15–25% of the 600 observations in each simulated dataset. The substantive model is a proportional hazards regression of survival time on Y_2. For MI the imputation model is

$$\text{logit}\{\Pr(Y_{i,2} = 1)\} = \beta_0 + \beta_1 Y_{i,3} + \beta_2 D_i + \beta_3 \log(T_i). \qquad (8.20)$$

They compare the following methods to estimate the exposure hazard ratio:

(a) use Y_3, the exposure measured with error;

(b) use Y_2, but only the subset of data where Y_2 is observed;

(c) use MI as described above;

(d) use regression calibration for measurement error (Spiegelman *et al.*, 2000); and

(e) analysis of the 'full' data on Y_2, (known, because this is a simulation study).

The relationship between Y_3 and Y_2 is defined by the sensitivity and specificity of Y_3 as a surrogate for error free Y_2. Eight scenarios are considered, with sensitivity 0.7, 0.9, specificity 0.7, 0.9, and validation study 15% and 25% of the study size. Across all 8 scenarios as expected (e) is unbiased, with greatest power and actual confidence interval coverage close to 95%. Methods (b)–(d) also have negligible bias. In six of the eight scenarios considered, regression calibration, (d), is slightly more powerful than (c) and substantially more powerful than (b). In the remaining two, (sensitivity = specificity = 0.7, proportion in validation study 15%, 25%) MI, (c), is more powerful than (b) which is more powerful than (d). Confidence interval coverage is close to the nominal 95% level for (b) but fractionally higher for (c) and (d), with a suggestion that it is higher for MI than regression calibration.

The results confirm that MI is a valid and practical alternative to regression calibration for measurement error, although as White (2006) points out, we might have expected MI to perform better, because unlike regression calibration it uses the true value when it is available. That it did not is most likely because (8.20) is missspecified: the discussion in Subsection 8.1.2 suggests that the cumulative hazard would be better choice than $\log(T_i)$, especially as the survival time is Weibull with shape parameter 2. □

Note that in some settings the validation study may not contain all the other variables in the substantive model. Reverting to our original example, it may be that in our principal dataset only response Y_1 and measured with error covariate Y_3 are available, while in a second, smaller dataset Y_3 and the gold standard Y_2 are measured. In this setting we may either

1. take Y_3 from the principal dataset, and Y_2, Y_3 from the validation dataset, impute Y_2 using only Y_3, creating K imputed vectors for $\mathbf{Y}_3$ in the principal data set, and then use these to fit the substantive model in each of the K principal datasets and combine the results for inference using Rubin's rules; *or*

2. put the principal and validation datasets together, impute missing values of all variables (Y_1 is missing on the validation portion, Y_2 missing in the principal portion), fit the substantive model to the imputed data sets and combine the results for inference using Rubin's rules.

However, under option 1, because the imputation model is uncongenial with the substantive model, indeed poorer than the substantive model, inference from Rubin's rules is likely to be unreliable. By contrast, under option 2, provided we fit the substantive model to the combined, imputed, principal and validation data, Rubin's rules should hold provided the imputation model is formulated appropriately with reference to the substantive model.

No gold standard available

Often, there is no gold standard available in measurement error problems. Instead, we have a number of observations on the same unit, typically individual, and can only recover the true measurement by hypothesising a model relating the true and observed values. We now discuss a simple version of such a model, and its implication for MI.

As before, we suppose that Y_1 is the outcome of interest, but now suppose both Y_2 and Y_3 are measured with error. A normal-theory measurement error model is:

$$\begin{aligned} Y_{i,j} &= \beta_0 + u_i + e_{i,j} \\ u_i &\overset{i.i.d.}{\sim} N(0, \sigma_u^2) \\ e_{i,j} &\overset{i.i.d.}{\sim} N(0, \sigma_e^2), \end{aligned} \tag{8.21}$$

for individuals $i = 1, \ldots, n$ and variable $j = 2, 3$. In this model the individual i's measurements have normally distributed error about their true value u_i which is in turn normally distributed about the population mean β_0.

The substantive model then relates the outcome to the estimate of the underlying value from (8.21), for example through a linear regression.

$$Y_{i,1} = \beta_0 + \beta_1 u_i + e_i, \quad e_i \overset{i.i.d.}{\sim} N(0, \sigma^2). \tag{8.22}$$

In this case we may extend our joint imputation model framework to incorporate both (8.21) and (8.22) as follows:

$$\begin{aligned} Y_{i,1} &= \beta_{0,1} + \beta_{1,1} u_{i,1} + e_{i,1} \\ Y_{i,j} &= \beta_{0,2} + u_{i,2} + e_{i,j}, \quad j = 2, 3 \end{aligned}$$

$$\begin{pmatrix} u_{i,1} \\ u_{i,2} \end{pmatrix} \overset{i.i.d.}{\sim} N_2 \left\{ \mathbf{0}, \sigma_u^2 \begin{pmatrix} 1 & 1 \\ 1 & 1 \end{pmatrix} \right\}$$

$$e_{i,1} \overset{i.i.d.}{\sim} N(0, \sigma^2); \text{ and independently } e_{i,j} \overset{i.i.d.}{\sim} N(0, \sigma_e^2), \quad i \in 1, \ldots, n. \tag{8.23}$$

The constrained covariance matrix for $(u_{i,1}, u_{i,2})$ ensures a correlation of 1, so that $u_{i,1} = u_{i,2}$ as desired. In this case, if our substantive model is (8.22), then there is no need to use MI. We can simply fit (8.23) for inference on $(\beta_{0,1}, \beta_{1,1})$. In general, however, we may have a number of other partially observed and/or auxiliary covariates, in which case developing (8.23) to incorporate these and impute may be attractive. Model (8.23) is an example of a multilevel, or hierarchical, model which we consider further in Chapter 9.

In conclusion, MI has potential in measurement error problems, not least because it holds out the hope of handling the missing data and 'dirty' data within a unified framework. We have sketched how this might work when validation data are, and are not, available. In the former case, our imputation model could readily be extended to allow for differential measurement error. The key point is that the validity of Rubin's rules requires the imputation model to include variables in the substantive model. In the latter case, if we adopt a Bayesian approach for fitting (8.23), we can use priors to incorporate information on the distribution of population means, or likely measurement error variance. In both cases, an MI approach provides a practical and accessible route for sensitivity analysis, as discussed in Chapter 10, which makes it attractive in applications.

8.8 Multiple imputation for aggregated scores

It often happens that a score to assess physical or mental functioning comprises a set of component subscores relevant to specific domains, which may then be summed to give the overall score. For example, the SF-36 score is a measure of state of health, and consists of 8 scaled scores relating to various specific aspects of health including physical, mental, social and emotional.

Such scores are derived from answers to a (typically quite substantial) number of questions. Frequently the score for an individual will be missing, either because an individual declined to answer any of the questions, or not infrequently because they started the questionnaire but broke off before completing it.

For our discussion, we consider the following simple set up. The extension to a weighted sum across domains with different numbers of questions is direct. Suppose we have $i = 1, \ldots, n$ individuals, $j = 1, \ldots, J$ domain scores and $l = 1, \ldots, L$ binary responses making up each domain score. Let patient i's response to question l domain j be $Y_{i,j,l}$, so that their domain score is

$$Y_{i,j,.} = \sum_{l=1}^{L} Y_{i,j,l},$$

and total score is

$$Y_{i,\ldots,} = \sum_{j=1}^{J} Y_{i,j,\cdot}.$$

Typically, the instructions for compiling the score have rather ad-hoc rules for handling missing data. For example, they may state that if more than half the items on a domain are missing, then that domain cannot be calculated. Conversely, if more than half are present, they can be summed in the usual way to give the score for that domain.

In general such ad-hoc rules will be biased, and may misrepresent the uncertainty caused by the missing data. To apply MI, we should first look for possible predictors of (i) the missing values and (ii) the missing values and the chance of them being missing. Any such variables are candidates for inclusion as auxiliary variables in the imputation model. Here, we assume MAR for imputation; the sensitivity to this can be investigated using one of the approaches outlined in Chapter 10.

The next decision is whether to impute the binary scores $Y_{i,j,l}$, or the domain scores, or the total score. The discussion of perfect prediction with binary data in Chapter 3 suggests that imputation of a large number of binary variables is likely to be problematic, and should be avoided if possible.

Fortunately, even for L as small as four or five, the domain averages, $\bar{Y}_{i,j.} = Y_{i,j.}/L$, will often be remarkably well approximated by the normal distribution. This suggests treating subdomain means as variables for imputation in a multivariate normal setup. Thus with $J = 3$ we would have

$$\begin{aligned}
\bar{Y}_{i,1} &= \beta_{0,1} + e_{i,1} \\
\bar{Y}_{i,2} &= \beta_{0,2} + e_{i,2} \\
\bar{Y}_{i,3} &= \beta_{0,3} + e_{i,3} \\
(e_{i,1}, e_{i,2}, e_{i,3})^T &\sim N_3(\mathbf{0}, \mathbf{\Omega}),
\end{aligned} \tag{8.24}$$

where each observed mean will lie between 0 and 1. This allows us to impute missing domain means, and once this is done we can convert them back to domain totals if desired. If the means have a skew distribution for some domains, these can – as usual – be transformed to be closer to normality before imputation and back transformed afterwards. When imputing we can reject values outside the permissible range; alternatively we can round values after imputation. In practice the difference is likely to be small.

For individuals with partially observed data in a domain, we can calculate the range of plausible total scores for their domain. We can use this to put bounds on the corresponding missing domain means in the imputation model. When imputing, we simply reject an imputed value that falls outside the bound, and draw again until one is accepted.

As these scores are often collected on a patient population repeatedly over time, and are likely to be highly correlated, extending model (8.24) to include all the domain means at each time may become unwieldy. One option is to use a multilevel model, as described in Chapter 9, possibly with a random intercept or random intercept and slope structure. Another is to have the response for each individual as the overall average at each time point, $\bar{Y}_{i,..,}$, and then apply (8.24) across time points. In either case, we can again use an individual's partial responses to provide bounds on their imputed values.

8.9 Discussion

In this chapter we have considered issues raised by more complex analyses where MI may be usefully applied. Principal among these is the analysis of survival data, were both time-to-event and censoring information need to be included appropriately when imputing missing values of covariates. Failure to do so can severely attenuate effect estimates towards the null, as was likely the case in Hippisley-Cox *et al.* (2007); see also related discussion in Sterne *et al.* (2009).

The range of situations considered in this chapter illustrate only some of the many adaptations of MI (Reiter and Raghunathan, 2007); for example, we have not discussed its use for creating synthetic imputations of confidential data for public release (see, e.g. Little, 1993). However, all the settings discussed are presently relatively under explored. The appropriateness of approximations made in the imputation model (e.g. to handle large datasets or survival data) and the error induced through applying Rubin's rules in broader settings than covered by the formal theory, are interesting topics for further research. Nevertheless, experience that Rubin's rules often work well away from the relatively narrow settings when they can be theoretically justified (e.g. Kang and Schafer 2007), together with the literature reviewed in this chapter, suggests that researchers may use MI in the situations discussed here with some confidence.

9

Multilevel multiple imputation

In this chapter we consider the imputation of data with a multilevel, or equivalently a hierarchical, structure. We extend our joint imputation model for a mix of discrete and continuous response types to the multilevel setting in Section 9.1, and describe the MCMC algorithm for fitting this model in Section 9.2.

We use an example to illustrate that, if data have multilevel structure, omitting this from the imputation model may give rise to misleading results, especially if the data are unbalanced. In Section 9.3 we consider the issues raised by the imputation of level-2 data, both for joint modelling and FCS approaches. We illustrate with the analysis of a dataset of paediatric hospital admissions from Kenya. Section 9.4 explores multiple imputation for multi-centre studies with individual patient data, e.g. individual patient meta-analyses.

In Section 9.5 we sketch out how the approach described here can be extended to more complex data structures, including random level-1 covariance matrices and cross-classified structures. We conclude with a discussion in Section 9.6.

9.1 Multilevel imputation model

Multilevel data structures arise when observations on individual units (typically individuals) cannot be considered independent, but instead are correlated because they are nested within groups or clusters of various kinds. For example, in educational research children are nested in classes within schools within educational authorities. In medical research, individual patients may be nested within general practices within health authorities, and repeated measurements nested within patients. Goldstein (2010) considers the analysis of multilevel data from a wide range of settings. The following is a typical educational example, which we use to highlight the issues raised by missing data in a multilevel setting.

Multiple Imputation and its Application, First Edition. James R. Carpenter and Michael G. Kenward.

Example 9.1 Class size data

Blatchford *et al.* (2002) report a study on the effects of class size on educational attainment among children in their first year of education in England. Each child's literacy and numeracy skills were assessed when they started school, and at the end of their first school year, known as the reception year. After adjustment for key confounders, the study found a nonlinear effect of class size on attainment, with falling attainment associated with class sizes above 25.

Our analyses here are merely illustrative. The version of the dataset we explore below was derived from the original; we restrict the analysis to a subset of complete records from 4873 pupils in 172 schools. School sizes vary greatly in these data and this is reflected in the number of pupils each school contributes to the analysis, which ranges from 1 to 88. The dataset is thus multilevel, and here we set aside class, and focus on children at level-1 belonging to schools at level-2.

Our substantive model is a regression of literacy score at the end of the first year on literacy measured when the children started school, eligibility for free school meals and gender. The pre- and post- reception year (i.e. first school year) literacy scores were normalised as follows. For each test, the children's results were ranked. Then for observation in rank order i, where n children sat the test, the normalised result was calculated as the inverse normal of $i/(n+1)$.

Let j denote school and i denote pupil. Our illustrative substantive model is:

$$\begin{aligned}
nlitpost_{i,j} &= \beta_{0,i,j} + \beta_1 nlitpre_{i,j} + \beta_2 gend_i + \beta_3 fsmn_i \\
\beta_{0,i,j} &= \beta_0 + u_j + e_{i,j} \\
u_j &\overset{i.i.d.}{\sim} N(0, \sigma_u^2) \\
e_{i,j} &\overset{i.i.d.}{\sim} N(0, \sigma_e^2),
\end{aligned} \tag{9.1}$$

where the u_j are independent of the $e_{i,j}$, *nlitpost* and *nlitpre* are respectively numerical post- and pre-reception year measures of attainment in literacy, and *gend* and *fsmn* are respectively indicators for boys and eligibility for free school meals.

Model 9.1 is a simple multilevel model known as a *random intercepts* model. While the effect of the covariates *nlitpre*, *gend* and *fsmn* is common across schools, we can think of every school, $j = 1, \ldots, J$ having a school-specific intercept $\beta_0 + u_j$. These are normally distributed with mean β_0 and variance σ_u^2.

Parameter estimates from fitting (9.1) are shown in column 2 of Table 9.1. The total variance is estimated as $\hat{\sigma}_u^2 + \hat{\sigma}_e^2 = 0.237 + 0.372 = 0.609$, of which $100 \times 0.237/0.609 = 39\%$ is between schools (i.e. between level-2 units). Estimates from the single-level model, where σ_u^2 is constrained to be 0, equivalent to a standard least squares regression, are shown in column 3. Now the level-1 (residual) variance estimate increases to 0.573.

Table 9.1 Parameter estimates (standard errors) from fitting model (9.1) to full and reduced data.

Parameter	Estimates (standard errors) from		
	Full data multilevel model (n = 4873)	Full data Single-level model (n = 4873)	Reduced data, Complete records (n = 3132)
β_0	0.088 (0.040)	0.065 (0.017)	0.016 (0.041)
β_1	0.733 (0.010)	0.662 (0.012)	0.712 (0.013)
β_2	−0.058 (0.018)	−0.086 (0.022)	−0.024 (0.023)
β_3	−0.068 (0.027)	−0.095 (0.030)	−0.038 (0.031)
σ_u^2	0.237 (0.028)	–	0.216 (0.027)
σ_e^2	0.372 (0.008)	0.573 (0.012)	0.369 (0.010)

Comparing the fixed effect estimates, we see that when the (substantial) component of variability between schools is omitted from the analysis, the gender coefficient in particular changes by more than one standard error. This is consistent with stronger gender differences in the larger (presumably urban) schools, which – as they contribute more pupils to the analysis – have a larger effect on the coefficients in the single-level (standard least squares regression) analysis.

We now make the data missing according to the following mechanism:

$$\text{logit}\{\Pr(\text{observe } \textit{nlitpre}_{i,j})\} = 1.5 + 0.5 \times \textit{nlitpost}_{i,j} - \textit{fsmn}_i - \textit{gend}_i. \quad (9.2)$$

This mechanism implies that we are more likely to see *nlitpre* for girls with higher *nlitpost* who are not eligible for free school meals. We then generate 4873 random numbers from a uniform distribution on [0, 1] and make each child's *nlitpre* observation missing if their corresponding draw from the uniform distribution is greater than the probability given by (9.2). This results in 3313 complete records. Fitting the multilevel substantive model to these, we see that the gender effect and the effect of eligibility for free school meals are diluted, so that they are no longer significant (column 4, Table 9.1).

After describing multilevel imputation below, we return to this example to illustrate its application. □

We know from the basic principles behind MI that the imputation model is derived from the conditional distribution of the missing data given the observed, congenial with the substantive model. This implies, in multilevel examples like this, that the conditional distribution of a missing observation will depend on any other variable with which it is correlated. For example, in a simple clustered setting, one observation from a cluster is correlated with all other observations in the same cluster, and the imputation model should take this into account. To achieve this we need to introduce the multilevel dependency structure into the imputation model. If we ignore such structure, the variance and covariance properties of the imputed data will not match those of the actual data. The implications of this error for the resulting analysis can be hard to predict. It depends on which parameter is being estimated, in particular whether the information on the estimator comes principally from within- or between-cluster information, on the actual design, and on the size of the correlations in the data.

Suppose we have $i = i, \ldots, I_j$ level-1 units observed on each of $j = 1, \ldots, J$ level-2 units. With two partially observed continuous variables, $Y_{1,i,j}$, $Y_{2,i,j}$ and fully observed variables $Y_{3,i,j}$, $Y_{4,i,j}$, the random intercepts imputation model is

$$\begin{aligned}
Y_{1,i,j} &= \beta_{0,1} + u_{1,j} + \beta_{1,1} Y_{3,i,j} + \beta_{2,1} Y_{4,i,j} + e_{1,i,j} \\
Y_{2,i,j} &= \beta_{0,2} + u_{2,j} + \beta_{1,2} Y_{3,i,j} + \beta_{2,2} Y_{4,i,j} + e_{2,i,j} \\
\begin{pmatrix} u_{1,j} \\ u_{2,j} \end{pmatrix} &\overset{i.i.d.}{\sim} N(\mathbf{0}, \mathbf{\Omega}_2) \\
\begin{pmatrix} e_{1,i,j} \\ e_{2,i,j} \end{pmatrix} &\overset{i.i.d.}{\sim} N(\mathbf{0}, \mathbf{\Omega}_1), \text{ independent of } (u_{0,j}, u_{1,j})^T.
\end{aligned} \tag{9.3}$$

Comparing with (9.1), we see that (9.3) is a joint random intercepts model for $Y_{1,i,j}$ and $Y_{2,i,j}$, where the fully observed variables are covariates and the partially observed variables responses. As discussed in Chapter 2, assuming MAR we obtain valid estimates of the parameters by fitting this model to the observed data. We can then impute missing data from the appropriate conditional distribution.

Thus if only $Y_{1,i,j}$ is missing for level-1 unit i belonging to level-2 unit j, it will be imputed from the conditional normal given $(Y_{2,i,j}, Y_{3,i,j}, Y_{4,i,j})$; if only $Y_{2,i,j}$ is missing it will be imputed from the conditional normal given $(Y_{1,i,j}, Y_{3,i,j}, Y_{4,i,j})$, and if both are missing they will be imputed from the bivariate normal given $(Y_{3,i,j}, Y_{4,i,j})$.

If we additionally assume a normal random intercepts model for $(Y_{3,i,j}, Y_{4,i,j})$ then $Y_{1,i,j}, Y_{2,i,j}, Y_{3,i,j}, Y_{4,i,j}$ have a joint random intercepts model:

$$\begin{aligned}
Y_{1,i,j} &= \beta_{0,1} + u_{1,j} + e_{1,i,j} \\
Y_{2,i,j} &= \beta_{0,2} + u_{2,j} + e_{2,i,j} \\
Y_{3,i,j} &= \beta_{0,3} + u_{3,j} + e_{3,i,j} \\
Y_{4,i,j} &= \beta_{0,4} + u_{4,j} + e_{4,i,j} \\
\begin{pmatrix} u_{1,j} \\ u_{2,j} \\ u_{3,j} \\ u_{4,j} \end{pmatrix} &\overset{i.i.d.}{\sim} N(\mathbf{0}, \mathbf{\Omega}_2) \perp \begin{pmatrix} e_{1,i,j} \\ e_{2,i,j} \\ e_{3,i,j} \\ e_{4,i,j} \end{pmatrix} \overset{i.i.d.}{\sim} N(\mathbf{0}, \mathbf{\Omega}_1),
\end{aligned} \tag{9.4}$$

where '$\perp$' denotes 'independent of'.

While model (9.4) is computationally slightly easier to fit than (9.3), with multilevel data (9.3) is more flexible, because we can extend it to allow $Y_{3,i,j}$

and $Y_{4,i,j}$ to have random coefficients at level-2. As we illustrate in Example 9.3 this aspect is useful when the covariate is observation time, and data are observed irregularly. More generally, a typical multilevel substantive model will have a number of covariates with random coefficients at level-2, and this should be reflected in the imputation model. This again points to including fully observed variables as covariates, in the form of (9.3).

Looking at (9.4) we see that while the mean of $Y_{1,i,j}, Y_{2,i,j}, Y_{3,i,j} Y_{4,i,j}$ varies across level-2 units, the covariance structure is common across all level-2 units. This means that the conditional distribution of any of the Y's given the others is the same across all level-2 units. This will not in general be true. Looking at (9.3) we see that if we extend the model to allow $Y_{3,i,j}$ and $Y_{4,i,j}$ to have random coefficients at level-2, then the conditional distribution of $(Y_{1,i,j}, Y_{2,i,j})$ given $(Y_{3,i,j}, Y_{4,i,j})$ varies by level-2 units: this is the distributional implication of introducing random coefficients at level-2. Nevertheless, the level-1 covariance matrix of $(Y_{1,i,j}, Y_{2,i,j})$ remains constant across level-2 units. If this is inappropriate, we may wish to allow the level-1 covariance matrix, $\mathbf{\Omega}_1$, to vary across level-2 units. We discuss this computationally more demanding option in Subsection 9.5.1. In practice, an approximation to this which will often prove adequate is to (i) have the partially observed variables as responses in the imputation model; (ii) have the fully observed variables as covariates and (iii) allow these covariates to have random coefficients if the data support this structure. In addition, as discussed in Chapter 7, this allows us to include nonlinear functions of the covariates if appropriate.

Example 9.1 Class size study *(ctd)*

Returning to the class size example, we now compare multilevel and single-level imputation for the missing *nlitpre* values (under missingness mechanism (9.2)). Having fitted the substantive model (9.1) to the partially observed data in `MLwiN`, we export the variables to `REALCOM-impute`, which proposes the imputation model shown in Figure 9.1.

This is an imputation model of the form of (9.4), which allows different means for the variables across schools, but imposes a common correlation. Thus, as discussed in the preceding paragraphs, this would not be appropriate if the substantive model (9.1), had random coefficients. In the latter case, we would need an imputation model of the form of (9.3), with only the partially observed variable as response, and the fully observed variables as covariates with random level-2 coefficients as supported by the data.

However, in this example, the substantive model has only random intercepts, so the imputation model shown in Figure 9.1, which treats all the variables as responses, is appropriate. This model can potentially allow for missing data in each variable (though in this case there is only missing data in *nlitpre*). The two continuous variables come first, each having its own intercept, random at the school level, and residual. The two binary variables we treat as unordered categorical, each with two levels. Thus each is associated with a single latent

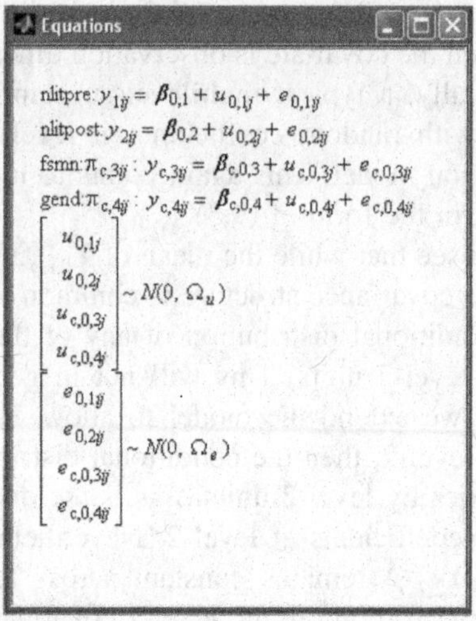

Figure 9.1 Imputation model for class size data, proposed by `REALCOM-impute` *following data export from* `MLwiN`.

normal, in exactly the way described in Chapter 5. Taking *fsmn*, this is shown by the notation

$$\text{fsmn:}\pi_{c,3,i,j} : Y_{c,3,i,j} = \beta_{c,0,3} + u_{c,0,3,j} + e_{c,0,3,i,j}$$

This indicates that the probability that $fsmn_{i,j}$ takes the value c is derived from the latent normal $Y_{c,3,i,j}$, which is modeled with a random intercept at the school level, and a residual at the pupil level which is constrained to have variance 1. The index '3' identifies this as the third of the four responses, and the index '0' identifies terms associated with constant (its fixed parameter, level-2 and 1 residuals). Additional fully observed auxiliary variables could be included on the RHS for each response variable if desired.

We use the `REALCOM-impute` software, which by default assumes a uniform prior over positive-definite inverse covariance matrices at level-1 and level-2. We fitted this model with a burn in of 2000, and imputed 20 datasets updating the MCMC sampler 500 times between each. We also created imputations ignoring the multilevel structure, effectively simply taking a linear regression model of *nlitpre* on the other variables as the imputation model. With single-level imputation we still fit the multilevel substantive model (9.1) to the imputed data. Table 9.2 shows the results.

By correctly taking into account the hierarchical nature of the data, multilevel MI gives point estimates close to the original, fully observed data, but with slightly increased standard errors (reflecting the lost information in the partially observed data). By contrast with single-level multiple imputation, the school

Table 9.2 Parameter estimates from original data, and with 20 imputations using multilevel MI and single-level MI.

Parameter	Estimates (std. errors) from		
	Full data multilevel model (n = 4873)	Multilevel MI	Single-level MI
β_0	0.088 (0.040)	1.04 (0.042)	0.121 (0.035)
β_1	0.733 (0.010)	0.732 (0.012)	0.651 (0.013)
β_2	−0.058 (0.018)	−0.052 (0.020)	−0.079 (0.023)
β_3	−0.068 (0.027)	−0.072 (0.029)	−0.105 (0.033)
σ_u^2	0.237 (0.028)	0.235 (0.029)	0.145 (0.019)
σ_e^2	0.372 (0.008)	0.376 (0.009)	0.435 (0.011)

level variance is dramatically underestimated, while the pupil level variance is overestimated. This has a direct impact on the standard errors of the linear model parameters. For coefficients that correspond to effects that that are wholly, or largely, between-cluster, such as the intercept, the standard errors will be too small from single-level MI analysis. By contrast, those estimated largely from within-subject information, that is, those that vary mainly within-clusters, in this example gender, eligibility for free school means and pre-reception attainment, will have standard errors that are too large. This is exactly the same impact that we see when a single-level substantive model is wrongly used for clustered data, albeit in a diluted form: the effect comes only from the inappropriate variance structure of the imputations not from an inappropriate variance structure applied to the entire data set. There is also an impact on the estimates themselves. We see that the gender and free school meal coefficients are overestimated (in absolute magnitude). This is because the effect of gender and free school meals is larger in the schools with more pupils (which are typically urban), which dominate the single-level imputation model. More discussion of this example is given in Carpenter *et al.* (2012b), and also Carpenter *et al.* (2011a) where imputation of the class size variable is also discussed. □

We now consider the more general setting, where the multilevel substantive model has covariates at level-1, and level-2. The latter are covariates that are constant for all level-1 units within a level-2 unit. For example, if level-1 is pupils and level-2 is classes, then characteristics of the class teacher (age, experience etc.) are constant for all pupils in the class. In general, data can be missing at both level-1 and level-2, and we wish to impute respecting the multilevel structure. We show how the multilevel imputation model described above can be extended to achieve this.

Example 9.2 Improving Medical Records

Ayieko *et al.* (2011) report the results of a cluster randomised trial involving eight hospitals to evaluate the effectiveness of a multifaceted intervention to improve admission paediatric care in Kenyan district hospitals. Overall, the results showed a marked benefit of the intervention, including improved completion of admission tasks, improved uptake of guideline recommended therapeutic practices and a reduction in inappropriate drug dosage.

Within this study was embedded the evaluation of a structured Patient Admission Record (PAR) form, designed to both systematise and improve the recording of essential paediatric admission information. This PAR form was made available to staff in all eight hospitals. Here, we give an illustrative analysis of how the completeness of paediatric admission records is affected by the use of this form, and some other relevant factors described below. A full analysis is given by Wagai *et al.* (2012).

Our analysis takes as a response the percentage completion of the desired admission tasks, and explores variation in this by use of the PAR form, child's gender, whether the hospital was one of the four randomised to receive the multifaceted intervention (hospitals numbered 1–4), the admitting clinician's gender and years of experience, and attendance of the admitting clinicians at short, ad-hoc refresher training sessions (termed Continuing Medical Education (CME) training) which were available in the four intervention hospitals.

For our analyses, we use the data which were collected every 6 months as part of hospital performance surveys. Each of these surveys sought to review 400 paediatric admission records from children admitted with an acute medical diagnosis in the preceding six months. This resulted in data from 8349 admissions, handled by 396 admitting clinicians in 8 hospitals, as shown in Table 9.3.

Table 9.3 Summary of data used for analysis of effectiveness of the PAR form. Denominators for proportions exclude admissions with missing values. Right column: proportion of total child-level or clinician-level records which are missing that variable. Hospitals 1–4 were randomised to receive a multifaceted intervention to improve admission paediatric care.

		Hospital								
		1	2	3	4	5	6	7	8	% missing
No. of admissions		1197	1210	1188	1007	798	798	1116	1035	
Mean completion	(%)	89	72	88	83	32	49	63	75	0
PAR use	(%)	97	82	96	92	22	52	60	97	0
Female child	(%)	42	39	41	39	44	38	44	41	6
Female clinician	(%)	76	60	52	70	64	92	58	54	14
Median years experience		0.5	0	0	4	3	3	0	0	20
Cont. Med. Ed.	(%)	46	20	35	59	Not offered				9

Table 9.3 also shows the proportion of missing observations. While around 6% of children did not have their sex recorded, most of the missing information is at the clinician level. Since each clinician was responsible for the admission of a number of children, this results in a complete records analysis of only 6775 out of 8349 (81%) of the available records. Moreover, preliminary analyses suggest clinician level data may not be MCAR.

Let i index child, j clinician and k hospital and '1[.]' denote an indicator random variable for the event in brackets. Our multilevel substantive model is the following:

$$\begin{aligned}
\text{completion}_{i,j,k} &= \beta_0 + u_{j,k} + \nu_k + \beta_1 1[\text{PAR use}_{i,j,k}] + \beta_2 1[\text{Female child}_{i,j,k}] \\
&\quad + \beta_3 1[\text{Female clinician}_{j,k}] + \beta_4(\text{years experience})_{j,k} \\
&\quad + \beta_5 1[\text{Intervention hospital}_k] + \beta_6[\text{Clinician takes CME}_{j,k}] \\
&\quad + \beta_7 1[\text{PAR use}_{i,j,k}] \times 1[\text{Clinician takes CME}_{j,k}] + \epsilon_{i,j,k} \\
\nu_k &\sim N(0, \sigma_\nu^2) \\
u_{j,k} &\sim N(0, \sigma_u^2) \\
e_{i,j,k} &\sim N(0, \sigma_e^2).
\end{aligned} \tag{9.5}$$

We return to this example after describing an appropriate multilevel imputation model. □

We now describe the extension of the imputation model (9.3) to include level-2 variables. As usual, we begin by considering continuous variables, which we model with the normal distribution, before extending the discussion to other data types via the latent normal structure described in Chapters 4–5. Let $j = 1, \ldots, J$ index level-2 units, and $i = 1, \ldots, I$ index level-1 units nested within level-2. For notational simplicity, we assume there are I level-1 units for each level-2 unit, but this is not required for any of what follows.

We suppose that in the multilevel dataset at hand there are p_1 partially observed level-1 variables observed on level-1 unit i nested within level-2 unit j, which we denote by the $p_1 \times 1$ column vector $\mathbf{Y}^{(1)}_{i,j}$. We also suppose there are f_1 fully observed level-1 variables, including the constant, which we use as level-1 covariates in our imputation model and thus denote by the $1 \times f_1$ row vector $\mathbf{X}^{(1)}_{i,j}$. In general, we will allow each of these f_1 variables, $(X^{(1)}_{i,j,1}, \ldots, X^{(1)}_{i,j,f_1})$ to predict each of the p_1 level-1 variables observed on unit i, j: $(Y^{(1)}_{i,j,1}, \ldots Y^{(1)}_{i,j,p_1})$, so there will be $f_1 p_1$ level-1 regression coefficients.

Further, let $\mathbf{Z}^{(1)}_{i,j}$ denote the $(1 \times q_1)$ row vector of covariates with random coefficients at level-2, including the constant. Typically, but not necessarily, a subset of the covariates $\mathbf{X}^{(1)}_{i,j}$ will have random coefficients at level-2, so that $\mathbf{Z}^{(1)}_{i,j}$ is a subset of $\mathbf{X}^{(1)}_{i,j}$. For each of the p_1 level-1 responses on unit i, j there are thus q_1 random effects; there are thus $p_1 q_1$ random effects for each level-1 unit i, j.

Using similar notation, let $\mathbf{Y}_j^{(2)}$ denote the $(p_2 \times 1)$ column vector of partially observed level-2 variables on unit j. Again, we also suppose there are f_2 fully observed level-2 variables, including the constant, which we use as level-2 covariates in our imputation model and denote by the $1 \times f_2$ row vector $\mathbf{X}_j^{(2)}$.

We note that some of the level-1 covariates included in $\mathbf{X}_{i,j}^{(1)}$ may be 'level-2 covariates' – that is, constant across all level-1 units i belonging to the same level-2 unit j. However the reverse is not allowed: level-2 covariates must take a single value for each level-2 unit, j.

The general form of the multivariate normal model we use for imputation is then

$$\begin{aligned}
\mathbf{Y}_{i,j}^{(1)} &= (\boldsymbol{I}_{p_1} \otimes \mathbf{X}_{i,j}^{(1)})\boldsymbol{\beta}^{(1)} + (\boldsymbol{I}_{p_1} \otimes \mathbf{Z}_{i,j}^{(1)})\boldsymbol{u}_j^{(1)} + \boldsymbol{e}_{i,j}^{(1)} \\
\mathbf{Y}_j^{(2)} &= (\boldsymbol{I}_{p_2} \otimes \mathbf{X}_j^{(2)})\boldsymbol{\beta}^{(2)} + \boldsymbol{u}_j^{(2)} \\
\boldsymbol{u}_j &= (\boldsymbol{u}_j^{(1)T}, \boldsymbol{u}_j^{(2)T})^T, \quad \boldsymbol{u}_j \sim N(\mathbf{0}, \boldsymbol{\Omega}_2) \\
\boldsymbol{e}_{i,j}^{(1)} &\sim N(\mathbf{0}, \boldsymbol{\Omega}_1)
\end{aligned} \tag{9.6}$$

As introduced above, the superscript (1) indicates level-1, and (2) level-2. The column vector $\boldsymbol{\beta}^{(1)}$ has $p_1 f_1$ elements, and the column vector $\boldsymbol{u}_j^{(1)}$ has $p_1 q_1$ elements. The column vector $\boldsymbol{\beta}^{(2)}$ has $p_2 f_2$ elements and the column vector $\boldsymbol{u}_2^{(2)}$ is simply the residuals at level-2 and thus a column vector of p_2 elements. $\boldsymbol{I}_p$ denotes the $(p \times p)$ identity matrix, and the symbol $\otimes$ is the Kronecker product, defined on p. 131. For example, if $\mathbf{X} = (X_1, X_2, X_3)$ then

$$\boldsymbol{I}_3 \otimes \mathbf{X} = \begin{pmatrix} X_1 & X_2 & X_3 & 0 & 0 & 0 & 0 & 0 & 0 \\ 0 & 0 & 0 & X_1 & X_2 & X_3 & 0 & 0 & 0 \\ 0 & 0 & 0 & 0 & 0 & 0 & X_1 & X_2 & X_3 \end{pmatrix}$$

Thus, for example, the notation $(\boldsymbol{I}_{p_1} \otimes \mathbf{X}_{i,j}^{(1)})\boldsymbol{\beta}^{(1)}$ is a concise way of writing that the mean of each of the p_1 responses from unit i, j is a different linear function of $\mathbf{X}_{i,j}^{(1)}$.

Example 9.3 Model for childhood and adult heights

To illustrate the multilevel multivariate-response model (9.6) we describe modelling childhood and adult heights. We have data from 108 children with height measured on up to six occasions around the age of 13, together with their adult heights. Altogether this gives 436 height measurements in childhood and 108 adult height measurements.

We therefore have a two level model, where level-1 is the repeated measures of childhood height, and level-2 is the adult height. As well as imputation of any missing childhood or adult data, such a model could be used to predict adult height from childhood height. At level-1, for each person j we have only one response at observation time $t_{i,j}$, namely the height. Although this is a relatively simple model, we write this using the notation for a multilevel multivariate response model set out above to illustrate its use. The model for the level-1 responses is a cubic in time, with random intercept and time terms. Adult height is modelled with a random intercept alone.

Let $t_{i,j}$ be the age of individual j when the ith height denoted $Y_{i,j}^{(1)}$ is measured, and $Y_j^{(2)}$ individual j's adult height. Under this model we have $\mathbf{X}_{i,j}^{(1)} = (1, t_{i,j}, t_{i,j}^2, t_{i,j}^3)$, $\boldsymbol{\beta}^{(1)} = (\beta_0^{(1)}, \beta_1^{(1)}, \beta_2^{(1)}, \beta_3^{(1)})^T$, $\mathbf{Z}_{i,j}^{(1)} = (1, t_{i,j})$, $\boldsymbol{u}_j^{(1)} = (u_{1,j}^{(1)}, u_{2,j}^{(1)})^T$, $\mathbf{X}_j^{(2)} = 1$, $\boldsymbol{\beta}^{(2)} = \beta_0^{(2)}$ and $\boldsymbol{u}_j^{(2)} = u_{1,j}^{(2)}$. Then

$$\begin{aligned} Y_{i,j}^{(1)} &= (\boldsymbol{I}_1 \otimes \mathbf{X}_{i,j}^{(1)})\boldsymbol{\beta}^{(1)} + (\boldsymbol{I}_1 \otimes \mathbf{Z}_{i,j}^{(1)})\boldsymbol{u}_j^{(1)} + e_{i,j}^{(1)} \\ Y_j^{(2)} &= (\boldsymbol{I}_1 \otimes \mathbf{X}_j^{(2)})\boldsymbol{\beta}^{(2)} + \boldsymbol{u}_j^{(2)} \end{aligned} \tag{9.7}$$

$$\begin{aligned} \begin{pmatrix} u_{1,j}^{(1)} \\ u_{2,j}^{(1)} \\ u_{1,j}^{(2)} \end{pmatrix} &\sim N(0, \boldsymbol{\Omega}_2) \\ e_{i,j} &\sim N(0, \boldsymbol{\Omega}_1). \end{aligned} \tag{9.8}$$

Because we only have one response for each individual j at time i, the matrix $\boldsymbol{I}_1 = 1$ (scalar), so that $(\boldsymbol{I}_1 \otimes \mathbf{X}_{i,j}^{(1)}) = \mathbf{X}_{i,j}^{(1)}$. With multivariate responses at each observation time, the notation gives the mean of each response as a different linear function of the same covariates.

Using the fitting algorithm described in Section 9.2 gives the parameter estimates in Table 9.4. Children are on average 153 cm at 13 years, and there is

Table 9.4 Parameter estimates from fitting model (9.8) to the growth data.

Coefficient	Estimate			Std. Err.
Level-1 model				
Intercept (cm)	153.05			0.69
Age (centred 13 years)	7.07			0.16
Age-squared	0.294			0.054
Age-cubed	−0.208			0.029
Level-2 model				
Intercept (cm)	174.7			0.80
Level-2 covariance matrix		57.77	1.30	50.01
		1.30	0.53	1.24
		50.01	1.24	69.42
Level-1 variance			3.12	

evidence of a linear, quadratic and cubic component of the growth curve. On average adults are 175 cm, and there is a strong association between childhood and adult height. □

The example shows how the multilevel imputation model (9.6) allows us to naturally handle irregular observation times, and if desired impute at a specific observation time for all individuals. Under model (9.6), if i indexes observation time, then we have an unstructured covariance matrix for all observations at a particular time, and the longitudinal correlation comes through the random structure at level-2. With random intercepts alone, we have an exchangeable structure (correlation is constant across time); if we include time as random at level-2 we allow the correlation to decline as time between observations increases, while the marginal variance may increase with time. If we have a dummy variable indexing time, random at level-2, we obtain an unstructured longitudinal covariance matrix. In applications, ideally the covariance structure in the imputation model should be consistent with that in the substantive model. In practice, unless the number of level-2 units is sufficiently large, an unstructured covariance over time may be poorly estimated and random intercepts and slopes will likely give adequate flexibility.

9.2 MCMC algorithm for imputation model

We now describe a general MCMC algorithm for fitting the multivariate multilevel imputation model (9.6). We have the following parameters: $\boldsymbol{\beta}^{(1)}, \boldsymbol{\beta}^{(2)}$, the random effects $\boldsymbol{u}_j^{(1)}, \boldsymbol{u}_j^{(2)}$, the level-1 residuals $\boldsymbol{e}_{i,j}^{(1)}$ and the covariance matrices $\boldsymbol{\Omega}_2, \boldsymbol{\Omega}_1$.

Taking an improper prior for the coefficients $\boldsymbol{\beta}$, and Wishart priors for the inverse covariance matrices, at update step r we update each of these in turn, conditional on all the others, as follows:

1. draw $\boldsymbol{\beta}^{(1)}$ from the $f_1 p_1$ variate normal distribution with mean

$$\left[\sum_{i,j}(\boldsymbol{I}_{p_1} \otimes \mathbf{X}_{i,j}^{(1)})^T (\boldsymbol{\Omega}_1)^{-1} (\boldsymbol{I}_{p_1} \otimes \mathbf{X}_{i,j}^{(1)})\right]^{-1} \times$$

$$\left[\sum_{i,j}(\boldsymbol{I}_{p_1} \otimes \mathbf{X}_{i,j}^{(1)})^T (\boldsymbol{\Omega}_1)^{-1} \left\{\mathbf{Y}_{i,j}^{(1)} - (\boldsymbol{I}_{p_1} \otimes \mathbf{Z}_{i,j}^{(1)})\boldsymbol{u}_j^{(1)}\right\}\right],$$

and covariance matrix

$$\left[\sum_{i,j}(\boldsymbol{I}_{p_1} \otimes \mathbf{X}_{i,j}^{(1)})^T (\boldsymbol{\Omega}_1)^{-1} (\boldsymbol{I}_{p_1} \otimes \mathbf{X}_{i,j}^{(1)})\right]^{-1}.$$

2. Partition the covariance matrix $\mathbf{\Omega}_2$ as

$$\mathbf{\Omega}_2 = \begin{pmatrix} \mathbf{\Omega}_2^{(1)} & \mathbf{\Omega}_2^{(1,2)} \\ \mathbf{\Omega}_2^{(2,1)} & \mathbf{\Omega}_2^{(2)} \end{pmatrix}, \tag{9.9}$$

where $\mathbf{\Omega}_2^{(1)}$ is the $p_1 q_1$ by $p_1 q_1$ variance matrix of the $\boldsymbol{u}_j^{(1)}$, $\mathbf{\Omega}_2^{(2)}$ is the p_2 by p_2 variance matrix of the $\boldsymbol{u}_j^{(2)}$, and $\mathbf{\Omega}_2^{(1,2)}$ is their $p_1 q_1$ by p_2 covariance matrix.

Sample $\boldsymbol{\beta}^{(2)}$ from the $p_2 f_2$ variate normal distribution with mean

$$\left[\sum_j (\boldsymbol{I}_{p_2} \otimes \mathbf{X}_j^{(2)})^T (\mathbf{\Omega}_2^{(2)})^{-1} (\boldsymbol{I}_{p_2} \otimes \mathbf{X}_j^{(2)})\right]^{-1} \sum_j (\boldsymbol{I}_{p_2} \otimes \mathbf{X}_j^{(2)})^T (\mathbf{\Omega}_2^{(2)})^{-1} \mathbf{Y}_j^{(2)},$$

and covariance matrix

$$\left[\sum_j (\boldsymbol{I}_{p_2} \otimes \mathbf{X}_j^{(2)})^T (\mathbf{\Omega}_2^{(2)})^{-1} (\boldsymbol{I}_{p_2} \otimes \mathbf{X}_j^{(2)})\right]^{-1}.$$

3. Calculate

$$\boldsymbol{u}_j^{(2)} = \mathbf{Y}_j^{(2)} - (\boldsymbol{I}_{p_2} \otimes \mathbf{X}_j^{(2)})\boldsymbol{\beta}^{(2)},$$

and form the conditional multivariate normal distribution of $\boldsymbol{u}_j^{(1)} | \boldsymbol{u}_j^{(2)}$ with mean

$$\boldsymbol{\mu}_j^{1|2} = \mathbf{\Omega}_2^{(1,2)} (\mathbf{\Omega}_2^{(2)})^{-1} \boldsymbol{u}_j^{(2)}$$

and variance

$$\mathbf{\Omega}_2^{1|2} = \mathbf{\Omega}_2^{(1)} - \mathbf{\Omega}_2^{(1,2)} (\mathbf{\Omega}_2^{(2)})^{-1} \mathbf{\Omega}_2^{(2,1)}.$$

4. For each $j = 1, \ldots, J$ sample $\boldsymbol{u}_j^{(1)}$ from the $p_1 q_1$ multivariate normal distribution with mean

$$\left[\sum_i (\boldsymbol{I}_{p_1} \otimes \mathbf{Z}_{i,j}^{(1)})^T (\mathbf{\Omega}_1)^{-1} (\boldsymbol{I}_{p_1} \otimes \mathbf{Z}_{i,j}^{(1)}) + (\mathbf{\Omega}_2^{1|2})^{-1}\right]^{-1} \times$$

$$\left[(\mathbf{\Omega}_2^{1|2})^{-1} \boldsymbol{\mu}_j^{1|2} + \sum_i (\boldsymbol{I}_{p_1} \otimes \mathbf{Z}_{i,j}^{(1)})^T (\mathbf{\Omega}_1)^{-1} \left\{\mathbf{Y}_{i,j}^{(1)} - (\boldsymbol{I}_{p_1} \otimes \mathbf{X}_{i,j}^{(1)})\boldsymbol{\beta}^{(1)}\right\}\right],$$

and covariance matrix

$$\left[\sum_i (\boldsymbol{I}_{p_1} \otimes \mathbf{Z}_{i,j}^{(1)})^T (\mathbf{\Omega}_1)^{-1} (\boldsymbol{I}_{p_1} \otimes \mathbf{Z}_{i,j}^{(1)}) + (\mathbf{\Omega}_2^{1|2})^{-1}\right]^{-1}.$$

5. Calculate

$$\boldsymbol{e}_{i,j} = \mathbf{Y}^{(1)}_{i,j} - (\boldsymbol{I}_{p_1} \otimes \mathbf{X}^{(1)}_{i,j})\boldsymbol{\beta}^{(1)} - (\boldsymbol{I}_{p_1} \otimes \mathbf{Z}^{(1)}_{i,j})\boldsymbol{u}^{(1)}_j$$

and form $\boldsymbol{u}_j = (\boldsymbol{u}^{(1)T}_j \boldsymbol{u}^{(2)T}_j)^T$.

6. Draw $(\boldsymbol{\Omega}_2)^{-1}$ from $\mathrm{W}(\nu_u, \mathbf{S}_u)$, where $\nu_u = J + \nu_{up}$, (J is the number of level-2 units),

$$\mathbf{S}_u = \left[\sum_j \boldsymbol{u}_j \boldsymbol{u}^T_j + \mathbf{S}^{-1}_{up} \right]^{-1},$$

and the prior for $(\boldsymbol{\Omega}_2)^{-1}$ is $\mathrm{W}(\nu_{up}, \mathbf{S}_{up})$.

7. Draw $(\boldsymbol{\Omega}_1)^{-1}$ from $\mathrm{W}(\nu_e, \mathbf{S}_e)$, where $\nu_e = IJ + \nu_{ep}$, (IJ is the total number of level-1 units),

$$\mathbf{S}_e = \left[\sum_{i,j} \boldsymbol{e}_{i,j} \boldsymbol{e}^T_{i,j} + \mathbf{S}^{-1}_{ep} \right]^{-1},$$

and the prior for $(\boldsymbol{\Omega}_1)^{-1}$ is $\mathrm{W}(\nu_{ep}, \mathbf{S}_{ep})$.

We note that the multilevel imputation model (9.6) naturally extends from 2 levels to any number of levels, including allowing coefficients to be random at the different levels. Likewise the fitting procedure described above extends to any number of levels without requiring any additional conceptual development.

Linear constraints on regression coefficients

In practice, we will quite often wish to have different covariates for different responses, both at level-1 and level-2. We focus on level-1, and the same approach applies to level-2 covariates. Computationally, this can be handled most easily by fitting a 'maximal' model, with f_1 covariates for all p_1 responses, within which certain coefficients are constrained to zero. Such a set of constraints is particular example of imposing l independent linear constraints on some, or all of the $f_1 p_1$ elements of $\boldsymbol{\beta}^{(1)}$. These constraints will involve $l^\star \geq l$ distinct elements of $\boldsymbol{\beta}^{(1)}$. The following computational procedure allows us to do this. For simplicity, we drop the superscript '(1)' on $\boldsymbol{\beta}$.

Re-order the elements of the coefficient vector $\boldsymbol{\beta}$ so that l of the $l^\star$ elements involved in the linear constraint appear first. We can write the set of constraints as

$$\mathbf{C}\boldsymbol{\beta} = \mathbf{k}, \tag{9.10}$$

where $\mathbf{C}$ is $l \times f_1 p_1$ and $\mathbf{k}$ is $l \times 1$.

We can write the QR decomposition of $\mathbf{C}$ as $\mathbf{C} = \mathbf{QR}$, where $\mathbf{Q}$ is an orthogonal $l \times l$ matrix, and $\mathbf{R}$ is $l \times f_1 p_1$. Further we can write $\mathbf{R} = (\boldsymbol{T}, \mathbf{V})$, where

$\boldsymbol{T}$ is an upper triangular $l \times l$ matrix and $\mathbf{V}$ is of dimension $l \times (f_1 p_1 - l)$. Let $\boldsymbol{\beta}^T = (\boldsymbol{\beta}_1^T, \boldsymbol{\beta}_2^T)$, where $\boldsymbol{\beta}_1$ contains the first l elements of the re-ordered coefficients, and $\boldsymbol{\beta}_2$ contains the remaining $f_1 p_1 - l$.

From (9.10) we have $\mathbf{Q}^T\mathbf{k} = \mathbf{Q}^T\mathbf{Q}\mathbf{R}\boldsymbol{\beta} = (\boldsymbol{T}, \mathbf{V})\boldsymbol{\beta}$, and we can construct

$$\begin{pmatrix} \boldsymbol{T} & \mathbf{V} \\ \mathbf{0} & \boldsymbol{I} \end{pmatrix} \boldsymbol{\beta} = \begin{pmatrix} (\boldsymbol{T}, \mathbf{V})\boldsymbol{\beta} \\ \boldsymbol{\beta}_2 \end{pmatrix} = \begin{pmatrix} \mathbf{Q}^T\mathbf{k} \\ \boldsymbol{\beta}_2 \end{pmatrix},$$

where $\boldsymbol{I}$ is $(f_1 p_1 - l) \times (f_1 p_1 - l)$, and $\mathbf{0}$ is $(f_1 p_1 - l) \times l$. Then, recalling $\boldsymbol{T}$ is upper triangular,

$$\begin{aligned} \begin{pmatrix} \boldsymbol{\beta}_1 \\ \boldsymbol{\beta}_2 \end{pmatrix} = \boldsymbol{\beta} &= \begin{pmatrix} \boldsymbol{T} & \mathbf{V} \\ \mathbf{0} & \boldsymbol{I} \end{pmatrix}^{-1} \begin{pmatrix} \mathbf{Q}^T\mathbf{k} \\ \boldsymbol{\beta}_2 \end{pmatrix} \\ &= \begin{pmatrix} \boldsymbol{T}^{-1} & -\boldsymbol{T}^{-1}\mathbf{V} \\ \mathbf{0} & \boldsymbol{I} \end{pmatrix} \begin{pmatrix} \mathbf{Q}^T\mathbf{k} \\ \boldsymbol{\beta}_2 \end{pmatrix} \\ &= \begin{pmatrix} \boldsymbol{T}^{-1}\mathbf{Q}^T\mathbf{k} - \boldsymbol{T}^{-1}\mathbf{V}\boldsymbol{\beta}_2 \\ \boldsymbol{\beta}_2 \end{pmatrix} \end{aligned} \tag{9.11}$$

It follows that if we first draw the $\boldsymbol{\beta}_2$ in the usual way – without any constraint – from their marginal distribution derived from step 1 on p. 214, we can apply (9.11) to calculate the corresponding values of β_1 under the linear constraint (9.10). Update steps for the other parameters remain unchanged.

If desired, though it is unlikely in the context of MI, we can use the same result to impose constraints on the random parameters $\boldsymbol{u}^{(1)}$. For further discussion see Goldstein (2010) pp. 176–7.

Ordered and unordered categorical data

So far we have only considered continuous data. We handle binary, ordinal or categorical data using the latent normal approach described in Chapters 4–5, which we can use at both level-1 and level-2.

Hence, for an M-level categorical level-1 variable, there will be $(M - 1)$ uncorrelated latent normal variables at level-1, each with variance constrained to 1, and constrained to be uncorrelated with the other $M - 2$ latent normals. Each of these may have a random intercept at level-2, and these intercepts may be correlated, although in applications with relatively few level-2 units we may need to restrict some of these correlations to zero in order to avoid over-parameterisation at level-2. We return to this point in Section 9.4.

For level-2 discrete variables, the associated latent normals may in principle be correlated with the level-2 random effects associated with level-1 variables.

As mentioned above, and discussed in more detail in Chapters 4–5, the latent normal structure for handling categorical variables imposes constraints on elements of the covariance matrices. When fitting the model using MCMC, this means we can no longer update the inverse covariance matrices using a draw from a Wishart distribution, as described in steps 6 and 7 on page 216. Instead, we need to update the elements of the covariance matrix individually using an appropriate MH step. This proceeds exactly as described in Chapter 4.

Imputing missing values

As described in Chapter 3, missing continuous responses are imputed from the appropriate conditional normal distribution, conditional on current parameter values and other data for the unit. With discrete data, again as described in Chapters 4–5, for each missing value we first draw the latent normal from the appropriate conditional distribution, and then draw the corresponding discrete variable value.

Example 9.2 Improving medical records *(ctd)*

We return to the hospital records example, and consider the appropriate imputation model. In line with the substantive model, this is multilevel, with patients at level-1 and clinicians at level-2. Ideally, we would have hospitals random at level-3, but our software does not accommodate this.

Because the data suggest that relations between variables may be different between the four hospitals randomised to receive the intervention (H1–H4) and those that did not (H5–H8), we impute separately in these two groups, always including a fixed effect of hospital. In addition, as we are interested in exploring the interaction between PAR use and whether or not a clinician undertakes CME, and PAR use is fully observed, within the randomised and control hospitals we further impute impute separately among those who do, and do not, use PAR. We therefore split the data into four groups, by hospital randomisation group and PAR use, and impute separately in all four groups. Thus, for PAR users among H5–H8 (where CME was not on offer), the imputation model is

$$\text{completion}_{i,j,k} = \beta_{1,0}^{(1)} + \sum_{l=2}^{4} \beta_{1,l}^{(1)} 1[k = 4 + l] + u_{1,j}^{(1)} + e_{1,i,j,k}^{(1)}$$

$$\Pr(\text{female child}_{i,j,k}) = \Pr\{\beta_{2,0}^{(1)} + \sum_{l=2}^{4} \beta_{2,l}^{(1)} 1[k = 4 + l] + u_{2,j}^{(1)} + e_{2,i,j,k}^{(1)} > 0\}$$

$$\text{years experience}_{j,k} = \beta_{1,0}^{(2)} + \sum_{l=2}^{4} \beta_{2,l}^{(2)} 1[k = 4 + l] + u_{1,j}^{(2)}$$

$$\Pr(\text{female clinician}_{j,k}) = \Pr\{\beta_{2,0}^{(2)} + \sum_{l=2}^{4} \beta_{2,l}^{(2)} 1[k = 4 + l] + u_{2,j}^{(2)} > 0\}$$

$$(u_{1,j}^{(1)}, u_{2,j}^{(1)}, u_{1,j}^{(2)}, u_{2,j}^{(2)})^T \sim N(\mathbf{0}, \mathbf{\Omega}_2),\ \mathbf{\Omega}_2 \text{ unconstrained except } \{\mathbf{\Omega}_2\}_{(4,4)} = 1,$$
$$\begin{pmatrix} e_{1,i,j,k}^{(1)} \\ e_{2,i,j,k}^{(1)} \end{pmatrix} \sim N\left\{\mathbf{0}, \begin{pmatrix} \sigma_{e,1}^2 & \sigma_{e,1,2} \\ \sigma_{e,1,2} & 1 \end{pmatrix}\right\}. \quad (9.12)$$

We fitted each of the four models, and imputed the missing values, using the `REALCOM-impute` software. To improve mixing of the MCMC chains, completion and years experience were, separately for each of the four imputation models, transformed to have mean 0 and variance 1 before imputation (and back transformed afterwards). Each imputation model was burned in for 5000 updates and the model was updated 500 times between each of the 10 imputations. Examination of the chains showed the sampler had converged and satisfactory mixing.

Table 9.5 shows the results. In both analyses, PAR dramatically increases the percentage of completeness in the hospital admission record, and the randomised intervention adds an additional 10% to completeness on average. However, whereas the complete records suggest clinicians with 3 years' experience will, on average, have about 1% less completion ($p < 0.05$), this effect is halved and no longer significant at the 5% level after imputation. More dramatically, after imputation, admissions records from children admitted by a clinician who had participated in continuing medical education (CME), but not used the PAR, have completion reduced by 5% ($p < 0.001$). Unsurprisingly, this is a small group of admissions (2.5% of those in H1–H4), yet still worth further investigation. Records from admissions by clinicians who took CME and used PAR show only a small and statistically nonsignificant increase in completion of (5.9–5.0) = 0.9% over those who only used PAR. Turning to the variance components, the complete records analysis substantially underestimates both between clinician and between child variability in record completeness, with complete record estimates of variance components lying outside the corresponding 95% confidence intervals from the MI analysis. Residuals are slightly heavy tailed relative to the normal distribution, but this is insufficient to substantively affect these inferences.

Table 9.5 Results of fitting (9.5) to complete records and after multilevel multiple imputation.

	Complete records			Multilevel MI		
Variable	Est.	SE	p-value	Est.	SE	p-value
PAR	50.20	0.43	< 0.001	48.71	0.41	< 0.001
female child	0.26	0.23	0.27	0.14	0.25	0.59
female clinician	0.15	0.88	0.86	0.46	1.09	0.68
years experience	−0.33	0.08	<0.001	−0.18	0.29	0.54
intervention hospital	9.99	3.10	0.001	11.03	3.48	0.002
CME	0.71	1.71	0.42	−5.00	1.76	0.005
PAR use × CME	−0.46	1.37	0.74	5.91	1.17	<0.001
constant	26.3	2.3	< 0.001	25.49	2.67	<0.001
Variance components		95% Conf. Int.			95% Conf. Int.	
hospital, σ_v^2	17.10	(5.02–58.25)		21.73	(6.37–74.14)	
clinician, σ_u^2	41.06	(33.41–50.46)		52.25	(42.57–64.13)	
child, σ_e^2	88.95	(85.93–92.07)		100.19	(97.08–103.41)	

The practically important difference between the complete records and MI analysis here is largely due to the additional information from the partially observed records (typically where the clinician did not report their gender or years of experience). Indeed there is very little information about the missing values of clinician's years of experience in the other variables. Auxiliary variables from the dataset could usefully be included to address this; since many clinicians report no experience, categorising this variable may also be appropriate. As usual, we make the assumption of MAR, and sensitivity analysis is appropriate to explore the robustness of the inferences to plausible MNAR mechanisms (see Ch. 10).

In conclusion, multilevel MI allows imputation of missing variables at the child and clinician level, respecting the multilevel structure. This confirms the substantive impact on completion of paediatric admission procedures of PAR and the randomised intervention, questions any effect of clinicians' years of experience and questions whether CME (at least as provided) is helpful in improving the completeness of admissions records. □

9.3 Imputing level-2 covariates using FCS

We now consider the conditional distribution of a level-2 variable given level-1 variables, when the joint distribution is bivariate normal. This gives some insight into the application of FCS to multilevel data. The algorithm we describe now was developed by Ian White (personal communication).

Consider a two level structure, where $Y_{i,j}^{(1)}$ is a level-1 variable, observed $i = 1, \ldots p$ times on each of the $j = 1, \ldots, J$ level-2 units, and $Y_j^{(2)}$ is a level-2 variable, observed once on each of the J level-2 units. Let $\mathbf{Y}_j^{(1)} = (Y_{1,j}^{(1)}, \ldots, Y_{p,j}^{(1)})^T$, and let $\mathbf{j}_p$ be a $p \times 1$ vector of 1's. Under an exchangeable correlation structure (i.e. random intercepts) for the $\mathbf{Y}_j^{(1)}$, we have

$$\begin{pmatrix} \mathbf{Y}_j^{(1)} \\ Y_j^{(2)} \end{pmatrix} \sim N\left[\begin{pmatrix} \beta_0^{(1)}\mathbf{j}_p \\ \beta_0^{(2)} \end{pmatrix}, \begin{pmatrix} \omega_1 \boldsymbol{J} + \sigma^2 \boldsymbol{I} & \omega_{1,2}\,\mathbf{j}_p \\ \omega_{1,2}\,\mathbf{j}_p{}^T & \omega_2 \end{pmatrix}\right],$$

where $\boldsymbol{J}$ is a $p \times p$ matrix of 1's and $\boldsymbol{I}$ is the $p \times p$ identity matrix. The distribution of $Y_j^{(2)}|\mathbf{Y}_1^{(1)}$ is thus normal, with mean $\beta_0^{(2)} + A(\mathbf{Y}_j^{(1)} - \beta_0^{(1)}\mathbf{j}_p)$, where $A = \omega_{1,2}\mathbf{j}_p^T(\omega_1 \boldsymbol{J} + \sigma^2 \boldsymbol{I})^{-1}$. This inverse is of form $(a\boldsymbol{J} + b\boldsymbol{I})$, where $a = -\omega_1/\{\sigma^2(p\omega_1 + \sigma^2)\}$ and $b = 1/\sigma^2$. Writing $e_{i,j} = Y_{i,j}^{(1)} - \beta_0^{(1)}$, we have

$$\begin{aligned} \mathrm{E}[Y_j^{(2)}|\mathbf{Y}_j^{(1)}] &= \beta_0^{(2)} + \omega_{1,2}(pa + b)\sum_{i=1}^{p} e_{i,j} \\ &= \left[\beta_0^{(2)} - p\omega_{1,2}(pa + b)\beta_0^{(1)}\right] + p\omega_{1,2}(pa + b)\bar{\mathbf{Y}}_j^{(1)}. \end{aligned}$$

Therefore, in the full conditional specification approach we need to include the mean of the level-1 responses as the covariate in the imputation of the level-2 variable, as our intuition would lead us to expect.

Now suppose we have no level-2 variables, but two groups of p variables observed at level-1, which for clarity we denote by $\mathbf{X}_j$, and $\mathbf{Y}_j$, both $(p \times 1)$ vectors. Again suppose a random intercepts model, so that the distribution is

$$\begin{pmatrix} \mathbf{X}_j \\ \mathbf{Y}_j \end{pmatrix} \sim N\left[\begin{pmatrix} \boldsymbol{\mu}_X \\ \boldsymbol{\mu}_Y \end{pmatrix}, \begin{pmatrix} \omega_X \boldsymbol{J} + \varsigma_X \boldsymbol{I} & \omega_{X,Y} \boldsymbol{J} + \varsigma_{X,Y} \boldsymbol{I} \\ \omega_{X,Y} \boldsymbol{J} + \varsigma_{X,Y} \boldsymbol{I} & \omega_Y \boldsymbol{J} + \varsigma_Y \boldsymbol{I} \end{pmatrix}\right] \tag{9.13}$$

Under this model,

$$\mathrm{E}[\mathbf{Y}_j|\mathbf{X}_j] = \boldsymbol{\mu}_Y + \boldsymbol{A}(\mathbf{X}_j - \boldsymbol{\mu}_X),$$

where

$$\boldsymbol{A} = \frac{1}{p}\left(\frac{\varsigma_X \omega_{X,Y} - \varsigma_{X,Y}\omega_X}{\varsigma_X(\omega_X + \varsigma_X/p)}\right)\boldsymbol{J} + \frac{\varsigma_{X,Y}}{\varsigma_X}\boldsymbol{I}.$$

Thus, since $\boldsymbol{J}\mathbf{X}_j/p$ is a $p \times 1$ vector each of whose elements is $\bar{\mathbf{X}}_j = \sum_{i=1}^{p} X_{i,j}/p$, $\mathrm{E}[\mathbf{Y}_j|\mathbf{X}_j]$ is a linear in both $\bar{\mathbf{X}}_j$ and $\mathbf{X}_j$.

So in FCS, under an exchangeable covariance matrix, we must include both mean and individual $X_{i,j}$ as covariates in the imputation model for $\mathbf{Y}_j$, and vice versa. Likewise, if have a joint imputation model and decide to include (fully observed) $\mathbf{X}_j$ as covariates, we need to include the mean, $\bar{\mathbf{X}}_j$ as well as the observations $\mathbf{X}_j$.

The above argument depends on the exchangeable correlation matrix in (9.13). In the case of random intercepts and slopes, instead of the mean of $\mathbf{X}_j$, we will have a function of the observations and observation time. We conclude that under FCS setting up appropriate conditional models is not straightforward, since the functions of the variables we condition on depend on the assumed covariance structure. Conversely, under a joint modelling approach, provided we include all variables as responses, we only need to specify the covariance structure for each response.

With a mix of data types at both levels, the appropriate specifications for FCS are thus awkward. In addition, with structured covariance matrices, estimation of the parameters of each conditional distribution gives information about the parameters of the marginal variance-covariance matrix. Thus the criterion for the validity of the FCS sampler is violated (see Subsection 4.5.1). Nevertheless, there are particular multilevel settings for which the FCS procedure is relatively easy to implement and hence convenient. Two important examples are

1. simple two-level multilevel designs with exchangeability within clusters, and

2. repeated measurements with common times of measurement, as is commonly met in clinical trials.

For these, and other particular settings, FCS is a convenient approach. However, once we move to the general multilevel setting, for example with unbalanced times of measurement and cross-classified structures, the FCS approach would appear to lose much of the simplicity and so loses its computational attraction. We therefore do not pursue it further in this setting.

9.4 Individual patient meta-analysis

An important application of multilevel imputation is individual patient meta-analysis, particularly when – as will usually be the case – not all contributing studies have followed the same protocol. For example, we may wish to estimate a risk model, but find that not all the contributing studies have collected the set of predictors we wish to include. Another issue that may arise alongside this is that studies may have recorded variables on different scales (e.g. continuous, ordinal). In addition to this, there will typically be missing data on variables that should have been recorded in a study, but for one reason or another were not.

The chief issue for applying multilevel MI using (9.6), using the latent normal structure to handle discrete variables, is that there are usually a large number of variables relative to the number of studies. If there are p continuous variables, then the level-2 (study level) covariance matrix will have $p(p+1)/2$ parameters; unless the number of studies comfortably exceeds this, estimation is likely to be extremely imprecise, and may not be possible. In practice there are therefore two options, which parallel those discussed in Section 8.5. We can either

1. stabilize the level-2 covariance matrix using a ridge-regression type approach, i.e., by adding a positive constant λ to the diagonal terms (variances) in the level-2 covariance matrix, or

2. restrict some of the level-2 covariance terms to zero, or restrict some of the partial correlation coefficients in the inverse level-2 covariance matrix to zero.

Given a (somewhat arbitrary) choice of ridge parameter λ, the first option is simpler computationally, especially if there are no categorical variables at level-2. In this case, the ridge-type approach still permits direct drawing of the level-2 inverse covariance matrix from the Wishart distribution.

The second option is perhaps less arbitrary. However, since it involves constraining (typically to zero) level-2 covariances (and possibly variances) for which there is little information, we then have to update the covariance matrix elementwise, as discussed on p. 218 and described in Chapter 4.

One approach to decide which study-level variances/covariances should be set to zero is as follows. First, for each variable in turn fit a multilevel model with component of variance at the patient and study level, and estimate the study level residuals. Then calculate the empirical covariances of the estimated study level residuals. Variables for which the between study component of variance is very small, or not estimable can be constrained to zero in the imputation model. Likewise, covariances which are practically unimportant can be constrained to zero in the imputation model. Such constraints can be imposed with the `REALCOM-impute` software.

In many examples it may suffice to simply set all the level-2 covariance terms to zero. To understand the implication of this, consider an imputation model for individuals (level-1) within a study (level-2), who have data on systolic and diastolic blood pressure (SBP, DBP). The imputation model is

$$\mathrm{SBP}_{i,j} = \beta_{0,1} + u_{0,1,j} + e_{1,i,j}$$

$$\mathrm{DBP}_{i,j} = \beta_{0,2} + u_{0,2,j} + e_{2,i,j}$$

$$\begin{pmatrix} u_{0,1,j} \\ u_{0,2,j} \end{pmatrix} \sim N\left[\begin{pmatrix} 0 \\ 0 \end{pmatrix}, \begin{pmatrix} \sigma^2_{u1} & \sigma_{u1,u2} \\ \sigma_{u1,u2} & \sigma^2_{u2} \end{pmatrix}\right]$$

$$\begin{pmatrix} e_{1,i,j} \\ e_{2,i,j} \end{pmatrix} \sim N\left[\begin{pmatrix} 0 \\ 0 \end{pmatrix}, \begin{pmatrix} \sigma^2_{e1} & \sigma_{e1,e2} \\ \sigma_{e1,e2} & \sigma^2_{e2} \end{pmatrix}\right]$$

Restricting $\sigma_{u1,u2} = 0$ does not formally affect the variance of SBP or DBP. The correlation of SBP and DBP from individual i in study j is

$$\frac{\sigma_{e1,e2}}{\sqrt{(\sigma^2_{u1} + \sigma^2_{e1})(\sigma^2_{u2} + \sigma^2_{e2})}} \text{ instead of } \frac{\sigma_{u1,u2} + \sigma_{e1,e2}}{\sqrt{(\sigma^2_{u1} + \sigma^2_{e1})(\sigma^2_{u2} + \sigma^2_{e2})}}$$

while for two different individuals in the same study the correlation is

$$0 \text{ instead of } \frac{\sigma_{u1,u2}}{\sqrt{(\sigma^2_{u1} + \sigma^2_{e1})(\sigma^2_{u2} + \sigma^2_{e2})}}.$$

However, because $\sigma_{e1,e2}$, i.e. the within individual covariance, typically dominates $\sigma_{u1,u2}$, this is unlikely to cause serious bias in practice. So, under the multilevel imputation model, even with constraints on the study level covariance matrix, imputation takes some account of the clustering within studies.

An alternative is to impute cross-sectionally, using a fixed effect for study. Such an imputation model does not take account of clustering within studies. In certain contexts this may be nontrivial: for instance when different studies recruit patients with different illness severity, or otherwise different backgrounds. Further, for systematically missing variables within a study, we have to choose another study (with the variable observed) as the reference, to obtain a mean value about which to impute. Again the appropriateness of this depends on the context of the various studies, but in general it is advisable to avoid this, especially if we wish to do study specific analyses and/or meaningful comparisons of summary statistics across studies. Nevertheless, in situations where the substantive model includes a common effect of covariates adjusted for study, it may be that imputing using a fixed effect for study, and not formally taking account of the multilevel structure, is practically equivalent for estimating the coefficients of such covariates. This is because differences in the mean of covariates between studies will be accounted for in the coefficients for the study indicator variables in the substantive model.

Different measurement scales

We consider two scenarios. First, a measurement of the same underlying quantity is rounded in some studies but not in others. Second, closely related yet different quantities are measured in different studies.

An example of the first is ejection fraction in patients with heart failure. Depending on how it is measured, this can be a percentage (between 0 an 100), but is quite often an ordinal score. If we wish to include the continuous variable in the substantive model, we can impute this for all patients, taking the ordinal values as bounds on the imputed values. For each patient, at each update of the imputation algorithm, the proposed imputed value is only accepted if consistent with the ordinal bounds. In the case of rejection, a new proposal is repeatedly drawn until one is accepted.

An example of the second is studies of lung function, which can be assessed, among other ways, using forced expiratory volume and forced vital capacity. Here the ideal is to have at least one study which has measured both, and to include both variables in the imputation model. The desired measure can then be imputed where it is missing and used in the substantive model.

9.4.1 When to apply Rubin's rules

Another issue in this context is the choice of the appropriate level at which Rubin's rules are applied in subsequent analysis. For example, suppose the goal of the analysis is estimation of a prognostic model. Then we can envisage two strategies:

Strategy 1: impute → meta-analysis → Rubin's rules.

This is appropriate when using a single multilevel imputation model across studies; we proceed as follows:

1. Fit the full imputation model, obtaining $k = 1, \ldots, K$ imputations of all the constituent studies;

2. For imputation k, fit the multilevel prognostic model to the data, with study at level-2;

3. Apply Rubin's rules to summarise the results of the $k = 1, \ldots, K$ prognostic models.

Strategy 2: impute → fit the prognostic model to each imputation for each study→ apply Rubin's rules within studies → meta-analysis.

This is appropriate when imputing within studies; we proceed as follows:

1. Fit the full imputation model, obtaining $k = 1, \ldots, K$ imputations of all the constituent studies *or* fit a separate imputation model within each study, again obtaining $k = 1, \ldots, K$ imputations of all the constituent studies;

2. For study $j = 1, \ldots, J$

   (a) fit the prognostic model to each of the $k = 1, \ldots, K$ imputations for the study;

   (b) apply Rubin's rules to obtain parameter estimates and standard errors for that study

3. Fit a meta-analysis to summarise the results across studies.

Strategy 1 is more consistent with the derivation of Rubin's rules, which are derived to summarise the posterior distribution of parameter estimates in models fitted to imputed data, and simulation studies by Wood *et al.* (2012) have confirmed this.

If the substantive model is a survival model, and we are interested in assessing the improvement in prediction through adding additional variables, it is worth remembering that many of the commonly used measures depend implicitly on the underlying event rate; so the same predictors will give different values of the predictive index with different underlying event rates. This is problematic with meta-analysis, because usually different studies will have very different event rates. It is thus more meaningful to apply such measures to a multilevel predictive model for all studies, than to apply them to individual studies and then attempt to summarise across studies.

9.5 Extensions

In principle we can extend the multilevel model of Section 9.1 from 2 levels to as many as required. The Gibbs sampling algorithm in Section 9.2 extends directly to this setting; we need to include separate random effects and associated covariate matrices for each additional level, and sample the associated parameters analogously to the level-2 random effects.

Cross classified, and associated multiple membership, structures occur when observations are grouped by two separate hierarchies. For example, in an educational setting, children are grouped in classes within schools, but children are also grouped by residential neighbourhood, which is typically linked to social class and hence academic achievement. Such structures are considered in detail in Goldstein (2010), Chapter 12. When modelling such data, omitting the cross-classified structure can result biased estimation of variance components, because groups of units in the second (crossed) classification are treated as independent when they could be highly correlated. This in turn can lead to misleading inference.

It follows that, when imputing such data, the model should allow for the cross classified structure. So far we have only considered hierarchical structure, and the full covariance matrix for the data has thus been block-diagonal. When modelling cross-classified data, we retain the block-diagonal structure for the first hierarchy, but the second hierarchy is captured through blocks of nonzero off-diagonal terms. It is computationally straightforward to update these terms one-at-a-time using Metropolis-Hastings steps. This proceeds in the way described, in the context of binary data, in Chapter 4.

9.5.1 Random level-1 covariance matrices

Yucel (2011) describes an extension to allow the level-1 covariance matrices to differ between level-2 units. An application where this may be useful is imputation for individual patient data meta-analysis. Here, the different entry criteria for the different studies may well result in different level-1 (within study) covariance matrices. However, we cannot impute each study separately, because – as discussed above – we need information from other studies to impute covariates that are not collected in specific studies. Another application arises in the context of multiple imputation with survey weights, discussed in Chapter 11.

In such situations, Yucel (2011) assumes that the level-1 precision (inverse covariance) matrices are drawn from a Wishart distribution. Hence the common precision matrix $\boldsymbol{\Omega}_1$ in (9.6) is replaced by $\boldsymbol{\Omega}_{1,j}$, with distribution

$$(\boldsymbol{\Omega}_{1,j})^{-1} \sim \mathrm{W}(a, A).$$

Here $a > p_1$ (the number of level-1 variables) is the degrees of freedom of the Wishart distribution, and A is the scale matrix.

In order to implement this, we need to extend the sampler described in Section 9.2. We first specify priors for $a \sim \chi^2_\eta$ and $A^{-1} \sim \mathrm{W}(\gamma, \Gamma)$. Here γ must be greater than the dimension of Γ, and the analyst needs to choose values of η, γ and Γ.

We first describe how to draw A, a and then describe how to draw $\boldsymbol{\Omega}_{1,j}$. Other parameters are updated as described in Section 9.2, but now respecting the different level-1 covariance matrices, $\boldsymbol{\Omega}_{1,j}$, for each of the level-1 units.

The inverse of A is drawn as follows:

$$A^{-1} \sim \mathrm{W}(\gamma + aJ, \Gamma^\star),$$

where J is the number of level-2 units, and $\Gamma^\star = (\Gamma^{-1} + \sum_j \boldsymbol{\Omega}_{1,j}^{-1})^{-1}$.

We update a using a Metropolis-Hastings step. First note that the conditional density of a is proportional to

$$f_1(a) \left\{ \prod_{j=1}^{J} f_{2,j}(a) \right\} f_3(a) = f(a), \text{ say,} \qquad (9.14)$$

where

1. $f_1(a)$ is the prior distribution of a, i.e. χ^2_η;

2. $f_{2,j}(a)$ is the $\mathrm{W}(a, A^{-1})$, distribution for the jth precision matrix, $\boldsymbol{\Omega}^{-1}_{1,j}$, as a function of a, and

3. $f_3(a)$ is the $\mathrm{W}(\gamma + aJ, \Gamma^\star)$ distribution for A^{-1}, again as a function of a.

We could use a Metropolis-Hastings sampler to update a. However, this will generally be awkward, as a has a skew distribution. Instead, Yucel (2011) proposes that since we must have $a > p_1$ we can write $u = \log(a + p_1)$, and then

$$f_U(u) = f(e^u - p_1)\left|\frac{\partial a}{\partial u}\right|,$$

where the function f on the right hand side is given by (9.14). We then use a Metropolis-Hastings step to update u, where the proposal is a t_4 distribution centred at the mode of $f_U(u)$, with the same curvature (second derivative) at the mode. Denote the mode by u_m, calculated, say, using a numerical or Newton-Raphson search and denote the second derivative at the mode by

$$d(u_m) = \frac{\partial^2}{\partial^2 u} f_U(u)\bigg|_{u=u_m}.$$

Then if we draw $T \sim t_4$, and set $U = \lambda T + u_m$, we have the proposal density

$$h(u) \propto \left[1 + \frac{(u - u_m)^2}{4\lambda^2}\right]^{-5/2}.$$

Since this has curvature $-5/(4\lambda^2)$ at the mode, to match the curvature of f_u, we choose

$$\lambda = \sqrt{-\frac{5}{4d(u_m)}}.$$

The Metropolis-Hastings sampler, currently at u, then accepts a proposed $u^\star$ with probability

$$\min\left\{1, \frac{f(u^\star)}{f(u)}\frac{h(u)}{h(u^\star)}\right\}.$$

Lastly, given draws of A, a, then for each j we draw

$$\boldsymbol{\Omega}^{-1}_{1,j} \sim \mathrm{W}(a + I, W_j^{-1}),$$

where $W_j = A^{-1} + \sum_{i=1}^{I} e_{i,j} e_{i,j}^T$ and

$$e_{i,j} = \mathbf{Y}^{(1)}_{i,j} - (\boldsymbol{I}_{p_1} \otimes \mathbf{X}^{(1)}_{i,j})\boldsymbol{\beta}^{(1)} - (\boldsymbol{I}_{p_1} \otimes \mathbf{Z}^{(1)}_{i,j})\boldsymbol{u}^{(1)}_j.$$

Yucel successfully applies this to impute data from a crime victimisation survey, where level-2 units are city blocks. At the time of writing there is no general software available for this method.

9.5.2 Model fit

Formal assessment of model fit is usually of secondary importance when constructing an imputation model, relative to selecting auxiliary variables and ensuring the structure in the substantive model is appropriately captured in the imputation model.

If desired, though, the Deviance Information Criterion (Spiegelhalter *et al.*, 2002) can be used to assess model fit. In order to calculate this, we need to calculate the log-likelihood at each cycle of the MCMC algorithm, say D_i, and also the log-likelihood at the final parameter estimates, say $D(\theta)$, where θ is usually obtained by averaging the post-convergence MCMC parameter chain. The deviance information criterion is then

$$\bar{D} + p_D, \text{ where } p_D = \{\bar{D} - D(\theta)\}.$$

Models with the smaller values of the deviance information criterion are then preferred. In applications with missing data we have to be careful to calculate the log-likelihood for the observed data, rather than the log-likelihood for the observed and imputed data, and it may be useful to do this in stages, i.e. calculate the log-likelihood for the continuous variables given the categorical variables, and add the log-likelihood for the categorical variables (Goldstein *et al.*, 2009).

9.6 Discussion

In this chapter we have considered imputation for multilevel data. We have proposed a general multilevel imputation model, and illustrated some of the issues that may arise if multilevel structure is ignored in imputation. We have illustrated the application of these methods to data with missing observations at level-2, and also considered the application to individual patient data meta-analysis, where some studies may not collect all of the variables we wish to include in the substantive model. Lastly, we have discussed extensions to more than two levels, cross-classified structures and random covariance matrices at level-1. As our applications illustrate, the class of multilevel imputation models described here allow congenial imputation for a range of models and data structures that are increasingly arising in applications, not least individual patient data meta-analysis.

10

Sensitivity analysis: MI unleashed

Up to this point we have applied MI under the assumption that data are MAR. In practice, we will usually wish to explore whether our inferences are robust to this assumption. To do this, we typically need to impute data under a MNAR mechanism, or approximate the results of so doing. This chapter explores both approaches. Unleashed from the restriction of MAR, MI provides a flexible, computationally straightforward route for inference under almost every conceivable MNAR assumption we may wish to explore.

While much of this book has been concerned with the details of choosing an imputation model, then fitting and imputing missing data under MAR, this should not detract from the practical importance of exploring the robustness of inference to the MAR assumption. This is because, as discussed at some length in Chapter 1, given a set of data we cannot definitively identify the missingness mechanism. In order to draw conclusions from partially observed data, we therefore need to understand the extent to which the data support such conclusions under a range of plausible missingness mechanisms, which will generally include some MNAR mechanisms.

In applications, it is important for all those who have an interest in inference from a partially observed dataset to understand both the range of plausible missingness mechanisms which support specific inferences, together with their relevance for the question at hand (Carpenter *et al.*, 2013). In other words, it is necessary to be comfortable with the implications of the assumptions about missing data underpinning an analysis, if one is to be comfortable with decisions based on the resulting inferences. This is particularly so in the context of analysing randomised clinical trials, which has consequently provided much of the impetus for sensitivity analysis.

Multiple Imputation and its Application, First Edition. James R. Carpenter and Michael G. Kenward.

For example, Section 7 of the new EMA guideline on missing data in confirmatory clinical trials (Committee for Medicinal Products for Human Use, 2010) is devoted to this, noting 'The sensitivity analyses should show how different assumptions influence the results obtained'. Recommendation 15 of the recent US National Research Council report entitled 'The prevention and treatment of missing data in clinical trials' (National Research Council, 2010) concurs, stating 'Sensitivity analyses should be part of the primary reporting of findings from clinical trials. Examining sensitivity to the assumptions about the missing data mechanism should be a mandatory component of reporting'. However, the final recommendation, 18, notes '...There remain several important areas where progress is particularly needed, namely: (1) methods for sensitivity analysis and principled decision making based on the results from sensitivity analysis...'.

The plan for this chapter is as follows. In Section 10.1 we review the theory underlying the analysis of data when missing values are MNAR, in particular focusing on the contrast between the pattern mixture and selection model approaches. Then in Section 10.2 we review some of the issues that have to be considered in framing sensitivity analyses. In Section 10.3 we outline the MI approach to pattern mixture modelling, illustrating its application to clinical and social examples we have considered before. An alternative, approximate, approach – which allows rapid exploration of local departures from MAR without re-imputing or re-analysing the imputed data – is described in Section 10.6. We conclude with a discussion in Section 10.7.

10.1 Review of MNAR modelling

Suppose we have two variables, $\mathbf{Y}_1, \mathbf{Y}_2$, with $\mathbf{Y}_1$ partially observed, and $\mathbf{R}$ the vector of response indicators for $\mathbf{Y}_1$ ($R_i = 1$ if $Y_{i,1}$ is observed and 0 otherwise). Then, as described in Chapter 1, for each unit i we have

$$f(Y_{i,1}, Y_{i,2}|R_i)f(R_i) = f(Y_{i,1}, Y_{i,2}, R_i) = f(R_i|Y_{i,1}, Y_{i,2})f(Y_{i,1}, Y_{i,2}). \quad (10.1)$$

The central expression is the joint distribution of the data, comprising the variables and the selection indicator. On the right-hand side, this is written as the product of density for selection given $Y_{i,1}, Y_{i,2}$ and a density of $Y_{i,1}, Y_{i,2}$. This is known in the literature as the *selection factorisation* or, more commonly, the *selection model* approach. A particular form of this relates $f(R_i|Y_{i,1}, Y_{i,2})$ and $f(Y_{i,1}, Y_{i,2})$ through a shared parameter; for a recent review see Albert and Follman (2009), and for an example of sensitivity analysis based on this see Kenward and Rosenkranz (2011).

By contrast, on the left-hand side we have a different distribution of $(Y_{1,i}, Y_{2,i})$ depending on whether $Y_{i,1}$ is observed. This is averaged over the probability that $Y_{i,1}$ is observed. In more realistic examples, there will be a number of *patterns* of missing observations, each potentially with a different joint distribution of partially observed and fully observed data, and then overall density as the average over these patterns, leading to the name *pattern mixture factorisation* or more commonly *pattern mixture model*.

The MAR assumption thus has two forms: the selection form,

$$f(R_i|Y_{i,1}, Y_{i,2}) = f(R_i|Y_{i,2}),$$

or the patten mixture form

$$f(Y_{i,1}, Y_{i,2}|R_i) = f(Y_{i,1}|Y_{i,2}).$$

In this simple case it is obvious that the one implies the other; however this holds true quite generally (e.g. Molenberghs *et al.*, 1998). This means that for sensitivity analysis we can either focus on modelling the different patterns, or on modelling the selection process. In a complex analysis we could do both, handling some aspects with a pattern mixture model and some aspects with a selection model.

If the focus is on pattern mixture modelling, then for each pattern we need to specify the joint distribution of the partially and fully observed variables. In turn, this implies the conditional distribution of partially observed data given the fully observed data within each pattern. This can take any form commensurate with the data type (continuous/ordinal/categorical). However, the majority of these forms will be extremely implausible, given the scientific context and the observed data. We therefore advocate starting from the conditional distribution implied by MAR, and then changing this to reflect assumptions (which could be based on contextual knowledge or expert belief) about the difference from the observed conditional distribution when the variable, or set of variables, is unobserved. Then a convenient starting point is

$$f(Y_{i,1}, Y_{i,2}|R_i) = f(Y_{i,1}|Y_{i,2}, R_i)f(Y_{i,2}|R_i),$$

keeping $f(Y_{i,2})$ (the marginal model for the fully observed variable) the same across patterns, and allowing $f(Y_{i,1}|Y_{i,2}, R_i)$ to differ with $R_i = 0, 1$

Under MAR we estimate the distribution $f(Y_1|Y_2)$ from the observed data, typically using a regression model of some form. A simple example is linear regression:

$$Y_{i,1} = \beta_0 + \beta_1 Y_{i,2} + e_i, \quad e_i \overset{i.i.d.}{\sim} N(0, \sigma^2); \tag{10.2}$$

fitting this gives estimates $\hat{\beta}_0, \hat{\beta}_1$, and $\hat{\sigma}^2$. To obtain the likelihood of the full data, we need to specify $f(Y_1|Y_2, R = 0)$. A natural suggestion is

$$Y_{i,1} = (\beta_0 + \delta_0) + (\beta_1 + \delta_1)Y_{i,1} + e_i, \quad e_i \overset{i.i.d.}{\sim} N(0, (\sigma + \delta_2)^2). \tag{10.3}$$

Using this model, once we have specified the joint distribution of $\boldsymbol{\delta} = (\delta_0, \delta_1, \delta_2)^T$, we have specified the distribution $f(Y_1|Y_2, R = 0)$. Since $f(R)$ is simply a Bernoulli distribution for the proportion of observed data, with say

$\Pr(R_i = 1) = \alpha$, given a density $f(Y_2; \gamma)$ we therefore have the full likelihood as the product of terms:

$$L_i = \begin{cases} (2\pi\sigma^2)^{-\frac{1}{2}} \exp\left\{-\left(\frac{Y_{i,1}-\beta_0-\beta_1 Y_{i,2}}{\sqrt{2}\sigma}\right)^2\right\} f(Y_{i,2}; \gamma)\alpha & \text{if } R_i = 1 \\ \iint f(\boldsymbol{\delta})\{2\pi(\sigma+\delta_2)^2\}^{-\frac{1}{2}} & \\ \quad \times \exp\left\{-\left(\frac{Y_{i,1}-(\beta_0+\delta_0)-(\beta_1+\delta_1)Y_{i,2}}{\sqrt{2}(\sigma+\delta_2)}\right)^2\right\} & \\ \quad \times f(Y_{i,2}; \gamma)(1-\alpha)\, dY_{i,1}\, d\boldsymbol{\delta} & \text{if } R_i = 0 \end{cases} \tag{10.4}$$

Given $f(\boldsymbol{\delta})$, whose parameters generally cannot be estimated from the observed data, we can then calculate the integral over the missing data to obtain the likelihood of the remaining parameters. Estimating these gives an estimate of the joint distribution of the data, hence any function of the data of interest. Depending on the details, we may wish to use maximum likelihood, the method of moments, or a Bayesian approach using MCMC. The latter is often convenient in practice, because having specified $f(\boldsymbol{\delta})$ and priors for $(\beta_0, \beta_1, \sigma^2)$, we can estimate any function of parameters or data from the MCMC draws from the posterior distribution. Examples of pattern mixture modelling include Little (1994); Molenberghs *et al.* (1998); Daniels and Hogan (2000); Thijs *et al.* (2002); Demirtas and Schafer (2003); Kenward *et al.* (2003). In Section 10.3 we describe the use of MI for pattern mixture modelling.

Now consider the selection model approach. Assuming a linear-logistic model,

$$\operatorname{logit}\{\Pr(R_i = 1)\} = \alpha_0 + \alpha_1 Y_{i,1} + \alpha_2 Y_{i,2}, \tag{10.5}$$

the likelihood of the data is the product of terms

$$L_i = \begin{cases} f(R_i | Y_{i,1}, Y_{i,2}) f(Y_{i,1} | Y_{i,2}) f(Y_{i,2}) & \text{if } R_i = 1 \\ \int f(R_i | Y_{i,1}, Y_{i,2}) f(Y_{i,1} | Y_{i,2}) f(Y_{i,2})\, dY_{i,1} & \text{if } R_i = 0. \end{cases} \tag{10.6}$$

The density $f(Y_{i,1}|Y_{i,2})$ is often a regression model such as (10.2); of course, the resulting parameter values and inferences differ in general to those from the subset of observed data.

Again, given the likelihood, we can estimate the parameters and draw inferences. We can often do this directly, using numerical integration (e.g. Diggle and Kenward, 1994; Verzilli and Carpenter, 2002) or using a Bayesian approach via MCMC (e.g. Carpenter *et al*., 2002).

Under the selection model approach, it may appear that we can estimate the parameter α_1 in (10.5), and hence test for MNAR. This is illusory, as estimation rests on assumptions about the distribution of the missing data (e.g. Kenward, 1998). Likewise in the pattern mixture approach, we cannot estimate the distribution of $\boldsymbol{\delta}$. In practice it is often preferable to explore sensitivity to different assumptions about the distribution of parameters controlling the pattern mixture distribution ($\boldsymbol{\delta}$, in (10.4)) or selection (α_1 in (10.5)).

Whichever approach is adopted, we reiterate that a useful sensitivity analysis must frame the assumptions in a way that is accessible to all those involved in the research, so they can in turn identify relevant, plausible departures from these assumptions to explore. In this respect, analysing data under MNAR models is qualitatively different than fitting a model to fully observed data, and then examining diagnostics. Further, the correspondence between the pattern mixture and selection approaches mentioned above implies that if we adopt a pattern mixture approach for framing assumptions, the selection consequences should be plausible, and vice-versa.

10.2 Framing sensitivity analysis

Analysis of partially observed data should consist of (i) a primary analysis, under a plausible primary missingness mechanism, and (ii) secondary analyses exploring the robustness of inference to departures from the primary missingness mechanism.

Framing both analyses requires careful consideration of the *estimand*, i.e. the quantity we wish to estimate and the population we wish to estimate it for, in conjunction with the reason for the missing data. While these issues are sharply defined in the analysis of clinical trials with missing outcome data, they are always present.

To focus our discussion, we initially consider the clinical trials setting, where we have randomised treatment allocation and longitudinal follow up. Missing data may arise due to, for example (i) poor compliance with, or withdrawal from, the treatment; (ii) unblinding, either of treatment or evaluation, and (iii) loss to follow up, so that no further information on the patient is available.

Estimands

Following Carpenter *et al.* (2013), for the population of eligible patients as defined by the trial inclusion criteria, let $\tilde{f}_{act}$ be the joint probability distribution function of baseline and post-randomisation responses for patients randomised to the *active* treatment, who follow the treatment regime exactly, withstanding all the rigours (including adverse events) without departing from the protocol. Define $\tilde{f}_{cont}$ analogously, for patients receiving the control treatment.

For response profile $\mathbf{Y}$, and any suitable function $g(.)$, we define the *de jure* (according to the rules) estimand as

$$\mathrm{E}_{\tilde{f}_{act}}[g(\mathbf{Y})] - \mathrm{E}_{\tilde{f}_{cont}}[g(\mathbf{Y})]. \tag{10.7}$$

De jure questions concern the magnitude of this quantity; in other words 'What would the expected treatment effect be in the eligible population if the treatment and control were taken as specified in the protocol', i.e. 'does the treatment work under the best case scenario?'

The function $g(.)$ defines the effect. For many choices of g, a more precise estimate of the quantity (10.7) can be obtained by conditioning on baseline, Y_0, say. Often $g(\mathbf{Y})$ is the last scheduled observation, so that if (i) there are no missing data and (ii) the observed data in the trial arms comes respectively from $\tilde{f}_{act}$, $\tilde{f}_{cont}$, then (10.7) can be efficiently estimated by regression of the final response on treatment group and baseline.

Now further define, for the population of eligible patients as defined by the trial inclusion criteria, f_{act} as the joint probability distribution function of baseline and post-randomisation responses that would be seen in the context of interest among patients randomised to the active arm. Define f_{cont} analogously for the control arm.

For response profile $\mathbf{Y}$, and any suitable function $g(.)$, we define the *de facto* (according to the fact) estimand as

$$\mathrm{E}_{f_{act}}[g(\mathbf{Y})] - \mathrm{E}_{f_{cont}}[g(\mathbf{Y})]. \tag{10.8}$$

De facto questions concern the magnitude of this quantity; in other words 'What would be the effect seen in practice if this treatment were applied to the population defined by the trial inclusion criteria?'

Our proposed terms, de facto and de jure, describe estimands in the sense defined by the National Research Council (2010). By contrast, the terms *effectiveness* and *efficacy*, besides causing confusion by their similarity, actually refer to different, loose concepts about the conditions under which the intervention is being used (National Institute for Clinical Excellence (NICE), 2011).

In some settings, patients may be unable to withstand the rigours of the regime. Thus, the distributions $\tilde{f}_{act}$, $\tilde{f}_{cont}$ may be counter-factual. By contrast, providing patients remain alive, their actual responses, with probability distributions f_{act}, f_{cont}, can almost always be observed given sufficient time and resources.

De jure questions parallel those asked in the early stages of drug development. Does the compound and its associated route of mechanism have the desired effect? While such questions are sometimes termed 'per protocol' this is unhelpful, as in some quarters 'per protocol' is linked with 'on-treatment' while in others it is not. Further the term 'on-treatment' is itself ambiguous, as it does not specify the extent of post-randomisation compliance.

De facto questions are relevant to a regulatory agencies wishing to understand the cost/benefit return for a specific treatment policy. For example, in England the National Institute for Health and Clinical Excellence (NICE, www.nice.org.uk/aboutnice/) provides national guidance on treating ill health, and often needs answers to de facto questions. De facto questions are sometimes referred to as 'Intention-to-treat' (ITT) questions. However, the latter term is sometimes used to refer to a set of patients and sometimes used to refer to an estimation method (e.g. Hollis and Campbell, 1999).

Implications for other settings

While the discussion above is focussed on randomised clinical trials, the issues apply to all analyses: for what population are we seeking to estimate the model, why are some of the data missing, and how (if at all) does the distribution of these missing data differ from what is predicted from the observed data, i.e. under MAR? For example, consider a survey of young people age 16, administered through schools. Are we interested in (i) inference for the population of pupils, if they attended and participated in school as they should, in school or (ii) inference for the population of pupils, taking account of those who may have been excluded from school, or whose attendance may be erratic? The former we would term a de jure estimand, the latter a de facto estimand.

We emphasise that, whatever the estimand, for inference we will generally wish to estimate the parameters under both MAR and MNAR mechanisms. However, the choices for latter will typically vary with the choice of estimand.

10.3 Pattern mixture modelling with MI

We motivate the discussion with an example, and then describe and illustrate a generic approach to pattern mixture modelling using MI.

Example 10.1 Peer review trial

Schroter *et al.* (2004) report a single blind randomised controlled trial among reviewers for a general medical journal. The aim was to investigate whether training improved the quality of peer review. The study compared two different types of training (face-to-face training, or a self-taught package) with no training.

We restrict ourselves to the comparison between those randomised to the self-taught package and no training. Each participating reviewer was pre-randomised into their intervention group. Prior to any training, each was sent a baseline article to review (termed paper 1). If this was returned, then according to their randomised group, the reviewer was either (i) mailed a self-training package or (ii) received no further training.

Two to three months later, participants who had completed their first review were sent a further article to review (paper 2); if this was returned, a third paper was sent three months later (paper 3). The analysis excluded all participants who did not complete their first review: this was not expected to cause bias since these participants were unaware of their randomised allocation.

Reviewers were sent manuscripts in a similar style to the standard *British Medical Journal* request for a review, but were told these articles were part of the study and were not paid. The three articles were based on three previously published papers, with original author names, titles and location changed. In addition, nine major and five minor errors were introduced. The outcome is the quality of the review, as measured by the Review Quality Instrument (RQI). This validated instrument contains eight items scored from 1 to 5. Rating was done

Table 10.1 RQI score of paper 1 by whether or not paper 2 was reviewed.

		Group		
		No intervention	Self-taught	Face-to-face
Returned review of	n	162	120	158
paper 2	mean	2.65	2.80	2.75
	SD	0.81	0.62	0.70
Did not return	n	11	46	25
review of paper 2	mean	3.02	2.55	2.51
	SD	0.50	0.75	0.73

independently by two editors. The response in our analysis is the mean of the first seven items, averaged over the two editors. This ranges between 1 and 5, where a perfect review would score 5.

We restrict attention to the second review. For this, analysis of the observed data showed a statistically significant difference at the 5% level in favour of the self-taught package. Table 10.1 breaks down the results of the baseline review (paper 1) by whether reviewers responded to the request to review paper 2. It suggests that the improved review quality on paper 2 in the self-taught group may be because poorer reviewers are disproportionately MNAR from this group, even after accounting for baseline. We consider the de facto estimand: what is the effect of being sent the self-taught package, compared with no training, regardless of whether it was used. Below, we explore the robustness of inference for this question to different assumptions about the missing review quality. □

Consider variables $\mathbf{Y}_1, \ldots, \mathbf{Y}_p$. For each unit, let $\mathbf{Y}_i^T = (Y_{i,1}, \ldots, Y_{i,p})$ and $\mathbf{R}_i^T = (R_{i,1}, \ldots, R_{i,p})$ be the vector of response indicators. Across all $i = 1, \ldots, n$ units, suppose there are $M \ll n$ distinct response patterns, indexed by $\mathbf{R}_m$, $m \in (1, \ldots, M)$. Each unit's missing and observed variables conform to one of these patterns, say $m(i)$, and one of the patterns corresponds to complete records on all p variables. Let $\mathbf{Y}_{\mathrm{O},m(i)}$, $\mathbf{Y}_{\mathrm{M},m(i)}$ be the observed and missing variables for unit i with response pattern $m(i)$.

For each unit, with missingness pattern $m(i) = m$ say, let η_m denote the parameters of the joint distribution of the observed and missing data. From this we can derive the conditional distribution of the missing given the observed data, denoted by

$$f(\mathbf{Y}_{\mathrm{M},m(i)} | \mathbf{Y}_{\mathrm{O},m(i)}, \eta_{m(i)}). \tag{10.9}$$

We have to estimate η_m before we can draw missing data from (10.9).

If data are MAR, then (10.9) does not depend on missingness pattern m; distributions are the same across all patterns, $\eta_m = \eta$, $m \in (1, \ldots, M)$, and we impute missing data from $f(\mathbf{Y}_{\mathrm{M},i} | \mathbf{Y}_{\mathrm{O},i}, \eta)$. However, if data are MNAR this distribution will differ with missingness pattern m, and could further differ for different units within missingness pattern m.

Suppose that $\hat{\theta} = \hat{\theta}(\mathbf{Y}) = \hat{\theta}(\mathbf{Y}_\mathrm{M}, \mathbf{Y}_\mathrm{O})$ is of interest. For example, θ may be a regression coefficient. With no missing data, we would estimate this from $\mathbf{Y}$, using the appropriate generalised linear model. For each missingness pattern m, let $\mathbf{Y}_{\mathrm{O},m}$ be the observed data from units i such that $m(i) = m$. Our approach is to define a form for (10.9), for each missingness pattern m, which reflects contextually relevant assumptions. Then we impute K 'complete' data sets by

MI1: taking a draw from the Bayesian posterior distribution of $f(\boldsymbol{\eta}_\mathrm{m}|\mathbf{Y}_\mathrm{O}, m)$ and then

MI2: imputing the missing data from (10.9) using the above draw of $\boldsymbol{\eta}_m$.

Both steps are repeated to create each imputed dataset. The parameter of interest is then estimated from each imputed data set in turn to give $\hat{\theta}_k$, with standard error $\hat{\sigma}_k$, $k = 1, \ldots, K$. These are then combined using Rubin's rules to give a single multiple imputation estimate and associated standard error.

To implement MI1 we need to choose a model for the observed data. To implement MI2 we need to specify (10.9). Taking the former first, our approach is to estimate a common parameter vector $\boldsymbol{\eta}$ from all the observed data assuming MAR. For the latter, we use specific rules or information to derive, or draw, $\boldsymbol{\eta}_m$. This is of necessity context specific. It could involve

1. explicitly specifying the distribution of $\boldsymbol{\eta}_m$ given $\boldsymbol{\eta}$, possibly using opinions elicited from experts, or

2. specifying how $\boldsymbol{\eta}_m$ is constructed from $\boldsymbol{\eta}$, for example in terms of rules across well-defined subsets of the data (such as treatment groups).

Consider now the pattern mixture model (10.2)–(10.3). In terms of the more general development here, $\boldsymbol{\eta}$, the parameters of the model for the observed data, are $(\beta_0, \beta_1, \sigma)$ and $\boldsymbol{\eta}_1$, the parameters of the model for the first (and only) missingness pattern, are $(\beta_0 + \delta_0, \beta_1 + \delta_1, \sigma + \delta_2)$. Thus $\boldsymbol{\delta} = \boldsymbol{\eta}_1 - \boldsymbol{\eta}$.

The examples we consider below illustrate approaches 1 and 2 above. We emphasise that we take MAR as our starting point for sensitivity analysis. It is not necessary to do this in order to use MI for pattern mixture modelling, and the approach we describe can readily be adapted accordingly if desired.

Example 10.1 Peer review trial *(ctd)*

Focusing on the baseline adjusted comparison of the self-taught training package with no training, the substantive model is

$$Y_i = \beta_0 + \beta_1 X_{1,i} + \beta_2 X_{2,i} + e_i, \quad e_i \overset{i.i.d.}{\sim} N(0, \sigma^2) \tag{10.10}$$

where i indexes participant, Y_i, $X_{1,i}$ are the mean RQI score for paper 2 and paper 1 respectively and $X_{2,i}$ is an indicator for the self-taught group. Inference for β_2

Table 10.2 Peer review trial: inference for comparison of self-taught package with no training, under various assumptions. Parameter estimates are differences in mean RQI score, on a scale of 0–5.

Analysis	Est	SE	MI df	p-value	95% CI
Complete records, MAR	0.237	0.070	N/A	<0.001	(0.099, 0.376)
MAR, $K = 20$	0.245	0.073	302	<0.001	(0.102, 0.389)
MAR, $K = 10,000$	0.237	0.070	$\approx \infty$	<0.001	(0.099, 0.375)
MNAR, $\rho = 0$, $K = 20$	0.209	0.178	27	0.25	(−0.158, 0.575)
MNAR, $\rho = 0$, $K = 10,000$	0.193	0.151	$\approx \infty$	0.20	(−0.102, 0.488)
MNAR, $\rho = 0.5$, $K = 20$	0.205	0.167	27	0.23	(−0.141, 0.234)
MNAR, $\rho = 0.5$, $K = 10,000$	0.190	0.137	$\approx \infty$	0.17	(−0.089, 0.459)
MNAR, $\rho = 1$, $K = 20$	0.213	0.134	34	0.12	(−0.059, 0.486)
MNAR, $\rho = 1$, $K = 10,000$	0.190	0.123	$\approx \infty$	0.12	(−0.050, 0.431)

from fitting (10.10) to the complete records, assuming review 2 is MAR given baseline review and intervention group, is shown in the first row of Table 10.2.

Analysis under MAR addresses the de jure question, because missing reviewer scores are imputed using information from participants who completed the second review and complied with the study protocol. We consider the de facto estimand: what would the effect of intervention be if it was rolled out to all reviewers by the *British Medical Journal*. Thus, White *et al.* (2007) devised a questionnaire which was completed by 2 investigators and 20 editors and other staff at the *British Medical Journal*. The questionnaire was designed to elicit the experts' prior belief about the de facto difference between the average missing and average observed review quality index. White *et al.* (2007) show that it was reasonable to pool information from the experts. The resulting distribution is negatively skewed, with mean −0.21 and SD 0.46 (on the review quality instrument scale). Suppose we denote by (δ_0, δ_1) draws from the distribution of the mean difference in review quality between observed and unobserved reviews, in respectively the control and self-taught groups. We adopt a bivariate normal model approximation to the prior:

$$\begin{pmatrix} \delta_0 \\ \delta_1 \end{pmatrix} \sim N\left[\begin{pmatrix} -0.21 \\ -0.21 \end{pmatrix}, 0.46^2 \begin{pmatrix} 1 & \rho \\ \rho & 1 \end{pmatrix}\right] \tag{10.11}$$

Unfortunately, it was not possible to elicit a prior on ρ from the experts; we therefore analyse the data with $\rho = 0, 0.5, 1$ below.

Given a draw (δ_0, δ_1) from this distribution the model is

$$
\begin{aligned}
Y_i &= \beta_0 + \beta_1 X_{1,i} + \beta_2 X_{2,i} + e_i && \text{if } Y_i \text{ observed,}\\
Y_i &= (\beta_0 + \delta_0) + \beta_1 X_{1,i} + (\beta_2 + \delta_1 - \delta_0) X_{2,i} + e_i && \text{if } Y_i \text{ unobserved,}\\
e_i &\overset{i.i.d.}{\sim} N(0, \sigma^2). && (10.12)
\end{aligned}
$$

Thus the mean review quality, relative to that in the observed data, is changed by δ_0 in the control arm and δ_1 in the self-taught arm.

Following the general approach for estimating pattern mixture models via MI described above, we proceed as follows, noting that the imputation model under MAR and the substantive model are the same in this example:

1. Fit the imputation model (10.10) to the observed data and draw from the posterior distribution of the parameters $\boldsymbol{\eta} = (\beta_0, \beta_1, \beta_2, \sigma^2)$.
2. Draw (δ_0, δ_1) from (10.11)
3. Using the draws obtained in steps 1 and 2, impute the missing Y_i using (10.12).

Steps 1–3 are repeated to create K imputed data sets. Then we fit the substantive model (10.10) to each imputed data set and apply Rubin's rules for inference.

The results are shown in Table 10.2. In line with theory, the results from MI under MAR agree with the complete records analysis, and this agreement is very close with $K = 10\ 000$ imputations (which in this example only take a matter of minutes). Imputing under MNAR, we see that the mean review quality instrument score in the self-taught group is no longer statistically significantly different from the no training group. The standard error is largest when $\rho = 0$, and decreases as $\rho \to 1$. We also see that $K = 20$ imputations is enough to clearly show this conclusion, to practically relevant precision. Results with 10 000 imputations agree extremely closely with both a theoretical approximation and a full Bayesian analysis reported by White *et al.* (2007), even though the latter allow for uncertainty in estimating the proportion with missing data, which is conditioned on in the pattern mixture approach.

We conclude that, taking experts' prior belief into account, there is no evidence that self-training improves the quality of peer review. □

This approach can also be applied to directly to discrete outcomes. The attractions of interpretability and computational simplicity remain. For example, it could be applied in the setting of Magder (2003), who framed departures from MAR through the response probability ratio. It could equally be applied to estimation and inference with bindary data using the 'Informative Missing Odds Ratio', proposed by Higgins *et al.* (2006). They framed departures from MAR through the ratio of the odds of response in patients whose data are observed to the odds of response in patients whose data are missing.

10.3.1 Missing covariates

We now consider sensitivity analysis for partially observed covariates in the substantive model. Exactly as above, we estimate the coefficients of the imputation model under MAR, but then modify them to reflect a departure from MAR before imputing the missing values. We illustrate with sensitivity analysis for the Youth Cohort Study.

Example 10.2 Youth Cohort Study

Consider again the youth cohort study (see, for example Chapter 5, p. 123). As shown there, the principle missing data pattern, in 11% of the records, is missing parental occupation but observed values for the other variables in our substantive model. The other, more complex patterns, account for $< 3\%$ of the missing records between them. Since imputing with or without the latter records makes no difference to the resulting inference, we restrict to the 61 609 records with either complete records or only parental occupation missing.

As before, the substantive model is a linear regression of GCSE score on ethnic group, adjusted for sex, parental occupation and cohort. Parental occupation is a three category variable, managerial, intermediate and working. We use a multinomial logistic imputation model, with managerial as the reference category. Let $\pi_{i,M}, \pi_{i,I}, \pi_{i,W}$ be the probability that pupil i's parental occupation is classed as managerial, intermediate or working, respectively, where $\pi_{I,i,M} + \pi_{i,I} + \pi_{i,W} = 1$. The imputation model is

$$\log(\pi_{i,I}/\pi_{i,M}) = \mathbf{X}_i \boldsymbol{\alpha}_I \tag{10.13}$$

$$\log(\pi_{i,W}/\pi_{i,M}) = \mathbf{X}_i \boldsymbol{\alpha}_W, \tag{10.14}$$

where $\mathbf{X}_i$ is a $(n \times q)$ matrix with columns corresponding to the constant, pupil's GCSE score centred at 38 points, and indicators for boys, ethnicity (6 variables) and cohort (3 variables).

For MAR imputation, we estimate the parameters of (10.13), (10.14) from the complete records and create proper imputations as described in Chapter 5. The results of the complete records analysis and MAR imputation are shown in the left two columns of Table 10.3. Of particular interest are the coefficients for Pakistani and Bangladeshi ethnicity, which under MAR become substantially more negative and statistically significant. Focusing on Bangladeshi ethnicity, we explore the sensitivity of this result to the MAR assumption, which addresses the de jure estimand, because missing parental occupation is imputed using information from those who comply with the study protocol. The MNAR analyses address de facto estimands under which the proportions imputed to the different parental occupation classes vary widely.

For MNAR we consider two scenarios: for pupils of Bangladeshi ethnicity (i) missing parental occupations are predominantly 'managerial', and (ii) missing parental occupation scores are predominantly 'working'. In the former

Table 10.3 Youth Cohort Study: model for the differences in GCSE points score (range 0–84) by ethnicity, adjusted for sex, parental occupation and cohort. Analyses used 20 imputations.

Covariate	Estimates (standard errors) from:			
	Complete records	MAR	MNAR ($\delta_I = \delta_W = -2$)	MNAR ($\delta_I = 0$, $\delta_W = 1.8$)
Black	−5.39 (0.57)	−6.88 (0.50)	−6.92 (0.49)	−6.88 (0.50)
Indian	3.83 (0.44)	3.25 (0.41)	3.22 (0.41)	3.22 (0.41)
Pakistani	−1.79 (0.59)	−3.55 (0.47)	−3.59 (0.47)	−3.53 (0.47)
Bangladeshi	0.69 (1.05)	−2.99 (0.72)	−4.93 (0.79)	−1.44 (0.70)
Other Asian	5.79 (0.69)	4.90 (0.63)	4.89 (0.62)	4.86 (0.63)
Other	0.37 (0.71)	−0.72 (0.65)	−0.71 (0.64)	−0.67 (0.64)
Boys	−3.47 (0.13)	−3.37 (0.13)	−3.37 (0.13)	−3.36 (0.13)
Intermediate parental occupation	−7.46 (0.15)	−7.80 (0.16)	−7.73 (0.17)	−7.77 (0.16)
Working parental occupation	−13.82 (0.17)	−14.33 (0.17)	−14.30 (0.17)	−14.37 (0.18)
1995 cohort	6.30 (0.18)	6.19 (0.17)	6.18 (0.17)	6.19 (0.17)
1997 cohort	4.96 (0.18)	5.01 (0.17)	5.01 (0.17)	5.01 (0.17)
1999 cohort	9.57 (0.19)	9.88 (0.18)	9.88 (0.18)	9.88 (0.18)
constant	4.81 (0.15)	4.11 (0.15)	4.07 (0.15)	4.10 (0.15)

case we add to the Bangladeshi coefficients in (10.13), (10.14) respectively ($\delta_I = -2, \delta_W - 2$), and in the latter ($\delta_I = 0, \delta_W = 1.8$). In the absence of prior information, in this example we do not follow (10.11) but instead set $\text{Var}(\boldsymbol{\delta}) = 0$. The resulting imputed parental occupations are then, respectively, predominantly managerial and predominantly working when combined with the observed occupations we obtain the proportions shown in Table 10.4. The rightmost columns of Table 10.3 show the corresponding effect on the coefficient for Bangladeshi ethnicity in the model of inference: under both scenarios, inference is remarkably robust.

We conclude that on average pupils of Bangladeshi ethnic origin have significantly lower GCSE scores than the complete records analysis would suggest, and this result is robust to plausible MNAR mechanisms. □

10.3.2 Application to survival analysis

We now consider the application of this approach to sensitivity analysis for nonrandom censoring, or loss to follow up, in survival analysis.

Table 10.4 Parental occupation of students of Bangladeshi ethnicity, in complete records and under MAR, NMAR. Twenty imputations were used.

	Complete	Imputation under		
	records	MAR	MNAR ($\delta_I = \delta_W = -2$)	MNAR ($\delta_I = 0, \delta_W = 1.8$)
Managerial	26 (12%)	48 (9%)	143 (26%)	34 (6%)
Intermediate	91 (41%)	215 (40%)	174 (32%)	126 (23%)
Working	104 (47%)	272 (51%)	221 (41%)	378 (70%)
Total	221	538	538	538

Example 10.3 Evaluation of antiretroviral treatment (ART) programmes in sub-Saharan Africa

HIV infection is a major cause of mortality and morbidity in sub-Saharan Africa, and between 2007 and 2010 the number of patients starting ART increased steeply (e.g. Boulle *et al.*, 2008), along with consequent interest in evaluating the efficacy of ART in this setting. However, during the same period there has been increasing concern about loss to follow up in these programmes (Brinkhof *et al.*, 2008), especially as those lost to follow up may have substantially worse mortality than those who are followed up, which will bias the evaluation (Bartlett and Shao, 2009; Brinkhof *et al.*, 2009).

Accordingly, Brinkhof *et al.* (2010) decided to use a pattern mixture approach, estimated through multiple imputation, to explore the robustness of inferences about mortality to nonrandom censoring. □

To show how the pattern mixture approach can be applied to survival data, suppose that T is the random variable representing the time-to-event and C the random variable representing loss to follow up (i.e. censoring). From each unit, or patient, we observe baseline covariates $\mathbf{X}_i$, and $Y_i = \min(T_i, C_i)$.

The Censoring at Random (CAR) assumption was introduced in Section 8.1, as the equivalent of the MAR assumption for survival data. Thus CAR assumes T_i and C_i are conditionally independent given the covariates $\mathbf{X}_i$. Under CAR, valid estimates for coefficients $\boldsymbol{\beta}$ relating covariates to survival time are obtained from modelling the observed data, where censored units contribute $\Pr(T_i > C_i|\mathbf{X}_i, \boldsymbol{\beta})$ to the likelihood.

Similarly, the Censoring Not at Random (CNAR) assumption is the MNAR assumption for survival data. Under CNAR, T_i and C_i are not independent, even given the covariates $\mathbf{X}_i$.

In order to obtain parameter estimates and inferences under CNAR, we adapt the strategy outlined on p. 236 to the survival setting. Specifically, we obtain an estimate of the hazard assuming CAR, and then introduce a sensitivity parameter defining the ratio of the hazard of censored individuals to those that are not censored. Using the notation of Chapter 8, the hazard under CNAR is

$$h(t_i|C_i, \mathbf{X}_i) = \begin{cases} h_{CAR}(t_i|\mathbf{X}_i) & \text{if } t_i < C_i \\ \exp(\delta)h_{CAR}(t_i|\mathbf{X}_i) & \text{if } t_i \geq C_i. \end{cases} \quad (10.15)$$

If $\delta = 0$, then given $\mathbf{X}_i$, the hazard is the same, irrespective of censoring; in other words CAR holds. Otherwise, the hazards are different. The parameter δ is once again the sensitivity parameter, but this time it is the log-hazard ratio of censored to uncensored units. As usual, the data at hand give no information on the distribution of δ. However information on this may be elicited from experts or other data sources; alternatively we may reanalyse the data with δ successively further from 0 and then assess the plausibility of the value of δ at which our conclusions change substantively.

For now we assume that we have a distribution of the log-hazard ratio

$$\delta \sim N(\mu_\delta, \sigma_\delta^2), \quad (10.16)$$

although in seeking prior information it will usually be better to work on the hazard ratio scale itself. We also assume a parametric model for survival. Then, given (10.16) and (10.15), we can apply the approach described on p. 236 directly, giving the following algorithm:

1. Assuming CAR, fit the survival model to the data, obtaining parameter estimates $\widehat{\boldsymbol{\beta}}$ relating the log-hazard to the covariates, with associated estimated covariance matrix $\widehat{\boldsymbol{\Sigma}}$, typically obtained from the observed information (Kenward and Molenberghs, 1998).

2. Draw $\widetilde{\delta}$ from (10.16) and $\widetilde{\boldsymbol{\beta}} \sim N(\widehat{\boldsymbol{\beta}}, \widehat{\boldsymbol{\Sigma}})$.

3. With these values, for each censored unit i impute the time-to-event from the hazard $\exp(\widetilde{\delta})h_{CAR}(t, \widetilde{\boldsymbol{\beta}}, \mathbf{X}_i)$. If a unit's imputed time is less than the censoring time we draw again, until it is greater than the censoring time. The observed and imputed event times together make the imputed dataset under CNAR.

Repeating steps 2–3, we can generate K imputed data sets, to each of which we fit the substantive model. This could be a parametric or semi-parametric survival model; at its simplest it could be the Kaplan-Meier estimate of survival at a specific time. This gives K point estimates and their standard errors, which can be combined for final inference by applying Rubin's rules on an appropriate scale. For example, for an estimate of the probability of surviving past time t, $\hat{S}(t)$, appropriate choices would be the probit, logit or complementary log-log scale. We would transform the estimate from each imputed data set, apply Rubin's rules, and then back transform the result.

In practice, in order to draw the survival times, we will often want to calculate the cumulative distribution function of the survival time, $F(t; \mathbf{X}, \widetilde{\boldsymbol{\beta}}, \widetilde{\delta})$, corresponding to the hazard $\exp(\widetilde{\delta})h_{CAR}(t; \mathbf{X}, \widetilde{\boldsymbol{\beta}})$. Once we have done this, then since

$$F(T; \mathbf{Y}, \widetilde{\boldsymbol{\beta}}, \widetilde{\delta}) \sim U[0, 1],$$

we can draw a survival time for censored unit i by drawing u_i from the uniform distribution on [0, 1] and then calculating

$$\tilde{t}_i = F^{-1}(u_i; \mathbf{X}_i, \widetilde{\boldsymbol{\beta}}, \widetilde{\delta}).$$

This approach is convenient under a parametric survival model. If we adopt a Cox proportional hazards model, then generating proper imputations is harder, as uncertainty in estimating both the coefficients in the relative hazard, as well as the baseline hazard, needs to be taken into account. We do not view this as a major limitation, since within the rich families of parametric survival models it is likely that an appropriate choice can be found for imputation. Of course, the proportional hazards model can be fitted to the imputed data. If there are concerns about inconsistencies between the imputation model and model of interest, a natural first check is to impute the censored data assuming CAR (i.e. $\delta = 0$), fit the substantive model to each imputed dataset and combine the results using Rubin's rules. Just as in Table 10.2 rows 1–3, the resulting inferences should be very close to those from the observed data.

Again, exactly as in the application to the peer review trial, it may well be appropriate to have different means and variances for δ in different treatment or other groups. In that case, values for the correlation between these also need to be selected. In trials, it is also possible to envisage piecing post-censoring hazards together by drawing on other trial arms, much as in the longitudinal trials discussion in Section 10.4.

Example 10.3 Evaluation of ART programmes in sub-Saharan Africa *(ctd)*

Brinkhof *et al.* (2010) apply the approach set out above to explore the robustness of inference about mortality of patients receiving ART in studies conducted in sub-Saharan Africa to CNAR. Their substantive model was the Kaplan-Meier estimate of survival 1-year following initiation of ART. They chose a Weibull model for imputation. Under this model, (10.15) becomes

$$h(t; \mathbf{X}, \boldsymbol{\beta}, C) = \begin{cases} \exp(\mathbf{X}^T\boldsymbol{\beta})\gamma t^{\gamma-1} & \text{if } t < C \\ \exp(\delta)\exp(\mathbf{X}^T\boldsymbol{\beta})\gamma t^{\gamma-1} & \text{if } t \geq C, \end{cases} \tag{10.17}$$

where $t > 0$, $\gamma > 0$, δ is unrestricted and the $p \times 1$ vector $\mathbf{X}$ includes the intercept. As discussed below, they explore sensitivity for fixed values of δ; they do not sample it as in (10.16).

To implement the algorithm described above, the Weibull model is first fitted to the observed data in the usual way. Then, using the observed information, to create each imputed data set we draw from the distribution of the parameters, $\widetilde{\boldsymbol{\beta}}, \widetilde{\gamma}$, then with these parameter draws, sample survival times for censored observations from $S(t|t > C, \mathbf{X}_i, \widetilde{\boldsymbol{\beta}}, \widetilde{\gamma}, \delta)$. Under the Weibull distribution, this is

$$S(t|t > C, \mathbf{X}_i, \widetilde{\boldsymbol{\beta}}, \widetilde{\gamma}, \delta) = \frac{S(t; \mathbf{X}_i, \widetilde{\boldsymbol{\beta}}, \widetilde{\gamma}, \delta)}{S(C; \mathbf{X}_i, \widetilde{\boldsymbol{\beta}}, \widetilde{\gamma}, \delta)} = \exp\{-e^{\delta}(t^{\widetilde{\gamma}} - C^{\widetilde{\gamma}}) \exp(\mathbf{X}_i^T \widetilde{\boldsymbol{\beta}})\}.$$

We can draw from this distribution as described above, since the cumulative distribution function $F = 1 - S$. In this application, the substantive model is simply the Kaplan-Meier estimate of 1 year survival. The results for two of the five studies analysed by Brinkhof *et al.* (2010) are shown in Table 10.5. The estimated 1-year survival probabilities from each imputed dataset, $\hat{S}(1)_k$, $k = 1, \ldots, K$, were transformed using the complementary log-log link, $Z_k = \log[-\log\{\hat{S}(1_k)\}]$ to be approximately normally distributed. Rubin's rules were applied to the transformed values to obtain point estimates and confidence intervals, which were then back transformed to the original scale.

The estimated 1-year survival in the observed data, and after CAR imputation ($\delta = 0$, $K = 10$ imputations) agree closely. This is what theory predicts: imputation of censored survival times under CAR should give the same results as the observed data CAR analysis.

For the sensitivity analyses, Brinkhof *et al.* (2010) used meta-regression of other studies available to them to estimate plausible values of δ for the Lighthouse and AMPATH studies. For each study, the sensitivity parameter δ was then fixed at the estimated value rather than drawn from a distribution as in (10.16). The results show a substantial, practically important, relative increase in mortality in these studies if the hazard ratio relating those lost to follow up to those remaining in follow up is consistent with that estimated in the meta-regression.

We conclude this example by noting that while, given δ, the point estimates in Table 10.5 could be approximated analytically, MI also provides estimates of the standard errors, and resulting confidence intervals. The ability to do this when δ has a distribution, and this distribution is allowed to differ by treatment arm or other subgroups, makes MI a very attractive method for estimation and inference. □

Table 10.5 Illustration of sensitivity analysis for increased mortality among patients lost to follow up, from Brinkhof *et al.* (2010).

Study	$\exp(\delta_{study})$	One year mortality			Relative increase
		in observed data	under (10.17) $\delta = 0$	under (10.17) $\delta = \delta_{study}$	
Lighthouse	6	10.9% (9.6–12.4%)	10.8% (9.4–12.3%)	16.9% (15.0–19.1%)	56%
AMPATH	12	5.7% (4.9–6.5%)	5.9% (5.1–6.9%)	10.2% (8.9–11.6%)	73%

10.4 Pattern mixture approach with longitudinal data via MI

We now extend this approach to longitudinal data, focusing particularly on longitudinal data arising from clinical trials, although the same ideas will typically be applicable to longitudinal data arising in other settings.

Suppose we intend to observe a response at baseline, and p follow up times, $Y_{i,0}, Y_{i,1}, \ldots, Y_{i,p}$. For a given estimand we define a *deviation from the protocol relevant to the estimand*, which we simply refer to as a *deviation*, as a violation of the protocol, such that post-deviation data (if available) cannot be directly used for inference about the estimand. Here we assume that post-deviation data are missing. If available, post-deviation data can naturally be incorporated within this framework to inform the analysis.

While the precise definition of an estimand and associated deviations will be trial specific, for de facto questions we typically regard the first instance of the following as deviations:

- unblinding, for example of treatment allocation, and
- loss to follow up (after which no data are available in any case);

whereas the following would typically not be deviations:

- moving to partial compliance with treatment, and
- withdrawal from treatment (e.g. following an adverse event).

For de jure questions, we typically regard the first instance of any of these as deviations:

- unblinding;
- moving to partial compliance with treatment;
- withdrawal from treatment, and
- loss to follow up.

We emphasise 'typically'; in applications, deviations need to be carefully defined in the protocol.

Having pre-specified the estimands and associated deviations, we are left with a dataset in which (i) each patient has longitudinal follow up data until either they deviate, or reach the scheduled end of the study, and (ii) the nature of each deviation is available. The approach we describe here is that, for each deviation (or – more likely – group of similar deviations occurring for similar reasons) we build an appropriate post-deviation distribution taking account of (i) the patient's pre-deviation definitions of observations; (ii) pre-deviation data from other patients in the trial; (iii) the nature of the deviation, and (iv) the reason for the deviation.

We stress that we do not advocate building the post-deviation distribution after unblinding. Instead, for a given estimand, and associated pre-specified definitions of deviations, we advocate pre-specifying (i) a *primary* and (ii) *one or more secondary* post-deviation distributions. The former gives the primary answer to the question; the latter provide sensitivity analyses.

10.4.1 Change in slope post-deviation

Suppose that post-deviation patients have a different, usually poorer response than predicted under MAR. For example in an asthma trial, FEV_1 might improve more slowly (or decline more quickly) after deviation. If the change in rate of decline post-deviation in arm a is denoted δ_a, then the MAR conditional mean for the first scheduled post-deviation observation is reduced by δ, the second by 2δ and so on. This is schematically illustrated in Figure 10.1.

As in Example 10.1, if possible we can elicit from experts the mean and variance of δ_a in the intervention arm a, which is assumed to be normally distributed, and Cor $(\delta_a, \delta_{a'})$, for all treatment groups a and a'. In practice, White *et al.* (2007) show the widest confidence intervals occur when the correlation is zero (assuming it is not negative), and often useful information can be obtained by assuming the distribution of δ is the same across arms.

Computationally, we follow the approach described on p. 236. First, separately within each treatment arm, we use the pre-deviation data to generate K imputations under MAR. Then, if we have two intervention arms, for each

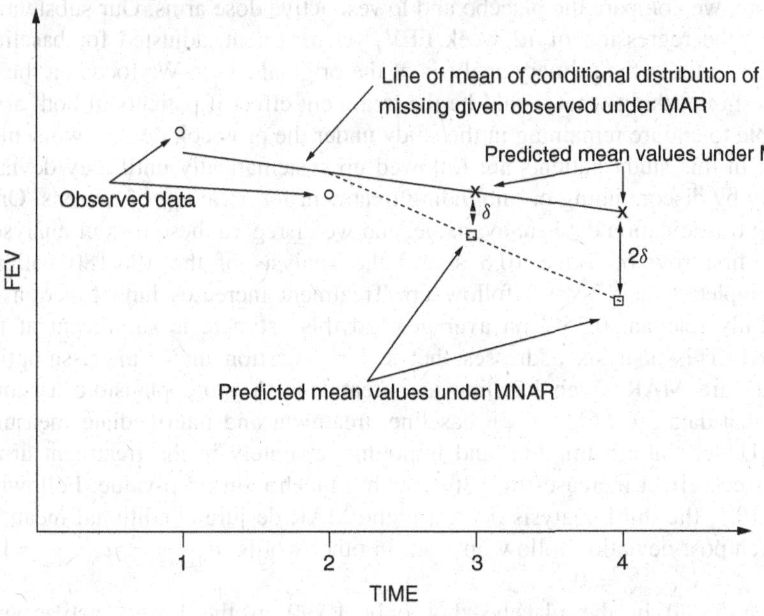

Figure 10.1 Schematic illustration of increasing the rate of decline by δ post-deviation.

imputation, $k = 1, \ldots, K$, we sample

$$\begin{pmatrix} \delta_{1,k} \\ d_{2,k} \end{pmatrix} \sim N\left[\begin{pmatrix} \mu_{\delta_1} \\ \mu_{\delta_2} \end{pmatrix}, \begin{pmatrix} \sigma_1^2 & \rho\sigma_1\sigma_2 \\ \rho\sigma_1\sigma_2 & \sigma_2^2 \end{pmatrix}\right].$$

For each patient, in each intervention arm $a = 1, 2$, for each imputation, we then decrease/increase the first MAR imputed observation by $\delta_{a,k}$, the second by $2\delta_{a,k}$ and so on. We then analyse the resulting datasets and combine the estimates using Rubin's rules. If the time between observations is not constant, we may want to change the multipliers of δ from $1, 2, 3, \ldots,$ to maintain a linear change. We can handle interim missing observations by decreasing them by δ_a, or simply leaving them with their MAR imputed values. The latter is consistent with a different mechanism driving interim missing data and patient deviation.

As discussed above the confidence intervals are going to be narrower the greater the correlation between the δ's for different treatment arms. In practice, information on this correlation is unlikely to be available, so as the correlation is unlikely to be negative, a conservative approach is to set $\rho = 0$. Likewise often, in the absence of prior information, we can set $\delta_1 = \delta_2$. Depending on the context, one approach may then be to increase δ until the treatment effect is no longer clinically relevant.

Example 10.4 Asthma study

We now illustrate this approach using the asthma study (see Chapter 7, p. 149). As before, we compare the placebo and lowest active dose arms. Our substantive model is the regression of 12 week FEV_1 on treatment, adjusted for baseline. This is essentially the primary analysis of the original study. We focus on the de jure question, asking what would be the treatment effect if patients in both arms were able to endure remaining in the study under the protocol, despite worsening asthma. In this study patients are followed up systematically until they deviate, typically by discontinuing or unblinding treatment for a variety of reasons. Only limited post-deviation data are available, and we disregard these for our analyses.

The first row of Table 10.6 shows the analysis of the 108/180 patients who completed the 12-week follow up. Treatment increases lung function by a clinically relevant 0.25 l on average, and this estimate is significant at the 5% level. This analysis addresses the de jure question under the assumption that data are MAR given baseline and treatment. A more plausible assumption is that data are MAR given baseline, treatment and intermediate measurements. Under this assumption, and imputing separately in the treatment arms, the 12 week effect increases to 0.36 l, with a much reduced p-value. Following Figure 10.1, the third analysis decreases the MAR de jure conditional mean by 0.1 l each post-deviation follow up visit. In other words, $\mu_{\delta_{\text{active}}} = \mu_{\delta_{\text{placebo}}} = 0.1$ and $\sigma_{\text{active}} = \sigma_{\text{placebo}} = 0$.

Since 53/90 in the placebo, but only 19/90 in the lowest active arm, deviate before 12 weeks, the consequence is to increase the treatment effect. The precision is unchanged from the randomised arm MAR analysis

Table 10.6 Asthma study: de jure estimates of the treatment effect under MAR, and MNAR with increasing post-deviation increments, δ. MI analyses used $K = 1000$ imputations.

Analysis	Treatment estimate (l)	Standard error	p-value
Complete records, de jure	0.247	0.100	0.0155
MI, de jure, randomised arm MAR	0.335	0.107	0.0017
MI, de jure, $\delta = 0.1, \sigma_\delta = 0$	0.361	0.108	0.0008
MI, de jure, $\delta = 0.1, \sigma_\delta = 0.1$	0.362	0.156	0.0207
MI, de jure, $\delta = 0.2, \sigma_\delta = 0.0$	0.388	0.110	0.0004
MI, de ure, $\delta = 0.2, \sigma_\delta = 0.1$	0.392	0.158	0.0132

because $\sigma_{\text{active}} = \sigma_{\text{placebo}} = 0$; with a relatively large $\sigma_{\text{active}} = \sigma_{\text{placebo}} = 0.1$, and $\rho = 1$, it is increased but the effect remains significant. Analysis with $\mu_{\delta_{\text{active}}} = \mu_{\delta_{\text{placebo}}} = 0.2$, retaining $\sigma_{\text{active}} = \sigma_{\text{placebo}} = 0.1$, $\rho = 1$, yields similar results. We conclude that, under the MNAR mechanism represented by this particular model for sensitivity analysis, the de jure inference is robust to MNAR. □

10.5 Piecing together post-deviation distributions from other trial arms

So far, our pattern mixture sensitivity analyses have all relied on specification of the distribution of the sensitivity parameter vector, $\boldsymbol{\delta}$. Carpenter *et al.* (2013) propose an alternative approach in the context of randomised clinical trials, which is to piece together the post-deviation distribution by making qualitative, not quantitative, reference to other arms. This is in the spirit of an approach to sensitivity analysis proposed by Little and Yau (1996); see also Kenward and Carpenter (2009), who provide an early implementation of this approach using sequential regression imputation. Thus, while the generic algorithm remains that described on p. 236, we now specify how the joint distribution of post-deviation data in the treatment arms is constructed, as follows:

1. Separately for each treatment arm, take all patients' pre-deviation data and – assuming MAR – fit a multivariate normal distribution with unstructured mean (i.e. a separate mean for each of the $1 + p$ baseline plus post-randomisation observation times) and unstructured variance-covariance matrix (i.e. a $(1 + p) \times (1 + p)$ covariance matrix), as described in Chapter 3.
2. Separately for each treatment arm, draw a mean vector and variance-covariance matrix from the posterior distribution.

3. For each patient who deviates before the end of the study, use the draws from step 2 to build the joint distribution of their pre- and post-deviation outcome data. Suggested options for constructing this are given below.

4. For each patient who deviates before the end, use their joint distribution in step 3 to construct their conditional distribution of post-deviation given pre-deviation outcome data. Sample their post-deviation data from this conditional distribution, to create a 'completed' data set.

5. Repeat steps 2–4 K times, resulting in K imputed data sets.

6. Fit the substantive model to each imputed data set, and combine the resulting parameter estimates and standard errors using Rubin's rules for final inference.

As usual, we use MCMC to sample from the appropriate Bayesian posterior in step 2, updating the chain sufficiently between successive draws to ensure they are effectively independent.

Constructing joint distributions of pre- and post-deviation data

We now give some examples of methods for constructing the joint distribution of each patient's pre- and post-deviation outcome data in step 3. Each option represents a difference between de jure and de facto behaviour post-deviation. Many others are possible but these are sufficient to explain our approach and illustrate its flexibility. Our experience is they are likely to prove appropriate in many settings.

Randomised-arm MAR
The joint distribution of the patient's pre- and post-deviation outcome data is multivariate normal with mean and covariance matrix from their randomised treatment arm.

Jump to reference
Post-deviation, the patient ceases their randomised treatment, and their mean response distribution is now that of a 'reference' group of patients (typically, but not necessarily, control patients). Such a change may be seen as extreme, and choosing the reference group to be the control group might be used as a worst-case scenario in terms of reducing any treatment effect since withdrawn patients on active will lose the effect of their period on treatment.
Post-deviation data in the reference arm are imputed under randomised-arm MAR.

Last mean carried forward
Post-deviation, it is assumed that the patient is expected, on average, to neither get worse nor better. So the mean of their distribution stays constant at the value of the mean for their randomised treatment arm at their last pre-deviation measurement. The variance-covariance matrix remains that for their randomised treatment arm.

Thus a patient who is well above the mean for their arm at the last pre-deviation measurement (giving a large positive pre-deviation residual) will tend to progress back across later visits to within random variation of the mean value for their arm at their pre-deviation measurement visit. The speed and extent of that progression will depend on the strength of the correlation between successive measurements.

Copy increments in reference
After the patient deviates, their post-deviation mean increments copy those from the reference group (typically, but not necessarily, control patients). Post-deviation data in the reference arm are imputed under randomised-arm MAR. If the reference is chosen to be the control arm, the patient's mean profile following deviation tracks that of the mean profile in the control arm, but starting from the benefit already obtained. This is what we might hope for in an Alzheimer's study where treatment halts disease progression. After stopping therapy the disease continues to progress again.

Copy reference
Here, for the purpose of imputing the missing response data, a patient's whole outcome data distribution, both pre- and post-deviation, is assumed to be the same as the reference (typically, but not necessarily, control) group. Post-deviation data in the reference arm are imputed under randomised-arm MAR. If the reference group is chosen as the control group, this mimics the case where those deviating are in effect nonresponders.

Perhaps surprisingly, this may often have a less extreme impact than 'jump to reference' above. This is because if a patient on active treatment is well above the control (i.e. reference) mean then this relatively large positive residual will feed through into subsequent draws from the conditional distribution of post-deviation data, to a degree determined by the correlation in the control (i.e. reference) arm. Thus, the patient's profile will decay back towards the mean for control at later visits relatively slowly.

Note that 'last mean carried forward' and 'copy increments in reference' have an important feature in common. For an active and a reference patient who deviate at the same time, the difference between their two post-deviation means is maintained at a constant value up to the end of the trial. In the former case the individual group mean profiles are held constant over time, in the latter they are allowed to vary across time. In this sense they both represent ways of implementing in a principled modelling framework the assumptions that might be implied by 'Last Observation Carried Forward' (LOCF) type methods.

Technical details

We now describe how step 3 works under 'jump to reference'. This leads to a brief presentation of the approach for the other options. Suppose there are two arms, active and reference.

In step 2, denote the current draw from the posterior for the $1 + p$ reference arm means and variance-covariance matrix by $\mu_{r,0}, \ldots \mu_{r,J}$, and $\mathbf{\Sigma}_r$. Use the subscript a for the corresponding draws from the other arm in question (which will depend on the arm chosen as reference for the analysis at hand).

Under 'jump to reference', suppose patient i is not randomised to the reference arm and their last observation, prior to deviating, is at time d_i, $d_i \in (1, \ldots, p - 1)$. The joint distribution of their observed and post-deviation outcomes is multivariate normal with mean

$$\boldsymbol{\mu}_i = (\mu_{a,0}, \ldots, \mu_{a,d_i}, \mu_{r,d_i+1}, \ldots, \mu_{r,p})^T;$$

that is post-deviation they 'jump to reference'.

We construct the new covariance matrix for these observations as follows. Denote the covariance matrices from the reference arm (without deviation) and the other arm in question (without deviation), partitioned at time d_i according to the pre- and post-deviation measurements, by:

$$\text{Reference } \mathbf{\Sigma}_r = \begin{bmatrix} \mathbf{R}_{11} & \mathbf{R}_{12} \\ \mathbf{R}_{21} & \mathbf{R}_{22} \end{bmatrix} \text{ and other arm: } \mathbf{\Sigma}_a = \begin{bmatrix} A_{11} & A_{12} \\ A_{21} & A_{22} \end{bmatrix}.$$

We want the new covariance matrix, $\mathbf{\Sigma}$ say, to match that from the active arm for the pre-deviation measurements, and the reference arm for the *conditional* components for the post-deviation given the pre-deviation measurements. This also guarantees positive definiteness of the new matrix, since $\mathbf{\Sigma}_r$ and $\mathbf{\Sigma}_a$ are positive definite. That is, we want

$$\mathbf{\Sigma} = \begin{bmatrix} \mathbf{\Sigma}_{11} & \mathbf{\Sigma}_{12} \\ \mathbf{\Sigma}_{21} & \mathbf{\Sigma}_{22} \end{bmatrix},$$

subject to the constraints

$$\begin{aligned} \mathbf{\Sigma}_{11} &= A_{11}, \\ \mathbf{\Sigma}_{21}\mathbf{\Sigma}_{11}^{-1} &= \mathbf{R}_{21}\mathbf{R}_{11}^{-1}, \\ \mathbf{\Sigma}_{22} - \mathbf{\Sigma}_{21}\mathbf{\Sigma}_{11}^{-1}\mathbf{\Sigma}_{12} &= \mathbf{R}_{22} - \mathbf{R}_{21}\mathbf{R}_{11}^{-1}\mathbf{R}_{12}. \end{aligned}$$

The solution is:

$$\begin{aligned} \mathbf{\Sigma}_{11} &= A_{11}, \\ \mathbf{\Sigma}_{21} &= \mathbf{R}_{21}\mathbf{R}_{11}^{-1}A_{11}, \\ \mathbf{\Sigma}_{22} &= \mathbf{R}_{22} - \mathbf{R}_{21}\mathbf{R}_{11}^{-1}(\mathbf{R}_{11} - A_{11})\mathbf{R}_{11}^{-1}\mathbf{R}_{12}. \end{aligned}$$

Under 'jump to reference' we have now specified the joint distribution for a patient's pre- and post-deviation outcomes, when deviation is at time d_i. This is what we require for step 4.

For 'copy increments in reference' we use the same $\mathbf{\Sigma}$ as for 'jump to reference' but now

$$\boldsymbol{\mu}_i = \{\mu_{a,0}, \ldots, \mu_{a,d_i-1}, \mu_{a,d_i}, \mu_{a,d_i} + (\mu_{r,d_i+1} - \mu_{r,d_i}), \mu_{a,d_i} + (\mu_{r,d_i+2} - \mu_{r,d_i}), \ldots\}^T.$$

For 'last mean carried forward', $\mathbf{\Sigma}$ equals the covariance matrix from the randomisation arm. The important change is the way we put together $\boldsymbol{\mu}$. Thus, for patient i in arm a under 'last mean carried forward',

$$\boldsymbol{\mu}_i = (\mu_{a,0}, \ldots, \mu_{a,d_i-1}, \mu_{a,d_i}, \mu_{a,d_i}, \ldots\ldots)^T; \quad \mathbf{\Sigma} = \mathbf{\Sigma}_a.$$

Finally for 'copy reference' the mean and covariance both come from the reference (typically, but not necessarily, control) arm, irrespective of deviation time.

A SAS macro implementing this approach, written by James Roger, can be downloaded from www.missingdata.org.uk

Example 10.4 Asthma study *(ctd)*

We return to the asthma study, and again focus on the placebo and lowest active dose arms, with the same definition of a deviation as before.

The first row of Table 10.7 (analysis DJ1) shows the complete records analysis (cf Table 10.6) by ANCOVA using the week 12 data, using the 108 patients with data at 12 weeks. It follows from the definition of deviation that the MAR assumption implies that, conditional on treatment and baseline, the distribution of unobserved and observed 12-week responses is the same. As the latter is estimated from on-treatment, protocol adhering patients, this analysis addresses the de jure question. However, there are only 37 out of 90 patients with 12-week data in the placebo arm, compared with 71 out of 90 in the active.

Thus analysis DJ2 includes all observed data in a Saturated Repeated Measurements (SRM) model. This fits a separate mean for each treatment and time, with a full baseline-time interaction and common unstructured covariance matrix. Analysis DJ3 further allows a separate, unstructured covariance matrix in each arm. The results show that inference from the primary analysis (DJ1: 0.247 l(itres), p = 0.0155), which addresses the de jure question, is robust to the different assumptions made by DJ2, DJ3; indeed DJ3 gives both the largest and most significant treatment estimate (0.346 l, p = 0.0013).

Analysis DJ4 makes the same MAR assumption as DJ3. In line with theory, the result from the SRM model with separate variance-covariance matrices agrees closely with that from using multiple imputation because the data are well modelled by the normal distribution. The only difference in underlying imputation model for DJ4 from the SRM model DJ3 is that the multiple imputation approach implicitly allows a full three-way interaction of baseline with treatment and time, whereas the SRM model has the same regression coefficients for baseline$\times$time in the two arms. Apart from this they are structurally equivalent.

Table 10.7 Estimated 12-week treatment effect on FEV_1 (litres), from ANCOVA, mixed models, multiple imputation and sensitivity analyses. All multiple imputation analyses used 1000 imputations, with a 'burn-in' of 1000 updates and 500 updates between imputations.

	Analysis		Treatment estimate (litres)	Std. Err.	DF (model)	t-statistic	p-value
De jure	DJ1	ANCOVA (Completers), joint variance	0.247	0.101	105	2.46	0.0155
De jure	DJ2	Mixed model, joint covariance matrix	0.283	0.094	131	3.02	0.0030
De jure	DJ3	Mixed model, separate covariance matrices	0.346	0.104	72.8	3.34	0.0013
De jure	DJ4	Macro Randomised-arm MAR	0.334	0.107	130.6	3.13	0.0022
De facto	DF1	Macro, last mean carried forward option	0.296	0.102	141.6	2.90	0.0043
De facto	DF2	Jump to reference (active)	0.141	0.119	102.7	1.18	0.2390
De facto	DF3	Jump to reference (placebo)	0.264	0.108	135.5	2.46	0.0153
De facto	DF4	Copy reference (active)	0.252	0.087	139.4	2.88	0.0046
De facto	DF5	Copy reference (placebo)	0.295	0.105	146.5	2.82	0.0055
De facto	DF6	Copy incr. in reference (active)	0.295	0.103	139.7	2.87	0.0048
De facto	DF7	Copy incr. in reference (placebo)	0.323	0.104	139.6	3.12	0.0022

We now consider the de facto question, and analyses DF1–DF7 in Table 10.7. Each of these assumes a different joint distribution for pre- and post-deviation data. For analyses DF2–DF7 the reference arm is always imputed using randomised-arm MAR.

Analysis DF1 corresponds to the underlying mean response remaining static after intervention stops. This would address the de facto question when after deviation patients took no further relevant medication and their condition was stable. If, allowing for the personal covariates such as baseline, they have a positive residual at their final pre-deviation visit, we expect that post-deviation their residuals will decrease (but continue to randomly vary), so on average they will get closer to their own conditional mean.

In the asthma setting, this flat mean profile post deviation may be plausible for a week or two after deviation, especially in the active treatment arm. In these data, the downward trend in the placebo arm (Table 1.5) suggests that LMCF is likely to yield higher estimates of the latter placebo means than the de jure analyses, while estimates for the lowest active arm will change in the other direction. This leads to a smaller treatment estimate (0.296 l), but not as low as that for DJ1.

We now apply the 'jump to reference' (DF2, 3), 'copy reference' (DF4, 5) and 'copy increments in reference' (DF6, 7) options. We discuss the implications for the interpretation of the choice of the 'reference' arm under these two approaches (in this example it could either be the placebo, or the lowest active dose arm).

Suppose we wish to address the de facto question corresponding to the assumption that, post-deviation, (i) patients on placebo obtain a treatment equivalent to the active, and (ii) the active treatment patients continue on treatment and adhere to the protocol, so that their post-deviation data can be imputed assuming randomised-arm MAR. In this case, we specify the *active arm* as 'reference'. The early part of the study suggests that 2–3 weeks are needed for a treatment to take effect. Further the patients have chronic asthma, so it is likely that they will seek an active treatment on deviation from the placebo arm. For the de facto question, this assumption is more plausible than considering placebo as 'reference'. Nevertheless, for discussion we also present results where the placebo is 'reference'; that is where post-deviation (i) patients on the active treatment switch to a placebo equivalent, and (ii) the placebo treatment patients continue on placebo adhering to the protocol, and their post-deviation data can be imputed assuming randomised-arm MAR. This latter assumption might be appropriate where no alternative treatment is generally available.

Analysis DF2 estimates treatment effect under 'jump to reference' when the 'reference' is the active arm. Of all the de facto analyses, this is the most extreme in terms of effect on the treatment difference, since the means prior to deviation follow the patients randomised arm and then abruptly switch to that of the specified 'reference' arm. The effect of this is shown in Figure 10.2; we find plots like this very useful tools for conveying the implications of assumptions to those we are collaborating with. This big change in placebo patients' post-deviation means results in a substantially reduced treatment estimate. (0.141 l, $p = 0.24$). We conclude that, if post-deviation medication has a comparable effect to the

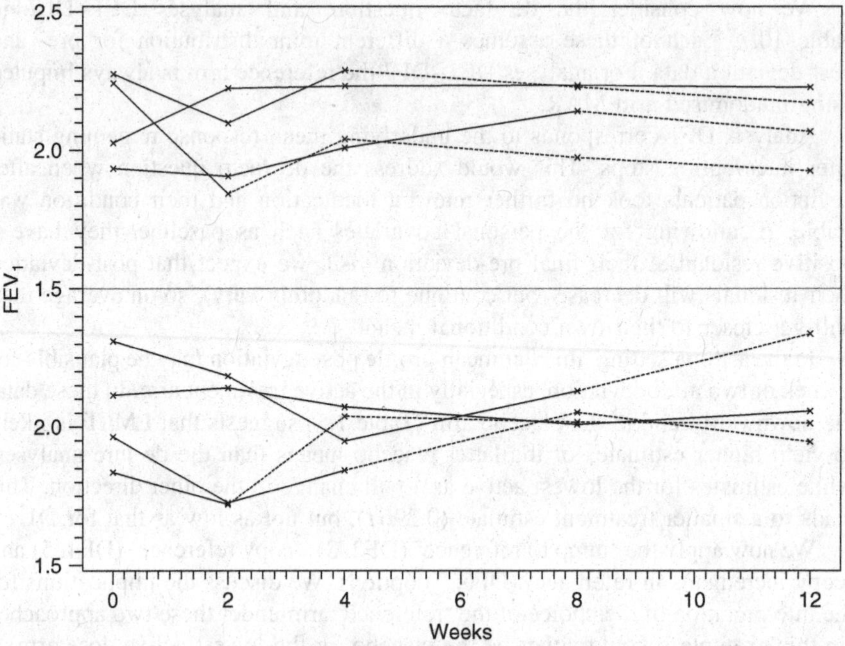

Figure 10.2 Mean FEV_1 (litres) against time for the four different deviation patterns. Solid lines join observed means (before deviation) and dotted lines join the means of the imputed data for that pattern. Top panel: lowest active dose, imputed under randomised-arm MAR; bottom panel: placebo arm imputed under 'jump to reference' (where 'reference' is lowest active dose).

lowest active dose, patients from both arms will have comparable lung function at the end of the study. This analysis mimics what we might expect from a *retrieved dropout analysis* (Committee for Medicinal Products for Human Use, 2010) where placebo patients are allowed to return to active treatment.

Analysis DF3 corresponds to the less plausible reverse option where after deviation the active patients now 'jump to reference' and the reference is the placebo. Since far fewer patients deviate in the active arm, the change from the de jure MAR analysis is much smaller: the treatment difference remains significant ($0.264\,l$, $p = 0.015$).

We now consider two further sets of assumptions for addressing the de facto question: 'copy reference' and 'copy increments in reference'. The former replaces both pre-deviation and post-deviation means with those of the specified 'reference', when constructing the joint distribution of pre- and post-deviation data in step 3 of the algorithm at the start of Section 10.5. The latter, 'copy increments in reference', has the randomised profile prior to deviation, but then the incremental changes in mean FEV_1 from visit to visit track those in the 'reference' arm.

When the active arm is specified as the 'reference', 'copy reference' (DF4) and 'copy increments in reference' (DF6) give 12 week treatment estimates of $0.252l$ and $0.295l$ respectively. In this case, 'copy reference' has a larger treatment effect than 'jump to reference' because under 'copy reference', pre-deviation placebo patients have relatively larger residuals (differenced from the mean for the active arm), which implies that after deviation they track to the active means more slowly; with 'jump to reference' pre-deviation placebo patients have smaller residuals (differenced from the mean for the placebo arm), so post-deviation they track to ethe active means more rapidly.

When placebo is specified as the 'reference', 'copy reference' (DF5) and 'copy increments in reference' (DF7) give much smaller changes from the randomised-arm MAR estimate, for the same reason as 'jump to reference' (DF3), discussed above.

In summary, the primary analysis addressing the de jure question assuming MAR is consistent with a significant beneficial effect of treatment relative to placebo. Addressing the de facto question with a conservative assumption about the effect of post-deviation (withdrawal) switching to active ('copy reference' or 'copy increments in reference') continues to show a significant improvement. However, if instead we use 'jump to reference' ('reference' is active treatment) then the treatment benefit is reduced by over 50% relative to randomised-arm MAR, and is no longer statistically significant. If the many placebo patients who deviate early switch to the active treatment, this is to be expected. □

10.6 Approximating a selection model by importance weighting

So far we have explored sensitivity analysis using a pattern mixture approach. In particular, having chosen a model for the observed data, we specified models for the various patterns of missing data relative to this. Missing data were then imputed from these models, then the substantive model fitted to each of the imputed data sets and the results combined using Rubin's rules.

While this approach involved no approximations, it did require that data be explicitly imputed under the MNAR model, and then the substantive model fitted to this imputed data. Assuming that imputation had previously been performed under MAR, this approach therefore entails a imputing a new set of data under each MNAR mechanism considered.

By contrast, here we describe an approximate approach, proposed by Carpenter *et al.* (2007), for exploring the sensitivity of conclusions to MNAR mechanisms without the need for imputing under the MNAR mechanism concerned. The idea is simple: having imputed K data sets under MAR, and fitted the substantive model to each, instead of averaging the results for the imputation estimate, we perform a weighted average, up-weighting imputations that are more likely under the MNAR mechanism we are considering.

This approach rests on the idea of importance sampling. Suppose we draw

$$Z_1, \ldots, Z_K \overset{i.i.d.}{\sim} g,$$

for some distribution g, but wish to estimate the expectation of some function, $h(Z)$ when Z is drawn from the distribution f. Provided the support of f is contained in that of g, and f/g is bounded, if we calculate $w_k = f(Z_k)/g(Z_k)$,

$$\mathrm{E}_f[h(Z)] \approx \frac{\sum_{k=1}^K w_k h(Z_k)}{\sum_{k=1}^K w_k}, \tag{10.18}$$

with the approximation tending to equality as $K \to \infty$.

Essentially, we apply this result to MI, identifying g with the imputation distribution under MAR, f with the imputation distribution under MNAR, k indexing imputations, Z_k with the kth imputation under MAR and $h(Z_k)$ with the estimate of the parameter in the substantive model obtained from imputation k.

To explore how this works, consider a very simple setting of two variables, $\mathbf{Y}_1, \mathbf{Y}_2$, and let the parameter of interest $\hat{\theta} = \hat{\theta}(\mathbf{Y}_1)$ be the mean of $\mathbf{Y}_1$. For this initial explanation, suppose further we have only a single observation pair, (Y_1, Y_2), but that Y_1 is missing. As usual, denote the missingness indicator by R, so that $R = 0$. Suppose, by some means, we were able to draw two imputations Y_1^1, Y_1^2 from the imputation model

$$f(Y_1|Y_2, R = 1). \tag{10.19}$$

This corresponds to imputing under MAR. However, suppose we wish to impute under MNAR, i.e. draw from

$$f(Y_1|Y_2, R = 0). \tag{10.20}$$

Earlier we took a pattern mixture approach and defined (10.20) by reference to (10.19) via sensitivity parameters. Here we consider a selection model, that is we define the relationship implicitly through the logistic regression of R on Y_1, Y_2 :

$$\operatorname{logit} \Pr(R = 1) = \alpha_0 + \alpha_1 Y_1 + \alpha_2 Y_2. \tag{10.21}$$

In this case, the weight is the ratio

$$\begin{aligned}\frac{f(Y_1|Y_2, R=0)}{f(Y_1|Y_2, R=1)} &= \frac{f(Y_1, Y_2, R=0)f(Y_2, R=1)}{f(Y_1, Y_2, R=1)f(Y_2, R=0)} \\ &= \frac{f(R=0|Y_1, Y_2)f(Y_2, R=1)}{f(R=1|Y_1, Y_2)f(Y_2, R=0)}.\end{aligned} \tag{10.22}$$

Now consider $f(R = 0|Y_1, Y_2)$. Under model (10.21), this is $\{1 + \exp(\alpha_0 + \alpha_1 Y_1 + \alpha_2 Y_2)\}^{-1}$, and $f(R = 1|Y_1, Y_2) = 1 - f(R = 0|Y_1, Y_2)$. So (10.22) is

$$\exp\{-(\alpha_0 + \alpha_1 Y_1 + \alpha_2 Y_2)\}\frac{f(Y_2, R=1)}{f(Y_2, R=0)}.$$

Therefore the weights for the two imputations, Y_1^1 and Y_1^2 are

$$\tilde{w}_1 = \exp(-\alpha_1 Y_1^1) \left\{ \exp[-(\alpha_0 + \alpha_2 Y_2)] \frac{f(Y_2, R=1)}{f(Y_2, R=0)} \right\} \text{ and}$$

$$\tilde{w}_2 = \exp(-\alpha_1 Y_1^2) \left\{ \exp[-(\alpha_0 + \alpha_2 Y_2)] \frac{f(Y_2, R=1)}{f(Y_2, R=0)} \right\}. \qquad (10.23)$$

Because the terms between the braces {} are common to both weights, the normalised weights, $w_1 = \tilde{w}_1/(\tilde{w}_1 + \tilde{w}_2)$ and $w_2 = \tilde{w}_2/(\tilde{w}_1 + \tilde{w}_2)$ are proportional to $\exp(-\alpha_1 Y_1^1)$ and $\exp(-\alpha_1 Y_1^2)$ respectively. In other words, we do not need estimates of α_0, α_2 to estimate the weights; all we need are the imputed values under MAR, and α_1. As with pattern mixture modelling, we do not estimate this parameter (cf Kenward, 1998). Instead, we explore the sensitivity of the results as α_1 varies from 0.

In fact, in the linear predictor '$\alpha_0 + \alpha_1 Y_1 + \alpha_2 Y_2$' we can have any function of the observed data; it will cancel out of the weights. This means that, in contrast to full joint modelling approaches, our inference is robust to possible mis-specification of the relationship between the probability of observing Y_i and the observed part of the data *provided* the relationship of the missingness process on the unseen data is correct.

So far we have considered only $n = 1$ units and 2 imputations. Now suppose we have $i = 1, \ldots, n_1$ units (out of a total of n) with Y_1 missing, and, for unit i, K values imputed assuming MAR, $Y_{i,1}^1, \ldots Y_{i,1}^K$. Since, given $Y_{i,1}^k, Y_{i',1}^k, Y_{i,2}, Y_{i',2}$ and $i' \neq i$, the probability of observing $Y_{i'}^k$ is independent of the probability of observing Y_i^k, it follows from (10.23) that the weight for imputation k is

$$w_k \propto \exp\left(-\alpha_1 \sum_{i=1}^{n_1} Y_{i,1}^k\right). \qquad (10.24)$$

In other words, the log-weight for imputation k is proportional to a linear combination of the imputed data. Lastly, we can replace $\theta(\mathbf{Y}_1) = \mathrm{E}(Y_1)$ with any general $\theta(\mathbf{Y}_1, \mathbf{Y}_2)$. Thus, in general we proceed as follows:

10.6.1 Algorithm for approximate sensitivity analysis by re-weighting

We write the data vector for unit i as $\mathbf{Y}_i = (\mathbf{Y}_{i,\text{obs}}, \mathbf{Y}_{i,\text{miss}})$. Let θ be the scalar quantity of interest, such as a treatment effect. Assume, as is usual with multiple imputation, that if there are no missing data the estimator of θ is approximately normally distributed. Given data, denote the estimated value of θ by $\hat{\theta}$. Assuming MAR, suppose we have imputed K versions of the missing data, $\mathbf{Y}_{\text{miss}}^1, \ldots \mathbf{Y}_{\text{miss}}^K$, and hence computed K estimates of the parameter of interest, $\hat{\theta}_1, \ldots, \hat{\theta}_K$ and their corresponding variances, $\hat{\sigma}_1^2, \ldots, \hat{\sigma}_K^2$.

Suppose we wish to explore sensitivity to MNAR on partially observed variable $\mathbf{Y}_1$, with corresponding missingness indicator $\mathbf{R}_1$. Consider the selection model

$$\operatorname{logit}\{\Pr(R_{i,1} = 1)\} = \alpha_1 Y_{i,1} + g(\mathbf{Y}_{i,\text{full}}), \tag{10.25}$$

where $\mathbf{Y}_{\text{full}}$ are those variables fully observed on all units.

To obtain an estimate of θ when data are MNAR, the analyst first chooses a plausible value of α_1. Suppose we re-order the data set so that units $i = 1, \ldots, n_1$ have missing $Y_{i,1}$. Let $Y_{i,1}^k$ denote the kth MAR imputation of $Y_{i,1}$. Then, for each imputation, k, compute

$$\tilde{w}_k = \exp\left(\sum_{i=1}^{n_1} -\alpha_1 Y_{i,1}^k\right), \quad \text{and} \quad w_k = \tilde{w}_k \Big/ \sum_{k=1}^{K} \tilde{w}_k. \tag{10.26}$$

Then, under the MNAR model implied by the analyst's choice of α_1, in (10.25), the estimate of θ and its variance are

$$\hat{\theta}_{\text{MNAR}} = \sum_{k=1}^{K} w_k \hat{\theta}_k, \tag{10.27}$$

with variance

$$\widehat{V}_{\text{MNAR}} \approx \widetilde{V}_W + (1 + 1/K)\widetilde{V}_B, \tag{10.28}$$

where now

$$\widetilde{V}_W = \sum_{k=1}^{K} w_m \hat{\sigma}_m^2, \quad \widetilde{V}_B = \sum_{k=1}^{K} w_m (\hat{\theta}_k - \hat{\theta}_{\text{MNAR}})^2. \tag{10.29}$$

$\hat{\theta}_{\text{MNAR}}$ and $\hat{V}_{\text{MNAR}}$ can then be used for inference.

Reliability of the approximation

The accuracy of the approximation justifying $\hat{\theta}_{\text{MNAR}}$ and $\widehat{V}_{\text{MNAR}}$ improves as the number of imputations, K increases, provided the two importance sampling conditions hold:

I1 the support of the MNAR distribution of missing data given observed is contained within the support of the MAR distribution, and

I2 the ratio of the MNAR distribution to the MAR distribution is bounded.

This has a number of practical implications.

First, for the full generality of MNAR models, I1 cannot hold. Thus, the method is suitable for exploring local departures from MNAR. In the example below we give some graphical diagnostics that can be used to assess 'local' in applications. Second, even locally, it may be that the ratio of the distributions is unbounded. For example, if the MAR imputation distribution is $N(1, 1)$ and the MNAR imputation distribution is $N(0.5, 1)$, this occurs in the left tail. Where this is a concern, a boundary can be imposed, for example through defining the MNAR distribution to be zero outside a given range.

Interestingly, in terms of under or over-estimating the difference between MNAR and MAR inference, I1 and I2 work in opposite directions. If I1 is violated, then as we move from the locality of the MAR model, the difference will be underestimated; if I2 is violated, then as the number of imputations increases $\hat{\theta}_{\text{MNAR}}$ will remain unstable. Despite this, simulation studies (Carpenter *et al.*, 2011b, 2007) have shown good performance in practically relevant situations, especially if care is taken to choose an appropriate imputation model under MAR when the sample size is small.

Taken together, these points suggest that when using this approach, often $K \geq 50$ will be needed; but this is not unduly burdensome for many problems. However, even for relatively large values of K, $\hat{V}_{\text{MNAR}}$ tends to slightly underestimate the variance, although the resulting confidence interval coverage is acceptable (Carpenter *et al.*, 2011b, supplementary material). One explanation is that after re-weighting the effective number of imputations is often considerably smaller than K. On possibility is to replace K in (10.29) by a measure of the effective sample size, such as the number of $\{Kw_k\}_{k=1}^{K}$ which are ≥ 1.

Lastly, we note that while the approach can be applied to longitudinal data, we then generally have more than one sensitivity parameter. For example, let $Y_{i,1}, Y_{i,2}, Y_{i,3}$ be three longitudinal measurements on subject i. Let $R_i = 1$ if $Y_{i,3}$ is observed. A general model for this is

$$\text{logit}\{\Pr(R_i = 1)\} = \alpha_0 + \alpha_1 Y_{i,1} + \alpha_2 Y_{i,2} + \alpha_3 Y_{i,3}.$$

If some subjects have $Y_{i,2}$, and/or $Y_{i,3}$ missing, then we need to specify both sensitivity parameters α_2, α_3, since no parameter in the selection model involving missing data cancels out when we normalise the weights. One possible approach to this would be to specify say α_3, and use an EM type approach to estimate other parameters; however given that typically there is relatively little information on these in the data, both a large number of imputations and a large number of observations are likely to be needed.

Example 10.5 Simulation study

Carpenter *et al.* (2007) report the following simulation study. Draw 100 pairs of observations $(X_1, Y_1), \ldots, (X_{100}, Y_{100})$ from

$$\text{N}\left\{\begin{pmatrix}0\\0\end{pmatrix}, \begin{pmatrix}1 & 0.5\\0.5 & 1\end{pmatrix}\right\},$$

and for each pair calculate

$$p = \frac{e^{X+Y}}{1 + e^{X+Y}}, \tag{10.30}$$

draw u from a uniform distribution on [0, 1], and set Y missing if $u > p$. This is equivalent to selecting observations using

$$\operatorname{logit} \Pr(\text{observe } Y_i) = \alpha_0 + \alpha_1 Y_i + \alpha_2 X_i.$$

We then estimate E(Y) (true value 0) using:

1. the average of the observed Y's, which assumes observations are missing completely at random;
2. K multiply imputed data sets, generated assuming observations are missing at random; and
3. by re-weighting the imputations drawn in 2.

In 3. we re-weight using the true value of $\alpha_1 = 1$, as we wish to see how close the estimated mean is to the true value of zero.

We performed 1000 such simulations, with various values of K, and averaged the resulting estimates of E(Y) obtained using methods 1, 2 and 3. Table 10.8 summarises the results. The first row gives the average of the 1000 estimates of E(Y) from the observed part of each simulated data set (i.e. the complete records). As this does not depend on the number of imputations, this is only shown in the second column. As (10.30) means we tend to observe larger values of Y, this estimate is biased upwards from the true value of 0.

Multiple imputation reduces the MCAR estimate by about 34%; although the precise estimates of E(Y) vary slightly with different choices of K, this is beyond the precision shown. As the underlying MAR model is wrong, no matter how large K the estimate will never converge to 0.

Re-weighting the MI estimates obtained under MAR is a simple calculation, hence fast computationally. It removes substantially more of the bias than MI under MAR. As the number of imputations increases, steadily more of the bias

Table 10.8 Results of simulation study. Estimated standard errors of $\widehat{EY}$ are all around 0.004 for method 2. and 0.005 for method 3.

	No. imputations, K				
	5	10	50	100	1000
Method 1: average observed data (assumes MCAR)	0.5				
Method 2: MI under MAR	0.33	0.33	0.33	0.33	0.33
Method 3: Re-weighting MAR imputations	0.20	0.16	0.1	0.06	−0.01
% bias of MAR estimates removed by method 3:	39	51	70	82	97

is removed. This makes sense, and is a direct consequence of the fact that the approximation in (10.18) improves as the number of imputations increases.

Clearly, $K = 1000$ imputations is more than would be used in many applications. However, the results suggest that even with, as here, typically 50% of the observations missing, useful results can be obtained with $K = 50$. Such values of K are not unusual today; indeed Meng (1994) (and some discussants therein) was calling for 30 imputations, instead of the conventional 4 or 5, to be commonplace over 15 years ago.

More subtly, the justification for the weights relies on (10.22), which has the true MAR distribution, in our notation $f(Y|X, R = 1)$, in the denominator. In practice, of course, this is estimated from the observed data. If the data set is very small, or there are many missing data, this estimate may be noisy, and in particular the resulting proper imputation distribution often has a considerably heavier tail than $f(Y|X, R = 1)$. This causes re-weighted estimates to overshoot the true MNAR value. This is because the imputed data drawn from the heavy tail of the imputation distribution gets disproportionately up-weighted. In our example, reducing $n = 100$ to $n = 20$ (with everything else identical) illustrated this. With $n = 20$ and $K = 100$ imputations, the estimated mean was −0.22 using the procedure above, whereas using the true weights, calculated from the known ratio of the MNAR distribution to the MAR distribution, gave a mean of 0.06. When data sets are small, the imputation distribution must therefore be chosen carefully (e.g. Carpenter *et al.*, 2011b). One possibility is to multiply the weight for each imputed dataset by the ratio of the improper to proper imputation density. However, in applications, apart from sensitivity analysis for meta-analysis with samll numbers of studies, and in line with the results in Table 10.8, we have found this error is of secondary importance. □

Example 10.1 Peer review trial *(ctd)*

We now perform a second sensitivity analyses for these data by imputing under MAR and re-weighting to explore sensitivity to MNAR. Specifically, we investigate the sensitivity of the results to the possibility that the RQI score from paper 2, Y_i, is missing not at random. Let $R_i = 1$ if Y_i is observed and 0 otherwise. We use the following selection model

$$\operatorname{logit} \Pr\{(R_i = 1)\} = \alpha_0 + \alpha_1 X_{1,i} + \alpha_2 X_{2,i} + \alpha_3 Y_i \tag{10.31}$$

where X_1 is the review of the baseline paper and X_2 is an indicator for the self-taught group. If $\alpha_3 = 0$, then Y is MAR. As α_3 increases from 0 the probability of Y being observed increases with Y (*i.e.*, increases with the review quality). If $\alpha_3 = 0$ we can fit this model using logistic regression. This gives the results shown in Table 10.9. Overall the probability of observing the RQI score from paper 2 decreases as baseline review quality increases, and is much higher in the self-taught arm.

The estimate $\hat{\alpha}_1 = 0.21$ suggests that each point rise in the baseline average RQI score multiplies the odds ratio of response by 1.23. In the light of this

Table 10.9 Parameter estimates (log odds ratios) for logistic regression for probability of observing the RQI score from paper 2, model (10.31), with $\alpha_3 = 0$.

	Parameter		
	α_0	α_1	α_2
Estimate	2.14	0.21	−1.75
Std. Err.	(0.64)	(0.22)	(0.35)

we carry out sensitivity analyses with $\alpha_3 = 0.3$ and $\alpha_3 = 0.5$ in (10.31). These correspond, on the odds-scale, to roughly 10% and 35% stronger adjusted association between the chance of seeing the second review and its quality.

We obtain estimates of the effect of the self-taught intervention vs. control using `winBUGS` by fitting models (10.10) and (10.31) jointly. We also obtain estimates and standard errors by re-weighting the imputations obtained under MAR, using (10.27) and (10.29). We do this using $K = 50$, 150, 250 and 1000 imputations. The results presented below are based on analyses including the face-to-face training group, with corresponding indicator variables added to (10.10), (10.31).

Table 10.10 shows the results. As expected, the estimated effect of the self-taught intervention is reduced, but it remains significant at the 5% level. The `winBUGS` estimates agree within at most 0.01 with the estimates obtained by re-weighting. The estimated standard errors are also similar, although for small K they appear to be underestimated (see p. 261). □

In applications, it is important to know whether we have enough imputations for a reasonably reliable answer, and also whether the range of parameter estimates from the MAR model is sufficiently wide to give acceptable support to the MNAR distribution – the key assumption for the method. We suggest two graphs for evaluating this. First, a graph of the parameters vs. the normalised weights, with a line at $1/K$, corresponding to equal weights. Second, a graph of the running re-weighted estimate,

$$\sum_{k=1}^{I} w_k \hat{\theta}_k \Big/ \sum_{k=1}^{I} w_k$$

for $I = 10, \ldots, K$. On the right of this plot, it is useful to show the original imputations. This gives a natural scale for the y-axis. More importantly, it shows whether the running mean is heading out of the range of the MI imputations, which suggests the MNAR distribution is not well supported by the MAR distribution.

Table 10.10 Peer review trial: estimated effects of the self-taught intervention versus the control. All models adjusted for baseline RQI score. Uncertainty in parameter estimates from winBUGS due to Monte Carlo estimation is less than ±0.001.

Method	Estimated effect of self-taught intervention vs. control	Standard error
Missing at random		
regression	0.236	0.070
multiple imputation, $M = 1000$	0.237	0.070
regression using winBUGS	0.236	0.070
Missing not at random, $\alpha_3 = 0.3$		
winBUGS	0.215	0.071
weighting, $M = 50$	0.209	0.066
weighting, $M = 150$	0.201	0.069
weighting, $M = 250$	0.205	0.068
weighting, $M = 1000$	0.205	0.069
Missing not at random, $\alpha_3 = 0.5$		
winBUGS	0.202	0.071
weighting, $M = 50$	0.205	0.063
weighting, $M = 150$	0.197	0.067
weighting, $M = 250$	0.199	0.066
weighting, $M = 1000$	0.195	0.067

Example 10.1 Peer review trial *(ctd)*

We consider these plots for $\alpha_3 = 0.5$, as this happens to throw up the highest weight of the 1000 imputations on imputation 18. Generally, the larger α_3 and smaller K, the greater the chance of extreme weights. Note too that, because all missing observations are weighted, there will not generally be a simple relationship between the imputation parameter estimate and its weight. In other words, two similar imputations may result from different combinations of the underlying data, one of which may be much more plausible under the MNAR model.

The plots are shown for (a) $K = 50$ and (b) $K = 250$ in Figure 10.3. The plot of the running means (left panels) shows the influence on the final outcome of rare estimates with high weights (right). These occur at visible 'steps' in the left plots. In this example it happens that a point of very high weight in the first 50 imputations (Figure 10.3 top right) is a cause for concern. Nevertheless, the change it causes to the running mean itself is small (Figure 10.3 top left); even omitting this point the mean over the first 49 imputations is 0.21. There is no evidence that the MNAR mean is not within the range of the MAR imputations. Moreover,

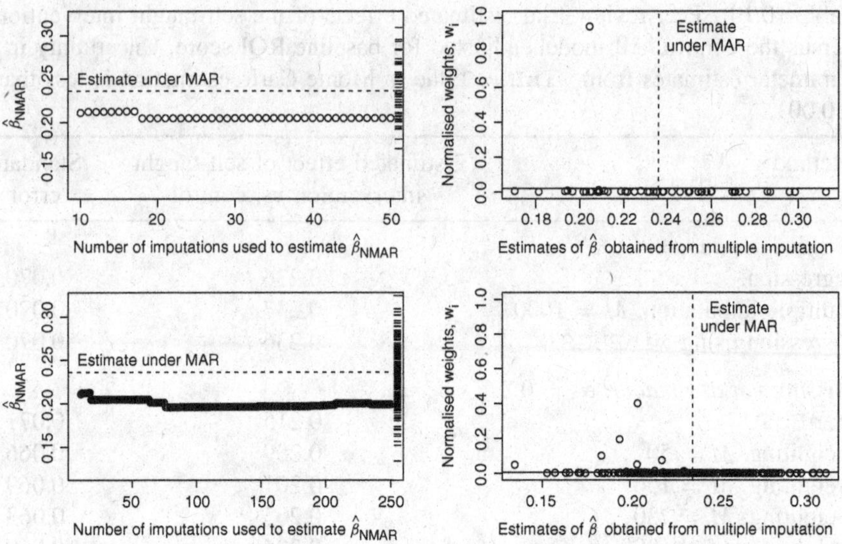

Figure 10.3 *Analysis with $\alpha_3 = 0.5$. Left panels: running estimate of $\hat{\beta}_{\text{MNAR}}$, using the first 50 (top) and 250 (bottom) imputations of a set of 1000 (shown in Figure 10.4). The distribution of the imputations is indicated by the 'rug' on the right of the plot. The dashed line shows the MAR estimate of β. Right panels: normalised weights using first 50 imputations (top) and 250 imputations (bottom). The solid line is 1/50 (top) and 1/250 (bottom).*

an estimate with very high weight is by definition very plausible under MNAR. Here the estimate with high weight is 0.204; the posterior mean from winBUGS (Table 10.7, $\alpha_3 = 0.5$) is 0.202. Of course, if possible we should include more imputations. Reassuringly (lower panels Figure 10.3), these do not change the conclusions. Finally, Figure 10.4 shows the results for all 1000 imputations. Notice that points in the region of imputation 18, 0.204, have the highest weights. We have virtually identical conclusions to those with only 50 imputations, but less concern over reliance on relatively few points of high weight.

In conclusion, this analysis by reweighting after MAR imputation confirms the results for the self-taught arm are sensitive to poorer reviewers not returning the second paper and hence withdrawing. Specifically, if the adjusted log odds of returning the second paper increases by 0.5 (OR 1.65) for every point increase in the RQI, the confidence interval for the self-taught intervention comes close to the null value. Analysis using winBUGS and weighting give similar conclusions. However, the latter is far quicker, even taking into account the time taken to draw the MAR imputations, and requires no specialist programming. In comparing the results of this analysis with those presented in Table 10.2, the principle difference is in the standard errors. The reason for this is that in the selection modelling we have fixed the sensitivity parameter α_3 at certain values, where as

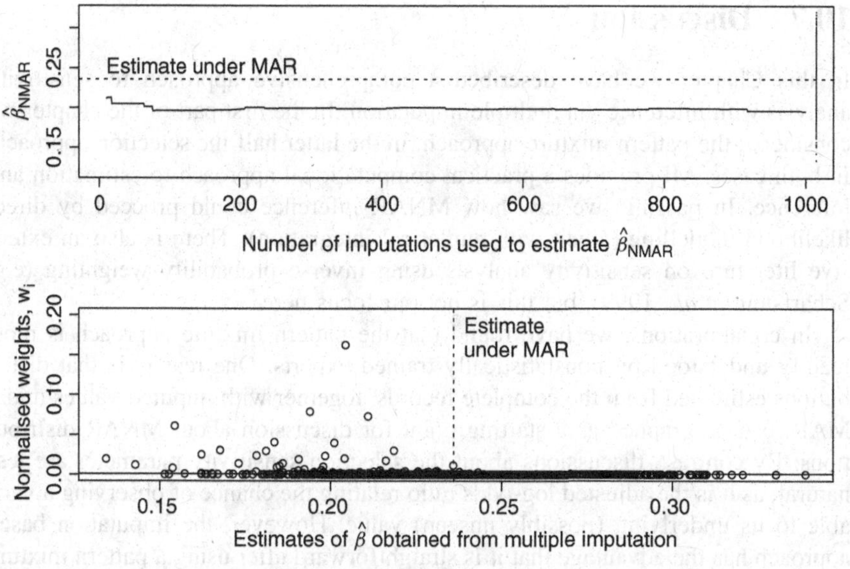

Figure 10.4 Analysis with $\alpha_3 = 0.5$. Running estimate of $\hat{\beta}_{\text{MNAR}}$ and normalised weights for $M = 1000$.

in the pattern mixture modelling, the corresponding sensitivity parameter, δ, had a distribution. □

Further developments

Carpenter *et al.* (2011b) apply this approach to publication bias in meta-analysis. Here, careful choice of imputation distribution is important, especially if there is marked asymmetry in the funnel plot. They report encouraging results from a simulation study and good agreement with a full Bayesian model where this is possible to fit using `winBUGS`. The advantage of the re-weighting approach in this context is its ability to rapidly handle otherwise computationally awkward (though practically relevant) selection mechanisms.

Bousquet *et al.* (2012) apply the method to sensitivity analysis for missing covariates. Here, after imputation under MAR, the selection model allows investigation of dependence of the missingness mechanism on the covariates. A separate sensitivity analysis performed for each covariate in turn. The substantive model is a logistic regression. In line with the theoretical results noted at the end of Chapter 1, where the complete records analysis suggests missingness does not involve the response, corresponding log-odds ratios are relatively unchanged by MAR imputation or sensitivity analysis. Where selection does involve the response, coefficients change after MAR analysis, and the method allows rapid exploration of sensitivity to MNAR.

10.7 Discussion

In this Chapter we have described a comprehensive approach to sensitivity analysis with inference via multiple imputation. In the first part of the chapter we considered the pattern mixture approach; in the latter half the selection approach. In both cases, MI provides a practical computational approach to estimation and inference. In passing, we saw how MNAR inference could proceed by direct likelihood modelling (albeit with numerical integration). There is also an extensive literature on sensitivity analysis using inverse probability weighting (e.g. Scharfstein *et al.*, 1999), but this is not our focus here.

In collaborations, we have found that the pattern mixture approach is most readily understood by nonstatistically trained experts. One reason is that distributions estimated from the complete records, together with imputed values under MAR, can be graphed as a starting point for discussion about MNAR distributions. By contrast, discussions about the selection sensitivity parameter are less natural, as it is the adjusted log-odds ratio relating the chance of observing a variable to its underlying (possibly unseen) value. However, the imputation based approach has the advantage that it is straightforward after using a pattern mixture approach to explore the selection implications, and vice-versa. For example, having created imputed datasets using the pattern mixture approach under MNAR, we can fit selection models to the imputed data, combine the results using Rubin's rules, and check with experts they are contextually plausible. Going in the reverse direction, Carpenter *et al.* (2011b) illustrate calculating weighted averages of the imputed data to graph the difference in mean between the observed and imputed data as selection increases.

A feature of our proposed pattern mixture approach for longitudinal data is the avoidance of explicit specification of sensitivity parameters by specifying instead patterns of profiles. This seems most natural in the clinical trials setting, where we have data in active and control arms and the appropriate approach to imputation depends on whether we are interested in de jure or de facto questions. As we argued above, in this setting, post-deviation distributions can be accessibly framed with reference to the various intervention arms.

In conclusion, as Rubin stressed in his original book (Rubin, 1987, ch. 6), the analysis of partially observed data involves untestable assumptions, and MI provides a natural framework for sensitivity analysis. The MAR assumption is a natural starting point, with its implication that conditional distributions of partially observed given fully observed data do not differ by missingness pattern. Moving to MNAR mechanisms, we have illustrated the flexibility, and hence broad utility, of an imputation based approach.

11

Including survey weights

Throughout this book we have been focussing on MI in the context of conventional model based statistical analysis, and we have used the Bayesian paradigm that sits at core of the technique to provide a broad justification for its use. In this chapter we make a brief departure from this framework, and consider settings that are common in survey sampling in which account must be taken of the sampling scheme, typically through appropriate weighting. A comprehensive reference for the use of model based analyses in this setting is provided by Särndal *et al.* (1992). The main problem with the justification of MI in the sample survey setting is the absence of methods for the construction of proper imputation schemes. Thus we cannot, in general, make recourse to the direct Bayesian arguments set out in Chapter 2. Hence exploration of the behaviour of MI schemes in the sample survey literature is usually based on direct assessment of the behaviour of the statistics involved, and it much harder to provide very general results. It has been known for a long time (e.g. Fay (1992, 1993); Kott (1995)) that a naive application of the MI variance formula in nontrivial survey settings will produce a biased estimator because the sets of multiply imputed data do not follow from the actual sampling mechanism. Kim *et al.* (2006) provide a recent exposition of the problem and derive some quite general results for the special case of estimators that are linear functions of the data. Much of Section 11.2 is based on their development. Before considering this in more detail, however, we first look at a special setting where these problems can be avoided.

11.1 Using model based predictions

We first consider a special setting, in which we are able to link the goal of our analysis, typically involving weights derived from the sampling scheme, directly to the model based analyses used in the rest of this book. The connection is made through model based *prediction* in a survey setting, see for example Royall (1992); Särndal *et al.* (1992). Suppose that the data are grouped or clustered, and we have a substantive model with parameter vector $\boldsymbol{\beta}_j$ in the jth of N clusters. Our goal is to estimate a weighted combination of some prediction $g(\boldsymbol{\beta}_j)$:

$$\theta = \sum_{j=1}^{n} w_j g(\boldsymbol{\beta}_j), \tag{11.1}$$

for weights w_j, $j = 1, \ldots, n$. It is important that we allow the substantive model parameters to differ in some way across clusters, otherwise the weighting is irrelevant as far as consistency of the estimator is concerned, although it may of course have a bearing on precision. An obvious and simple example occurs when we want to estimate a weighted average of the cluster means, where $g(\boldsymbol{\beta}_j) = \beta_j$ is the mean for the jth cluster:

$$\theta = \sum_{j=1}^{n} w_j \beta_j.$$

If sampling is completely random within clusters, and missing data are MAR, then we can apply the conventional MI procedure *separately* within each cluster, to produce a set of MI estimators $\widehat{\boldsymbol{\beta}}_{\mathrm{MI},j}$ and corresponding MI variance estimators $\widehat{\mathbf{V}}_{\mathrm{MI},j}$, $j = 1, \ldots, n$. A consistent estimator of θ is then given by:

$$\widehat{\theta} = \sum_{j=1}^{n} w_j g(\widehat{\boldsymbol{\beta}}_{\mathrm{MI},j}),$$

and a consistent estimator of the variance of this can obtained from Rubin's variance estimators, $\widehat{\mathbf{V}}_{\mathrm{MI},j}$, using standard steps. This is particularly simple when $g(\boldsymbol{\beta}_j) = \boldsymbol{\beta}_j$, for then

$$\widehat{\theta} = \sum_{j=1}^{n} w_j \widehat{\boldsymbol{\beta}}_{\mathrm{MI},j},$$

with variance estimator

$$\sum_{j=1}^{n} w_j^2 \widehat{\mathbf{V}}_{\mathrm{MI},j}.$$

The justification for this stems from the valid MI procedures within each cluster. The resulting combination of information follows conventional steps.

The applicability of this approach is limited however. The data structure may be more complex than simple clustering and, even with a single set of clusters, these need to be of sufficient size to support MI within each. There are many situations, for example when the weights are inverse response probabilities, where the weights can be unique to each unit. Clearly this approach cannot then be applied without forming groups defined by the weights in some *ad hoc* way. If we eschew this approach, one might consider instead an overall MI procedure, but here the survey structure causes problems with the variance combination formula which must be then be applied across clusters. If the sampling structure of the imputations does not match that of the data, then the Rubin's variance formula will be biased. We explore this below, and consider how corrections can be made. Finally in Section 11.3 we consider another route in which a clustered sampling structure is introduced directly into the imputation model using a multilevel approach.

11.2 Bias in the MI variance estimator

Kim *et al.* (2006) derive quite general conditions for approximate unbiasedness of the MI variance estimator, which we give shortly. They confine their development to linear estimators of the form

$$\widehat{\theta}_{\mathrm{C}} = \mathbf{a}_O{}^T\mathbf{Y}_O + \mathbf{a}_M{}^T\mathbf{Y}_M \tag{11.2}$$

for known coefficient vectors $\mathbf{a}_O$ $(n_O \times 1)$ and $\mathbf{a}_M$ $(n_M \times 1)$, the elements of which are assumed to contain weights and other relevant quantities from the survey design, as well as covariate values. For example, the estimator of any linear function $\mathbf{c}^T\boldsymbol{\beta}$ of the linear regression parameter $\boldsymbol{\beta}$ can be expressed in this form.

Recall that, in the scalar setting, the conventional MI variance estimator of $\widehat{\theta}_{\mathrm{MI}}$ can be written

$$\widehat{V_{\mathrm{MI}}} = \widehat{W} + (1 + 1/K)\,\widehat{B}$$

for $\widehat{W}$ the average of the within-imputation set variance estimators, and $\widehat{B}$ the between-imputation variance

$$\widehat{B} = \frac{1}{K-1}\sum_{k=1}^{K}(\widehat{\theta}_k - \widehat{\theta}_{\mathrm{MI}})^2.$$

We are interested in the bias in $\widehat{V_{\mathrm{MI}}}$ when survey weights are introduced into the complete data estimator $\widehat{\theta}_{\mathrm{C}}$. The MI estimator can be partitioned as follows

$$\widehat{\theta}_{\mathrm{MI}} = \widehat{\theta}_{\mathrm{C}} + (\widehat{\theta}_{\mathrm{MI},\infty} - \widehat{\theta}_{\mathrm{C}}) + (\widehat{\theta}_{\mathrm{MI}} - \widehat{\theta}_{\mathrm{MI},\infty}) \tag{11.3}$$

where $\widehat{\theta}_{\mathrm{MI},\infty}$ is the limiting form of the MI estimator as the number of imputations increases:

$$\widehat{\theta}_{\mathrm{MI},\infty} = \lim_{K\to\infty} \widehat{\theta}_{\mathrm{MI}}.$$

Given a set of assumptions that will be satisfied in typical survey settings, Kim *et al.* (2006) show that the three components on the right of (11.3) need to be uncorrelated for Rubin's variance estimator to be approximately unbiased. One implication of this is that

$$\mathrm{Var}(\widehat{\theta}_{\mathrm{MI},\infty}) \simeq \mathrm{Var}(\widehat{\theta}_{\mathrm{C}}) + \mathrm{Var}(\widehat{\theta}_{\mathrm{MI},\infty} - \widehat{\theta}_{\mathrm{C}})$$

which is another way of expressing the self-efficiency requirement of Meng (1994), discussed on p. 66. Kim *et al.* (2006) also show that this is equivalent to the requirement that the average covariance of $\widehat{\theta}_{\mathrm{C}}$ and the difference $(\widehat{\theta}_k - \widehat{\theta}_{\mathrm{C}})$ be zero when the expectation is taken over the entire sampling process, for $\widehat{\theta}_k$ the estimator from the kth imputed data set. From this we can see that, if this holds approximately, then

$$\mathrm{E}(\widehat{B}) \simeq \mathrm{Var}(\widehat{\theta}_{\mathrm{MI},\infty} - \widehat{\theta}_{\mathrm{C}}).$$

For the congenial setups considered in Chapter 2, with completely random sampling, we can see that this will be true exactly, at least when the expectation of the imputed values consists of linear functions of the observed data, that is,

$$\mathrm{E}(\widetilde{\mathbf{Y}}_{M,k} \mid \mathbf{Y}_O) = \mathbf{H}\mathbf{Y}_O,$$

for some fixed $n_M \times n_O$ matrix $\mathbf{H}$.

As a simple example of this consider the linear regression imputation model whose properties were explored Section 2.7. We have

$$\widehat{\boldsymbol{\beta}}_{\mathrm{MI}} = \widehat{\boldsymbol{\beta}}_O + (\mathbf{X}^T\mathbf{X})^{-1}\mathbf{X}_M^T(\mathbf{X}_M\bar{\boldsymbol{b}}_. + \bar{\boldsymbol{e}}_.),$$

from which

$$\widehat{\boldsymbol{\beta}}_{\mathrm{MI},\infty} = (\mathbf{X}_O^T\mathbf{X}_O)^{-1}\mathbf{X}_O^T\mathbf{Y}_O$$

and

$$\widehat{\boldsymbol{\beta}}_{\mathrm{C}} = (\mathbf{X}^T\mathbf{X})^{-1}\mathbf{X}_O^T\mathbf{Y}_O + (\mathbf{X}^T\mathbf{X})^{-1}\mathbf{X}_M^T\mathbf{Y}_M$$

The difference of these is

$$\widehat{\boldsymbol{\beta}}_{\mathrm{MI},\infty} - \widehat{\boldsymbol{\beta}}_{\mathrm{C}} = \left\{(\mathbf{X}_O^T\mathbf{X}_O)^{-1} - (\mathbf{X}^T\mathbf{X})^{-1}\right\}\mathbf{X}_O^T\mathbf{Y}_O - (\mathbf{X}^T\mathbf{X})^{-1}\mathbf{X}_M^T\mathbf{Y}_M$$

and so

$$\begin{aligned}\mathrm{Var}(\widehat{\boldsymbol{\beta}}_{\mathrm{MI},\infty} - \widehat{\boldsymbol{\beta}}_{\mathrm{C}}) &= \sigma^2\left\{(\mathbf{X}_O^T\mathbf{X}_O)^{-1} - (\mathbf{X}^T\mathbf{X})^{-1}\right\}\mathbf{X}_O^T\mathbf{X}_O\left\{(\mathbf{X}_O^T\mathbf{X}_O)^{-1} - (\mathbf{X}^T\mathbf{X})^{-1}\right\}\\ &\quad + \sigma^2(\mathbf{X}^T\mathbf{X})^{-1}\mathbf{X}_M^T\mathbf{X}_M(\mathbf{X}^T\mathbf{X})^{-1}\\ &= \sigma^2\left\{(\mathbf{X}_O^T\mathbf{X}_O)^{-1} - (\mathbf{X}^T\mathbf{X})^{-1}\right\}.\end{aligned}$$

which is, as shown in Section 2.7, is equal to $\mathrm{E}(\widehat{\mathbf{B}})$.

However, when survey weights enter the definition of $\widehat{\theta}_C$ the conventional MI variance estimator will typically be biased. Kim *et al.* (2006) show that this bias can be expressed as a function of the covariance between $\widehat{\boldsymbol{\theta}}_C$ and $\widehat{\boldsymbol{\theta}}_{MI,\infty}$,

$$E(\widehat{\mathbf{V}}_{MI}) - \mathrm{Var}(\widehat{\boldsymbol{\theta}}_{MI}) \simeq -2\,E\left\{\mathrm{Cov}(\widehat{\boldsymbol{\theta}}_k - \widehat{\boldsymbol{\theta}}_C, \widehat{\boldsymbol{\theta}}_C)\right\}.$$

In the particular case in which the observations Y_i are independent with common variance σ^2, this expression takes a particularly simple form:

$$\mathrm{Cov}(\widehat{\boldsymbol{\theta}}_k - \widehat{\boldsymbol{\theta}}_C, \widehat{\boldsymbol{\theta}}_C) = \sigma^2 \mathbf{a}_M{}^T(\mathbf{H}\mathbf{a}_O - \mathbf{a}_M),$$

giving the bias

$$\mathrm{Bias} = E(\widehat{\mathbf{V}}_{MI}) - \mathrm{Var}(\widehat{\boldsymbol{\theta}}_{MI}) = 2\sigma^2 \mathbf{a}_M{}^T(\mathbf{a}_M - \mathbf{H}\mathbf{a}_O). \qquad (11.4)$$

As an illustration, consider again the situation in which the imputation model is a linear regression, this time with simple inverse probability weighting, with weights the elements of $\mathbf{w}_O$ and $\mathbf{w}_M$ for the observed and missing data respectively. That is the substantive and imputation models are both based on the same linear regression model

$$\mathbf{Y} \sim N(\mathbf{X}\boldsymbol{\theta}, \sigma^2\mathbf{I}), \qquad (11.5)$$

but, because of the sampling design, we need to use the weighted least squares estimator

$$\widehat{\boldsymbol{\theta}} = (\mathbf{X}^T\mathbf{W}\mathbf{X})^{-1}\mathbf{X}^T\mathbf{W}\mathbf{Y}, \qquad (11.6)$$

for $\mathbf{W}$ the diagonal matrix of weights w_i. In the notation we have used earlier, the bias in the MI variance estimator (11.4) for this setup can be written

$$\mathrm{Bias} = 2\sigma^2\left[\mathbf{w}_M^T\mathbf{w}_M - \mathrm{tr}\left\{\mathbf{w}_O^T\mathbf{X}_O(\mathbf{X}_O^T\mathbf{X}_O)^{-1}\mathbf{X}_M^T\mathbf{w}_M\right\}\right]. \qquad (11.7)$$

A practically important consequence follows from this expression: if the weights are included in the space spanned by the variates in the regression model, that is, if we can write

$$\mathbf{w}_O = \mathbf{X}_O\mathbf{d} \quad \text{and} \quad \mathbf{w}_M = \mathbf{X}_M\mathbf{d},$$

for some fixed $\mathbf{d}$ then

$$\begin{aligned}\mathrm{Bias} &= 2\sigma^2\left[\mathbf{d}^T\mathbf{X}_M^T\mathbf{X}_M\mathbf{d} - \mathrm{tr}\left\{\mathbf{d}^T\mathbf{X}_O^T\mathbf{X}_O(\mathbf{X}_O^T\mathbf{X}_O)^{-1}\mathbf{X}_M^T\mathbf{X}_M\mathbf{d}\right\}\right]\\ &= 2\sigma^2\left[\mathbf{d}^T\mathbf{X}_M^T\mathbf{X}_M\mathbf{d} - \mathbf{d}^T\mathbf{X}_M^T\mathbf{X}_M\mathbf{d}\right] = 0.\end{aligned}$$

This points to an important technique for correcting for the bias in Rubin's variance estimator when using such weights, at least with linear regression: introduce these into the linear predictor. We now consider the implications of this in more detail for the special case of simple weighted estimation schemes.

11.2.1 MI with weights

Seaman *et al.* (2012b) apply the results of Kim *et al.* (2006) to the general regression setting, and much of this section follows their development. We begin by moving from the direct expression of the estimator as given in (11.2) to its representation as a solution of set of estimating equations. We suppose that, in the absence of weights, the required estimator of $\boldsymbol{\theta}$ from the substantive model is the solution the unbiased estimating equation

$$\sum_{i=1}^{n} \mathbf{U}(\widehat{\boldsymbol{\theta}}; \mathbf{Y}_i) = \mathbf{0}.$$

We now introduce the design weights w_i, $i = 1, \ldots, n$. In the absence of missing data we would estimate $\boldsymbol{\theta}$ by solving

$$\sum_{i=1}^{n} w_i \mathbf{U}(\widehat{\boldsymbol{\theta}}; \mathbf{Y}_i) = \mathbf{0}.$$

Now suppose that for units (typically individuals) $i \in \mathcal{M}$ one or more component variables are missing, and denote by $\widetilde{\mathbf{Y}}_{i,k}$ the set of observations for the ith of these completed by the kth imputation. Seaman *et al.* (2012b) give conditions under which multiple imputation will give consistent parameter estimators. These are

1. The design weights are correct;
2. Given the variables used to calculate the weights, the probability of an individual i being included in the sample does not depend on their data $\mathbf{Y}_i$;
3. Within the sample observations, $i = 1, \ldots, n$, data are missing at random given the weights and observed data; and
4. The imputation model includes the weights and is correctly specified.

Then if $\boldsymbol{\theta}_k$ is the estimate obtained by using the kth set of imputed data to solve

$$\sum_{i \in \mathcal{O}} w_i \mathbf{U}(\widehat{\boldsymbol{\theta}}; \mathbf{Y}_i) + \sum_{i \in \mathcal{M}} w_i \mathbf{U}(\widehat{\boldsymbol{\theta}}; \widetilde{\mathbf{Y}}_{i,k}) = \mathbf{0},$$

we have, as usual, the MI estimator

$$\widehat{\boldsymbol{\theta}}_{\text{MI}} = \frac{1}{K} \sum_{k=1}^{K} \widehat{\boldsymbol{\theta}}_k \tag{11.8}$$

is consistent for $\boldsymbol{\theta}$ when $K = \infty$.

In the context of design weights, condition 2 above will hold if the data have been collected according to the design. Conditions 3 and 4 are sufficient to ensure the imputed data comes from the correct distribution, taking into account the weights and the missingness mechanism. For condition 4 to hold, we will have to include not only the weights in our imputation model, but also all necessary interactions with the weights. Thus we may, in general need to include interactions between the weights and partially observed variables, using one of the approaches discussed in Chapter 7. In many settings though, including relevant interactions between the weights and the fully observed variables will be sufficient. Including all, or too many, interactions in the imputation model risks losing efficiency or inducing model fitting problems. Below, we discuss a random effects approach which may avoid such issues.

In other settings, we may wish to use estimated weights; for example we may wish to weight for unit nonresponse and impute for item nonresponse (the motivation for Seaman *et al.*, 2012b). Provided our weight model is correct, (11.8) is again consistent. Further, if desired we can work with weights calculated from the design weights and estimated weights.

While the condition requiring $K = \infty$, i.e. an infinite number of imputations, is required for mathematical convergence, in practice it does not appear that more imputations are needed in this than in other settings.

Notice that this result applies whether the covariate or response is missing, and for any probability model or link function that give rise to the score equations.

However, for these results to be of use in practice we also need to be able to use Rubin's variance formula. To justify the use of this we confine ourselves to the linear regression setting with auxiliary variables. Suppose that the substantive model, and accompanying weighted estimator, follow (11.5) and (11.6). We assume as well that for complete data the estimator of the covariance matrix of $\hat{\boldsymbol{\theta}}$ is

$$(\mathbf{X}^T\mathbf{W}\mathbf{X})^{-1}\{\mathbf{X}^T\mathbf{W}(\mathbf{Y}-\mathbf{X}\hat{\boldsymbol{\theta}})(\mathbf{Y}-\mathbf{X}\hat{\boldsymbol{\theta}})^T\mathbf{W}\mathbf{X}\}(\mathbf{X}^T\mathbf{W}\mathbf{X})^{-1}. \tag{11.9}$$

We now introduce auxiliary variables into the imputation model. We assume that the setting of the problem provides p additional variables $\mathbf{Z}$ and we add to this two generated sets of variables $\mathbf{WX}$ and $\mathbf{WZ}$. The requirement for these follows the same argument used in eliminating the bias in (11.7). Hence the imputation model is the regression

$$\mathbf{Y} \sim \mathrm{N}(\mathbf{V}\boldsymbol{\beta}, \sigma^2\mathbf{I}), \tag{11.10}$$

for $\mathbf{V} = (\mathbf{X}, \mathbf{WX}, \mathbf{Z}, \mathbf{WZ})$. Using conventional imputation procedures based on this model, with unknown σ^2, we obtain the kth estimate of $\boldsymbol{\theta}$

$$\hat{\boldsymbol{\theta}}_k = (\mathbf{XWX})^{-1}(\mathbf{X}_O\mathbf{W}_O\mathbf{Y}_O + \mathbf{X}_M\mathbf{W}_M\tilde{\mathbf{Y}}_{M,k})$$

for $\mathbf{W}_O$ and $\mathbf{W}_M$ the partitions of $\mathbf{W}$ corresponding to the observed and unobserved observations respectively, and associated covariance estimator

$$\tilde{\mathbf{V}}_k = (\mathbf{XWX})^{-1}\begin{bmatrix} \boldsymbol{A}_O\boldsymbol{A}_O^T & \boldsymbol{A}_O\boldsymbol{A}_M^T \\ \boldsymbol{A}_M\boldsymbol{A}_O^T & \boldsymbol{A}_M\boldsymbol{A}_M^T \end{bmatrix}(\mathbf{XWX})^{-1}$$

for $\boldsymbol{A}_O = \mathbf{X}^T \mathbf{W}_O(\mathbf{Y}_O - \mathbf{X}_O\widehat{\boldsymbol{\theta}}_k)$ and $\boldsymbol{A}_M = \mathbf{X}_M^T \mathbf{W}_M(\widetilde{\mathbf{Y}}_{M,k} - \mathbf{X}_M\widehat{\boldsymbol{\theta}}_k)$. We can then define the MI estimator and covariance estimator in the usual way:

$$\widehat{\boldsymbol{\theta}}_{\mathrm{MI}} = \frac{1}{K}\sum_{k=1}^{K}\widehat{\boldsymbol{\theta}}_k,$$

$$\widehat{\boldsymbol{\theta}}_k = \frac{1}{K}\sum_{k=1}^{K}\widetilde{\mathbf{V}}_k + \frac{K+1}{K(K-1)}\sum_{k=1}^{K}(\widehat{\boldsymbol{\theta}}_k - \widehat{\boldsymbol{\theta}}_{\mathrm{MI}})(\widehat{\boldsymbol{\theta}}_k - \widehat{\boldsymbol{\theta}}_{\mathrm{MI}})^T.$$

Seaman *et al.* (2012b) show that

1. $\widehat{\boldsymbol{\theta}}_{\mathrm{MI}}$ is consistent for $\boldsymbol{\theta}$;
2. $\widehat{\mathbf{V}}_{\mathrm{MI}}$ is asymptotically unbiased for $\mathrm{Var}(\widehat{\boldsymbol{\theta}}_{\mathrm{MI}})$ as $n \to \infty$ and
3. at $K = \infty$, $\widehat{\mathbf{V}}_{\mathrm{MI}}$ is consistent for $\mathrm{Var}(\widehat{\boldsymbol{\theta}}_{\mathrm{MI}})$.

If we omit **WZ** from (11.10) in general then consistency (3) no longer holds.

We note that this result only holds for linear regression, where the response has missing observations. With missing covariates, there will be an asymptotic upward bias in the variance; Seaman *et al.* (2012b) use Theorems 1 and 2 of Robins and Wang (2000) to derive this for their simulation study, and find it is $< 4\%$ for all parameters, and $< 1\%$ for the majority.

Up to now we have assumed the weights are known. If they are estimated, then we need to replace (11.9) with a sandwich variance estimator that accounts for uncertainty in the weights (Robins *et al.*, 1994); otherwise the variance will be biased upwards.

Seaman *et al.* (2012b) further explore the performance of this approach when the substantive model is logistic, with missing response or missing covariate. In the latter case there is a small, but practically negligible, upward bias in the variance estimate.

11.2.2 Estimation in domains

On occasion analysts are interested in estimating summary statistics, or relationships between variables, in a specific subset or domain of the data. Perhaps this is most common in the analysis of survey data, where for example economic data are summarised within social and ethnic groups.

In terms of handling missing data by MI, summarising variables within domains not recognised within the imputation model does not result in a biased estimate within those domains. However, the corresponding MI variance estimate will, generally, be too large. This is the same issue identified and explored in some detail by Meng (1994) (see the discussion in Section 2.8), who concludes that the MI variance is still usually smaller than the complete records variance, and that the resulting confidence intervals (though they may over-cover) and inferences are therefore preferable.

By contrast, Kim *et al.* (2006) cite the issues raised by MI and domain estimation – particularly the need to include in the imputation model both the domain indicator and potentially its interactions with the other variables – as sufficient reason to conclude that MI 'is not generally recommended for public use data'. However, we find this conclusion unduly negative.

First, we would argue that those imputing data and subsequently releasing it for public use should also publish the imputation model, so that users can see for which domains Rubin's variance formula will be hold, and for which it will likely be an overestimate. Second, as pointed out by Meng (1994), the fact that the MI variance will, even if an overestimate, still likely be smaller than the complete records variance needs to be remembered. In many settings, the dataset is large, and the importance of effects is clear. Third, the practicality and flexibility of MI for many analysts who will be unfamiliar with the more technical alternatives is a key advantage. In any case, releasing imputed data sets does not preclude analysts adopting other approaches, such as the jack-knife (Rao and Shao, 1992) if desired.

Further, the continuing increase in desktop computing power means that, increasingly, the imputer and the analyst are the same individual. In addition, it is relatively fast to create additional sets of imputations, consistent with weights and specific domains, as required. In this case, the MI variance formula should apply; the above criticisms are not relevant.

11.3 A multilevel approach

We have seen above that, with design weights, estimated weights, or their combination, for Rubin's variance formula to be valid the weights, and potentially a full interaction with the other variables, must be included in the imputation model. Further, the imputation model must be correctly specified. In other words, the above discussion implicitly assumed that the imputation model gave a valid estimate for the mean, so that including a linear effect of weight (as a continuous covariate) and linear interactions with the other variables allowed Rubin's rules to give a valid estimate of the variance. However, it could be the case that in addition to this we need to include a nonlinear effect of weight, or inverse weight.

In such cases, the consequence is likely to be a complex imputation model. Even if it is not formally over-specified, the resulting imputations are likely to be noisy.

A natural alternative in this setting is shrinkage via a random effect model. Consider continuous variables and cross-sectional imputation of partially observed $\mathbf{Y}_1$ given fully observed $\mathbf{Y}_2$, and weights $\mathbf{W}$. Instead of the the imputation model

$$Y_{i,1} = \beta_0 + \beta_1 Y_{i,2} + \beta_2 W_i + \beta_3 Y_{i,2} W_i + e_i, \quad e_i \sim N(0, \sigma^2), \tag{11.11}$$

we may use distinct weight values to define level-2 units, $l = 1, \ldots, L$, say and use the imputation model

$$\begin{aligned} Y_{i,1,l} &= (\beta_0 + u_{0,l}) + (\beta_1 + u_{1,l})Y_{i,2,l} + e_{i,l} \\ (u_{0,l}\ u_{1,l}) &\sim N(0, \mathbf{\Omega}_u) \\ e_{i,l} &\sim N(0, \sigma_e^2). \end{aligned} \tag{11.12}$$

This random intercept and slope model allows a different linear imputation within each weight stratum, for the price of one more parameter than (11.11). Furthermore, in strata with small numbers of observations, the relationship will be shrunk to the overall mean, while reflecting the variability across the dataset. In practice, with many unique weights, we may need to form level-2 units from groups of units with similar weights. We anticipate that Rubin's rules are asymptotically valid in this framework, because asymptotically (11.12) will tend to imputing separately in strata defined by each weight, which is equivalent to the imputation model allowing for (i) a linear effect of weight, (ii) departures from that linear effect, (iii) a linear interaction of weight with other variables and (iv) departures from that linear interaction. Thus asymptotically the justification of Rubin's variance formula discussed above, which stems from including a linear effect of weight and its interaction with other variables in the imputation model, should hold. Alternatively, if after imputation we can apply Rubin's rules within each stratum, then we are in the setting described in Section 11.1, which gives valid inference.

Some additional simulations we have carried out confirm that it remains important to get the imputation model right in this setting. For example, it may be that to get the mean model right we need to include the inverse weights as a covariate, as well as including the weights to ensure that Rubin's rules give a valid estimate of the variance. Our simulations also gave promising results for using weights to define level-2 units, both in terms of variance estimation and confidence interval coverage.

Now consider two partially observed continuous covariates, $\mathbf{Y}_1$, $\mathbf{Y}_2$, and fully observed $\mathbf{Y}_3$. Again using weights to define the second level units, $l = 1, \ldots, L$ the natural joint multilevel imputation model is

$$\begin{aligned} Y_{i,1,l} &= (\beta_0 + u_{0,l}) + (\beta_1 + u_{1,l})Y_{i,3,l} + e_{1,i,l} \\ Y_{i,2,l} &= (\beta_2 + u_{2,l}) + (\beta_3 + u_{3,l})Y_{i,3,l} + e_{2,i,l} \\ (u_{0,l}, u_{1,l}, u_{3,l}, u_{4,l})^T &\sim N_4(0, \mathbf{\Omega}_u) \\ (e_{1,i,l}, e_{2,i,l})^T &\sim N_2(0, \sigma_e^2). \end{aligned}$$

This model allows for a different linear relationship across strata between the two partially observed variables and $\mathbf{Y}_3$. However, given this, the correlation of $\mathbf{Y}_2$ and $\mathbf{Y}_3$ is the same. One way to address this would be to have a random covariance matrix at level 1, and possibly level 2, in the spirit proposed by Yucel (2011), and described in Subsection 9.5.1.

Another issue that frequently arises, particularly if weights are estimated, is that some variables involved in the derivation are partially observed, and the corresponding weights are missing. If we use weight as a covariate in the imputation model, missing values can be imputed, in the usual way, as part of the imputation process. While the theory does not extend to this setting, imputation of a minority of weights is unlikely to affect inferences. Alternatively, it may be preferable to substitute a 'best guess' of the missing weight, using for example the calibration procedure proposed by Carpenter and Plewis (2011). Within the multilevel approach, missing weights correspond to missing level-2 identifiers. Within a Bayesian approach, we can postulate a distribution and/or model for these, and thus include the corresponding units.

Example 11.1 Youth cohort study

To illustrate this approach, we return to the Youth Cohort study (see p. 240 and 123). These analyses showed (i) that the missingness mechanism depends on the response and ethnic group, so that under MAR the complete records analysis gives biased estimation of the coefficients for ethnic group, which is corrected by MI and (ii) that this correction is robust to plausible MNAR mechanisms.

We now complete the analysis by including the survey weights, supplied with each cohort of the data, in the imputation model. These weights were derived to adjust for student nonresponse (i.e. missingness at the unit level). Ideally, the variables used to derive these weights would be available, and included in the imputation model. However, this is not the case, and neither is there any documentation about how the weights were calculated.

We therefore compare a number of analyses here:

1. an unweighted complete records analysis;

2. a weighted complete records analysis;

3. standard MI, but including the weight as a covariate; and

4. multilevel MI, with the weights defining level-2 units.

In these analyses, we restrict attention to the subset of 61 609 records where only parental occupational group is missing, with 54 872 complete records. Across these 61 609 records, the weights supplied with the data range between 0.2 and 3.6, with mean 1.0. For the random effects approach, strata are formed by students with identical weights, regardless of cohort. This assumes that the weights can be interpreted similarly across cohorts, which seems reasonable. It gives over 850 weight strata, with a minimum of 10 observations in each.

We fitted the multilevel imputation model and imputed 10 datasets using the REALCOM-impute software. There was strong evidence that the intercept varied between level 2 units defined by weights, but no evidence for a random

Table 11.1 Estimated coefficients (standard errors) for ethnic groups in the YCS analysis, with the weights handled in various ways. Ten imputations were used.

Analysis	Ethnicity (reference: white)				
	Black	Indian	Pakistani	Bangladeshi	Other Asian
Complete records	−5.6	3.6	−2.0	0.3	5.5
(unweighted)	(0.6)	(0.4)	(0.6)	(1.0)	(0.7)
Complete records	−5.4	4.1	−2.1	0.3	6.2
(weighted)	(0.6)	(0.5)	(0.7)	(1.3)	(0.9)
MI including weights	−6.9	3.4	−3.6	−3.3	5.0
(substantive model weighted)	(0.5)	(0.5)	(0.5)	(0.8)	(0.8)
Multilevel MI	−6.8	3.4	−3.6	−3.3	4.9
(substantive model weighted)	(0.5)	(0.5)	(0.5)	(0.8)	(0.8)

coefficient of GCSE score. As before the substantive model regresses GCSE score on cohort, sex, parental occupation and ethnic group. The weighted substantive model was fitted to each imputed dataset, and then the results were combined using Rubin's rules in the usual way.

As the results for other coefficients are little changed on those given on p. 125, Table 11.1 gives the results for ethnic group. We see from the first four rows that weighting makes little difference to the complete records analysis. In rows 5–6 are the results from the usual cross-sectional MI, including the weights as a continuous covariate in the imputation model. Rows 7–8 give the results for multilevel MI with weights defining strata at level 2 and a random intercept. We see that the results from including the weights as a covariate, and the multilevel approach, are virtually identical. However, comparing with results on p. 125, weighting makes no substantive difference to the results. □

11.4 Further developments

Valid imputation in conjunction with estimated weights unlocks the possibility of a two-stage approach, which was the motivation of Seaman *et al.* (2012b). Under this approach, the handling missing data can be broken down into two parts. A natural (but not the only) way to do this is unit nonresponse and item nonresponse. Unit nonresponse can be handled by weighting, and then item nonresponse through multiple imputation which takes appropriate account of the weights.

The usefulness of dissecting the problem this way is that weighting and/or imputation models are simplified, and thus more likely to be correctly specified. Of the two-stage approaches, using MI in both stages will be most efficient, and this will thus be attractive for the final analysis. Exploring robustness by using weighting for the first stage is however an attractive, relatively straightforward diagnostic. Practically relevant differences between the two point estimates suggest further investigation into the structure of the data, particularly possible interactions, is warranted.

A question that has not been tackled in the literature thus far, but is relevant to the analysis of complex surveys, is imputation with weights in a multilevel setting when weights are attached to both level-1 units and level-2 units. Here, a generalisation of the random covariance matrix approach mentioned above may be useful. We can have random covariance matrices at level-2, identified by level-2 weights; within level-2 units we could have random covariance matrices at level-1, identified by level-1 weights.

11.5 Discussion

In this chapter we have explored some of the issues raised by design weights, and estimated weights, in the context of MI. In both settings, if our imputation model excludes the weights, but we fit a weighted substantive model to each imputed dataset and apply Rubin's rules for inference, in general our point estimates will not be consistent and our standard errors (usually upwardly) biased.

The extent to which this is a practically relevant issue in any specific analysis is hard to predict. Nevertheless, if there is little difference in the complete records analysis when design weights are included/omitted, concerns about specifying the imputation model to appropriately include the design weights are secondary.

In settings where it is important to include the weights in the imputation model, this needs to be done with care so that the number of interactions is limited. In this context, the multilevel approach with random covariance matrices is an attractive route for further development.

12

Robust multiple imputation

12.1 Introduction

A key assumption in many routine implementations of MI is that the missing data are MAR. We have seen in Chapter 10 how the impact of departures from this assumption can be assessed through appropriate sensitivity analyses, for example using pattern mixture models or reweighting. In this chapter we take a rather different approach to this issue. We develop a modification of the basic MI procedure that has certain robustness properties, to be spelled out in detail below. We will refer to this approach as Robust Multiple Imputation (RMI). We envisage this being used to target particular incomplete variables, to see if the robust form of imputation changes the conclusions in a nontrivial way: if it *does* then we have evidence of sensitivity to the assumptions surrounding the role of this particular variable. The material in this chapter is drawn from Daniel and Kenward (2012).

We begin by making some definitions. We use the term *full data assumptions* to refer to the assumptions we would have made when analysing the full data were they to have been completely observed. As we have seen repeatedly, when analysing incomplete data further assumptions are usually necessary, in addition to the full data assumptions and MAR. Broadly speaking, these additional assumptions fall into two categories: (1) those regarding the form of the conditional distribution of the missing data given the observed data, which, for this chapter, we term the *partially-observed data* (POD) model, and (2) those regarding the form of the conditional probability of observing the partially-observed variables given the observed data, which, again for this chapter, we term the *probability of missingness* (POM) model. As before we use we use the *substantive model* model to refer to the model (fully-, semi- or nonparametric) which would

Multiple Imputation and its Application, First Edition. James R. Carpenter and Michael G. Kenward.

have been used for the analysis if the data had been completely observed. Often, the POD model is not fully specified by the substantive model. For example, suppose that the substantive model is a linear regression of the outcome Y on explanatory variables X_1 and X_2, but that X_1 is MAR conditional on X_2 and Y. In this case, a model for X_1 conditional on X_2 and Y is not implied by the substantive model, and thus further assumptions will be necessary if, say, a maximum likelihood or MI analysis of the incomplete data is to be conducted: namely, the POD model must be specified. As we have already seen, misspecification of the POD model generally induces inconsistency in the resulting estimators.

If a POM model is needed, this is clearly not implied by the substantive model. So methods based on inverse probability weighting (dating back to Horvitz and Thompson, 1952), for example, require the additional specification of a POM model. Again, misspecification of the POM model, in general, induces inconsistency in the resulting estimators.

An exception occurs when a maximum likelihood (or Bayesian) analysis is planned and the substantive model implies a POD model. This occurs, for example, in a repeated measurements setting when the repeated outcomes are MAR and follow a monotone pattern and a multivariate normal model is assumed. In practice, however, the model for the full data is unlikely to be precisely correct, and the consequences of departures from this model are potentially more serious when the data are incomplete. In addition, the fit of the substantive model can only be assessed for the observed data. Even if the substantive model appears to fit the observed data well, the assumption that it also fits the unobserved data well obviously cannot be assessed from the data at hand, and can rely on considerable extrapolation when the observed and unobserved data differ substantially on the values of some variables. Even apparently mild misspecification of the substantive model can lead to inconsistency in the resulting estimators.

So-called *doubly robust* (DR) methods (Robins *et al.*, 1994; Scharfstein *et al.*, 1999; Bang and Robins, 2005; Tsiatis, 2006) specify (in addition to MAR and a substantive model) *both* a POD and POM model, and the results from such an analysis have been shown to be valid when (in addition to the assumptions of MAR and the substantive model) *at least one* of the POD and POM models is correctly-specified. In particular, they have principally been proposed in situations in which the substantive model is either semi- or even nonparametric, thus increasing the chances of correctly specifying the substantive model. This (partial) protection against model misspecification makes DR methods attractive in many settings. Until recently, however, the absence of a general method for deriving DR estimators coupled with the complex underlying mathematical theory has meant that – although introduced in this context in the 1990s – DR estimators have not been very widely used in practice. However, Bang and Robins (2005) introduced a general method for calculating DR estimators that requires only the use of existing statistical software, for both cross-sectional univariate missing data and longitudinal data with monotone dropout. In this chapter we develop the ideas in Bang and Robins (2005) within the MI framework with the aim of improving the robustness of

MI estimators. In certain settings we see that the resulting estimators are DR. More generally, for example when the pattern of missingness is nonmonotone, and using the fully conditional specification, it has been conjectured that the approach can lead to improved robustness, and this is supported using results from simulation studies. The approach is motivated from two different perspectives. First, to reduce the reliance of MI on the correct specification of the imputation model. Second, because MI is a method that can easily deal with nonmonotone patterns of missingness, it is a natural starting point when seeking doubly robust estimators for incomplete data with such missingness patterns.

The outline of this chapter is as follows. We start, in Section 12.2, with an overview of some of the relevant theory from the missing data literature that has not already been covered in earlier chapters. In particular, we introduce randomised monotone missingness (RMM) processes and augmented inverse probability weighted (AIPW) estimating equations. In Section 12.3, we describe the method, before demonstrating its properties in Section 12.4, using simulation studies. In Section 12.5, we apply this method to data from a clinical trial comparing three different anti-glycaemic drugs for type II diabetes patients. This dataset contains repeated measurements of a measure of long-term glucose control, HbA_{1c}, subject to nonmonotone missingness.

12.2 Theoretical background

12.2.1 Simple estimating equations

Suppose that we intend to collect J measurements from each of $i = 1, \ldots, n$ units. As before we define $\mathbf{Y}_i = (Y_{i,1}, Y_{i,2}, \ldots, Y_{i,J})^T$ to be the full data vector on unit i, $(i = 1, \ldots, n)$, with corresponding missing value indicator $\mathbf{R}_i = (R_{i,1}, R_{i,2}, \ldots, R_{i,J})^T$, with $R_{i,j} = 1$ if Y_{ij} is observed and 0 otherwise. It will be convenient in the following to have an indicator for $\mathbf{Y}_i$ fully observed. We use C_i for this, with $C_i = 1$ when $\mathbf{R}_i = (1, 1, \ldots, 1)^T$ and 0 otherwise.

In the absence of missing data, we suppose that the following unbiased estimating equation

$$\sum_{i=1}^{n} U(\mathbf{Y}_i; \widehat{\boldsymbol{\theta}}^{\text{FULL}}) = \mathbf{0}$$

would be solved to estimate $\boldsymbol{\theta}$ from the substantive model.

When the data are incomplete, the complete records (CR) estimator $\widehat{\boldsymbol{\theta}}^{\text{CR}}$ is the solution to

$$\sum_{i=1}^{n} C_i U(\mathbf{Y}_i; \widehat{\boldsymbol{\theta}}^{\text{CR}}) = \mathbf{0}$$

Even when it is assumed that the full data model is correct, it is easily shown that for $\widehat{\boldsymbol{\theta}}^{\text{CR}}$ to be consistent, the missing data must be MCAR.

To correct for the bias in the CR estimator whenever data are not MCAR, we can weight the contributions to the estimating equation according to the true inverse probability of $C_i = 1$ given $\mathbf{Y}_i$. The resulting inverse probability weighted complete record (IPW) estimating equation is

$$\sum_{i=1}^{n} \frac{C_i}{\mathrm{P}(C_i = 1 \mid \mathbf{Y}_i)} U(\mathbf{Y}_i; \widehat{\boldsymbol{\theta}}^{\text{i-IPW}}) = \mathbf{0}, \tag{12.1}$$

and this estimating equation is unbiased whenever the substantive model is correct. Intuitively, we assign a high weight to units with a low conditional probability of being fully observed, so that they represent units with similar characteristics who were not fully observed and thus are not included in the CR analysis. We refer to this estimator as $\widehat{\boldsymbol{\theta}}^{\text{i-IPW}}$ as the *infeasible* IPW estimator (Robins *et al.*, 1992) because, in most practical settings $\Pr(C_i = 1 \mid \mathbf{Y}_i)$ is unknown and must be estimated from the data, using the POM model under the MAR assumption.

12.2.2 The Probability Of Missingness (POM) model

Consider first the simple setting in which only the jth variable $\mathbf{Y}_{(j)}$, say, is incomplete, where $\mathbf{Y}_{(j)} = (Y_{1,j}, Y_{2,j}, \ldots, Y_{n,j})^T$. Given the MAR assumption $\Pr(R_{i,j} = 1|\mathbf{Y}_i)$ can, in principle, be estimated from the data, for example by fitting a logistic regression model with potentially all variables except the jth in the linear predictor. From this fitted probabilities, $\widehat{\pi}_i$ can be calculated that estimate $\Pr(R_{i,j} = 1|\mathbf{Y}_i)$ for all i.

We now extend this to *monotone* missing data. We suppose that monotone missingness patterns occur for the first block of p variables $\mathbf{Y}_{i,1}$ say, and the remaining q variables $\mathbf{Y}_{i,2}$ are always observed ($p + q = J$). The POM model for this setup can be defined in a straightforward sequential extension of the univariate POM model just described. Suppose that the ith unit is missing data on variables from $r + 1, \ldots, p$. Then we need the probability of observing the first r variables for this unit. This can be estimated sequentially as follows. Let $\widehat{\pi}_{i,1}$ be the fitted probability for unit i from the appropriate (logistic say) regression of $R_{i,1}$ of $\mathbf{Y}_{i,2}$, in the same way as for the univariate setting above. Next, for $j = 2, \ldots, r$, $\widehat{\pi}_{i,j}$ is the fitted conditional probability from the appropriate regression of $R_{i,j}$ on $\{Y_{i,1}, \ldots, Y_{i,j-1}, \mathbf{Y}_{i,2}\}$. As formally shown by Molenberghs *et al.* (1998) the product of these probabilities

$$\widehat{\pi}_{i(r)} = \prod_{j=1}^{r} \widehat{\pi}_{ij}$$

is a consistent estimator of the probability that the first r variables are observed on unit i, provided that the POM model is correctly specified, and MAR holds.

Finally we consider estimating the POM model in the case of *nonmonotone* missingness. This raises a complication in that doubts have been cast over the appropriateness of the MAR assumption for nonmonotone missing data (Robins and Gill, 1997). These authors introduce a new mechanism, *randomised monotone missingness* (RMM), a subset of MAR, and argue that this is the only plausible *nonmonotone* MAR mechanism that is not MCAR. They show (Gill and Robins, 1997) that there exist mechanisms that are MAR but not RMM, but that for a computer to generate data under such a mechanism, it requires knowledge of the unobserved data which is then 'concealed' later in the process. They call this phenomenon 'MAR is more than it seems' and say:

> 'We have been unable to conceive of a plausible social, economic, physical or biological process that would generate MAR processes that are not RMM representable, due to the subtle and precise manner in which the data must be "hidden" to ensure that the process is MAR. That is, we believe that natural missing data processes that are not representable as RMM processes will be [MNAR].'

Gill and Robins (1997) define a subset of RMM mechanisms called *Markov* RMM (MRMM) mechanisms in which the probability of observing a given variables conditional on the previous variables observed is independent of the order in which these variables were observed, and prove that any MAR mechanism representable as RMM is also representable as MRMM. Robins and Gill (1997) describe a method for estimating the required probabilities of observing particular missing value patterns under a MRMM mechanism using an EM algorithm in which the unobserved orderings are treated as missing data. As the number of time-points increases, the computation involved in this procedure increases geometrically. When the number of potential patterns is large, Robins and Gill (1997) propose a simulated EM algorithm that greatly diminishes this computational burden.

In the case of *nonmonotone* longitudinal data, there exists only one plausible (*i.e.*, temporal) ordering and MRMM reduces to a very special setting in which, in the $p = 3$ case for example, the probability of observing Y_3, say, is dependent on Y_2 if and only if Y_2 has been observed. As Vansteelandt *et al.* (2007) argue, it is implausible in most settings that the probability of observing Y_3 only depends on Y_2 if Y_2 happens to have been observed, and therefore MAR is rarely a sensible assumption for *nonmonotone* repeated measurements. However, as a point of departure for sensitivity analyses it is useful to be aware of the form of this MAR mechanism. For such longitudinal settings, obtaining the required probabilities is then much more straightforward than in the general case, since the order in which the variables were observed is always known. For further details we refer to the papers cited above and Subsection 2.4.3 of Daniel and Kenward (2012).

12.2.3 Augmented inverse probability weighted estimating equation

Although $\widehat{\boldsymbol{\theta}}^{\text{i-IPW}}$, the solution of (12.1), is consistent for $\boldsymbol{\theta}$ provided the relevant assumptions hold, it is, in general, inefficient (Robins *et al.*, 1995). Its efficiency can be particularly poor when the complete records account for only a small proportion of the observed data. Robins *et al.* (1995) show that, by considering estimating equations of the form

$$\sum_{i=1}^{n}\left\{\frac{C_i}{\widehat{\pi}_i}U(\mathbf{Y}_{i,O};\widehat{\boldsymbol{\theta}}^{\text{AIPW}})+\left(1-\frac{C_i}{\widehat{\pi}_i}\right)\phi(\mathbf{R}_i,\mathbf{Y}_{i,O};\widehat{\boldsymbol{\theta}}^{\text{AIPW}})\right\}=\mathbf{0} \qquad (12.2)$$

for some suitable function $\phi(\cdot)$, where $\mathbf{Y}_{i,O}$ is the observed part of $\mathbf{Y}_i$, the efficiency can be increased. Using the semiparametric theory based on influence functions and Hilbert spaces (Tsiatis, 2006), Robins *et al.* (1995) show that, for a particular $U(\mathbf{Y}_i;\boldsymbol{\theta})$, if there is only one variable subject to missingness, the most efficient choice for $\phi(\cdot)$ is

$$\phi(\mathbf{R}_i,\mathbf{Y}_{i,O};\boldsymbol{\theta}) = \mathrm{E}\left\{U(\mathbf{Y}_i;\boldsymbol{\theta}) \mid \mathbf{Y}_{i,O}\right\}$$

When there are many variables subject to missingness, in a monotone pattern, the same theory shows that the most efficient choice of $\phi(\mathbf{R}_i,\mathbf{Y}_{i,O};\boldsymbol{\theta})$ is

$$\sum_{j=1}^{J}\frac{R_{i,j-1}}{\widehat{\pi}_{i(j)}}\left(\frac{\widehat{\pi}_{i(j)}}{\widehat{\pi}_{i(j-1)}}-R_{i,j}\right)\mathrm{E}\left\{U(\mathbf{Y}_i;\boldsymbol{\theta}) \mid \mathbf{Y}_{i,O}\right\}.$$

In both cases above, $\phi(\mathbf{R}_i,\mathbf{Y}_{i,O};\boldsymbol{\theta})$ is a function of $\mathrm{E}\left\{U(\mathbf{Y}_i;\boldsymbol{\theta}) \mid \mathbf{Y}_{i,O}\right\}$. Because $U(\cdot)$ is a function of the missing and observed data, we can specify its conditional expectation given the observed data using a model for the missing data given the observed, that is, a POD model. Thus it can be seen that DR estimators involve *both* a POM and POD model. Scharfstein *et al.* (1999) were the first in the biostatistical setting to show that, when MAR and the assumptions of the substantive model hold, the DR estimator is consistent if, in addition, *at least one* of the POM and POD is correctly specified. Thus DR estimators offer two advantages over their IPW counterparts: increased efficiency, and double robustness.

12.3 Robust multiple imputation

12.3.1 Univariate MAR missing data

We now suppose that the full data for unit i consists of a univariate outcome Y_i that may be missing with indicator R_i, and a fully observed vector of covariates $\mathbf{X}_i$. For simplicity, it is assumed that interest lies in estimating the mean μ of Y_i over the sample, but this approach could be applied more generally (e.g. for estimating the coefficients of a generalised linear model).

Following the idea proposed by Bang and Robins (2005), a suitable regression model (such as logistic regression) is first chosen for R, conditional on $\mathbf{X}$, the POM model. Let $\widehat{\boldsymbol{\alpha}}$ be the parameter estimates from this regression and let $\widehat{\pi}_i = \pi(\mathbf{X}_i,\widehat{\boldsymbol{\alpha}})$ be the predicted probability (that $R_i = 1$) from this model for unit i.

Next, a suitable regression model for Y conditional on $\mathbf{X}$ and $\widehat{\pi}^{-1}$ is fitted to those subjects who have complete data. We call the corresponding model *without* the inverse probability weights, i.e.,

$$E(Y_i \mid \mathbf{X}_i, R_i = 1) = \Psi\{s(\mathbf{X}_i, \boldsymbol{\beta})\}, \tag{12.3}$$

the POD model, where $\Psi^{-1}(\cdot)$ is the canonical link function from an appropriate GLM and $s(\mathbf{X}_i, \boldsymbol{\beta})$ is a known function of $\boldsymbol{\beta}$ and $\mathbf{X}$. We call

$$E(Y_i \mid \mathbf{X}_i, \widehat{\pi}_i^{-1}, R_i = 1) = \Psi\{s(\mathbf{X}_i, \boldsymbol{\beta}) + \phi\widehat{\pi}_i^{-1}\}, \tag{12.4}$$

the *extended* POD model.

Define

$$\hat{e}\left(\mathbf{X}_i, \widehat{\boldsymbol{\beta}}, \widehat{\phi}, \widehat{\pi}_i^{-1}\right) = \Psi\{s(\mathbf{X}_i, \widehat{\boldsymbol{\beta}}) + \widehat{\phi}\widehat{\pi}_i^{-1}\} \tag{12.5}$$

to be the predictions from the extended POD model.

Next, K proper imputations are drawn, $\widetilde{Y}_{i,k}$, $k = 1, \ldots, K$ for each of the missing Y_i's based on the extended POD model. Finally, the proposed estimator is the solution $\widehat{\mu}_{\text{RMI}}$ of

$$\sum_{k=1}^{K}\sum_{i=1}^{n}(Y_{i,k}^* - \widehat{\mu}_{\text{RMI}}) = 0,$$

for $Y_{i,k}^* = R_i Y_i + (1 - R_i)\widetilde{Y}_{i,k}$. Daniel and Kenward (2012) Theorem 3.1 show that the estimator $\widehat{\mu}_{\text{RMI}}$ is DR.

An obvious next step would be to use Rubin's variance formula to estimate the variance of $\widehat{\mu}_{\text{RMI}}$. However, this variance estimator has two drawbacks in this setting. First and, most importantly, it is not DR. Provided the POD model is correctly specified it will behave in the way expected, but it does not preserve the DR properties of $\widehat{\mu}_{\text{RMI}}$. That is, when the POD model is misspecified but the POM model is correct, it will not, in general, provide an acceptable estimator of the variance of $\widehat{\mu}_{\text{RMI}}$. If the RMI procedure is used as a sensitivity analysis, then the limitations above may be acceptable; otherwise, a bootstrap estimator of variance may be preferred.

The second issue is that we are treating the weights as though they are known in this formula, and ignoring the variability in these. This is unlikely to be a major problem unless the sample is small. More seriously, the consistency of $\widehat{\mu}_{\text{RMI}}$ when the POD model is correctly specified (but not necessarily the POM model) relies on the fact that the true value of ϕ (as defined in (12.4)) in this situation is zero. In finite samples, however, the value of $\hat{\phi}$ in (12.5) will not be exactly zero. When the weights are very variable (which can happen, for example, if the conditional probability of having Y_i observed given $\mathbf{X}_i$ is close to zero for some i), $\hat{\phi}$ could be nonnegligibly far from zero leading to large finite sample bias and instability in the estimator $\widehat{\mu}_{\text{RMI}}$. This problem, along with some proposed solutions, have received considerable attention in the recent IPW literature. We return to this point at the end of the chapter, noting that this issue applies to all the RMI estimators discussed below.

It is of interest to compare this estimator with that from Bang and Robins (2005), who introduce what they call the outcome regression (OR) estimator, which is the solution to

$$\sum_{i=1}^{n}\{\widehat{e}(\mathbf{X}_i,\widehat{\boldsymbol{\beta}})-\widehat{\mu}_{\mathrm{OR}}\}=0,$$

where $\widehat{e}(\mathbf{X}_i,\widehat{\boldsymbol{\beta}})$ are the predictions from the (nonextended) POD model (12.3). This is equivalent to maximum likelihood estimation, when the estimating equations are score equations.

The doubly robust estimator proposed by Bang and Robins (2005) is the solution to

$$\sum_{i=1}^{n}\{\widehat{e}(\mathbf{X}_i,\widehat{\boldsymbol{\beta}},\widehat{\phi},\widehat{\pi}_i^{-1})-\widehat{\mu}_{\mathrm{DR}}\}=0,$$

where the $\widehat{e}(\mathbf{X}_i,\widehat{\boldsymbol{\beta}},\widehat{\phi},\widehat{\pi}_i^{-1})$ are as defined in (12.5).

12.3.2 Longitudinal MAR missing data

The same idea can be extended to the case of multivariate missing data and, in contrast to the Bang and Robins (2005) approach, the pattern need not be monotone.

Suppose now, that in addition to the fully observed covariates $\mathbf{X}_i$ we have T partially observed outcome variables $\mathbf{Y}_i=(Y_{i,1},\ldots,Y_{i,T})^T$. To simplify the exposition we assume that interest lies in estimating the mean of the final observation, $\mu=\mathrm{E}(Y_{i,T})$. A similar development can be used for other estimands. As before let $\mathbf{R}_i=(R_{i,1},\ldots,R_{i,T})^T$ be the vector of missingness indicators with $R_{i,j}=1$ indicating that $Y_{i,j}$ is observed.

We first describe the RMI method for monotone longitudinal data before moving to the case of nonmonotone longitudinal data.

Monotone longitudinal data

When the missingness pattern is monotone, we can easily estimate

$$\hat{\pi}_{i,t}=\Pr(R_{i,t}=1\mid\mathbf{X}_i,\overline{\mathbf{Y}}_{i,t-1}),\quad i=1,\ldots,n,$$

for $\overline{\mathbf{Y}}_{i,t-1}=(Y_{i,1},\ldots,Y_{i,t-1})^T$.

The POD model is postulated sequentially by first specifying a model for Y_1 given $\mathbf{X}$, and then a model for Y_2 given Y_1 and $\mathbf{X}$ and so on. To construct an extended POD model, for each $t=1,\ldots,T$, $\widehat{\pi}_{i,t}^{-1}$ is included as a covariate, additionally to $\mathbf{X}$ and $\overline{\mathbf{Y}}_{i,t-1}$, in the model for $Y_{t,i}$. In what is essentially a modification of sequential regression imputation, starting with Y_1, any missing values in Y_1 are multiply imputed, with the imputations drawn from the extended POD model for Y_1 conditional on $\mathbf{X}$ and $\widehat{\pi}_1^{-1}$. Next, any missing values in Y_2 are multiply imputed, with the imputations drawn from the extended POD model for Y_2 conditional on Y_1, $\mathbf{X}$ and $\widehat{\pi}_2^{-1}$; for subjects with Y_1 also missing, the imputed value of Y_1 from the jth imputed dataset is used to impute Y_2 in the jth imputed dataset, and so on.

By starting with Y_1 and working forwards in this way, a problem is encountered that does not arise in the method proposed by Bang and Robins (2005), which starts with Y_T and works backwards. The problem is that $\widehat{\pi}_{t,i}$ can only be calculated for subjects who have $Y_{i,t-1}$ observed, but (unlike Bang and Robins, 2005), it is now required that $\hat{\pi}_{i,t}$ be known for all subjects.

Suppose a particular subject, i, drops out after being observed at time $t-2$. At time $t-1$, in the kth imputed dataset, a value $\widetilde{Y}_{i,t-1,k}$ is imputed, based on $\mathbf{X}_i$, $\overline{\mathbf{Y}}_{i,t-2}$, and $\widehat{\pi}_{i,t-1}$, which are all observed. But at the next time point, t, it is necessary to impute the missing $Y_{i,t}$ using $\mathbf{X}_i$, $\overline{\mathbf{Y}}_{i,t-2}$, $\widetilde{Y}_{i,t-1,k}$, and $\widehat{\pi}_{i,t}$. The marginal probability $\widehat{\pi}_{i,t}$ is the product

$$\widehat{\pi}_{i,t-1}\widehat{\pi}(t \mid \mathbf{X}_i, \overline{\mathbf{Y}}_{i,t-1})$$

for $\widehat{\pi}(t \mid \mathbf{X}_i, \overline{\mathbf{Y}}_{i,t-1})$ the estimate of the conditional probability that $R_{i,t} = 1$ given $\mathbf{X}_i$, $\overline{\mathbf{Y}}_{i,t-1}$ and $R_{i,t-1} = 1$. It is this latter conditional probability which cannot be estimated directly for this subject. However, as a function of the missing $Y_{i,t-1}$, it is known. Thus the RMI method works by imputing a value for $\widehat{\pi}_{i,t}$ based on $\widehat{\pi}_{i,t-1}$, $\widehat{\pi}(t \mid \mathbf{X}_i, \overline{\mathbf{Y}}_{i,t-1})$ and $\widetilde{Y}_{i,t-1,k}$ as follows:

$$\widetilde{\pi}_{i,t,k} = \widehat{\pi}_{i,t-1}\widehat{\pi}(t \mid \mathbf{X}_i, \overline{\mathbf{Y}}_{i,t-2}, \widetilde{Y}_{i,t-1,k}).$$

In other words, no additional model is fitted to obtain the imputation $\widetilde{\pi}_{i,t,k}$, and no additional draws from the Bayesian posterior distribution are made. Rather, $\widetilde{\pi}_{i,t,k}$ is imputed as a deterministic function of $\widehat{\pi}_{i,t-1}$ (i.e. a passive imputation) and $\widehat{\pi}(t \mid \mathbf{X}_i, \widetilde{Y}_{i,t-1,k})$, which, as a function of $\mathbf{X}_i$ and $\overline{\mathbf{Y}}_{i,t-1}$, is estimated using subjects who have Y_{t-1} observed, as previously.

Similarly, for subject i at time $t+1$, the method works by first imputing a value for $\widehat{\pi}_{i,t+1}$, based on $\widetilde{\pi}_{i,t,k}$, $\widehat{\pi}(t+1 \mid \mathbf{X}_{i_1}, \overline{\mathbf{Y}}_{i,t})$, $\widetilde{Y}_{i,t-1,k}$ and $\widetilde{Y}_{i,t,k}$ as follows:

$$\widetilde{\pi}_{i,t+1,k} = \widetilde{\pi}_{i,t,k}\widehat{\pi}(t+1 \mid \mathbf{X}_{i_1}, \overline{\mathbf{Y}}_{i,t-2}, \widetilde{Y}_{i,t-1,k}, \widetilde{Y}_{i,t,k}),$$

and then $Y_{i,t+1}$ is imputed using $\mathbf{X}_{i_1}$, $\overline{\mathbf{Y}}_{i,t-2}$, $\widetilde{Y}_{i,t-1,k}$, $\widetilde{Y}_{i,t,k}$ and $\widetilde{\pi}_{i,t+1,k}$.

Finally, $\widehat{\mu}_{\text{RMI}}$ is calculated as the solution to

$$\sum_{k=1}^{K}\sum_{i=1}^{n}(\widetilde{Y}_{i,T,k} - \widehat{\mu}_{\text{RMI}}) = 0. \tag{12.6}$$

Daniel and Kenward (2012), Theorem 3.2, show that the estimator $\widehat{\mu}_{\text{RMI}}$ as defined in (12.6) is doubly robust.

A variance estimator analogous to Rubin's variance estimator used in the univariate setting can be obtained, but the same caveats apply to this estimator as in the univariate case: it is only singly robust, requiring the POD model to hold, and does not incorporate the uncertainty in the estimates of the probabilities.

Again it is of interest to compare this estimator with the corresponding estimator from Bang and Robins (2005). The OR estimator is now the solution to

$$\sum_{i=1}^{n}\{H_0(\mathbf{X}_i, \widehat{\boldsymbol{\beta}}_0) - \widehat{\mu}_{\mathrm{OR}}\} = 0,$$

where $H_0(\mathbf{X}_i, \widehat{\boldsymbol{\beta}}_0)$ is as defined by Bang and Robins (2005). Briefly, their sequential regression estimator is built as follows. They write $H_T = Y_T$ for those who have Y_T observed. Then, for $t = T-1, \ldots, 0$, $H_t(\mathbf{X}, Y_1, \ldots, Y_t) = E(H_{t+1} \mid \mathbf{X}, Y_1, \ldots, Y_t)$ is defined for everyone for whom Y_t is observed. They calculate each H_t using regression models which together constitute the POD model and show that, if this model is correct and the MAR assumption holds, then $E\{H_0(\mathbf{X})\} = E(Y_T) = \mu$, leading to the estimating equation above.

The DR estimator proposed by Bang and Robins (2005) is the same as the OR estimator but with the POD model replaced with the extended POD model.

Nonmonotone longitudinal data

For nonmonotone missingness patterns, we recommend first examining the assumption that the missing data mechanism belongs to the randomised monotone missingness (RMM) subclass described above, using the test described by Robins and Gill (1997). If the data do not support this hypothesis, then MAR should be rejected as implausible; even in this case, however, an analysis which assumes ignorability might be appropriate as a point of departure for subsequent sensitivity analyses. Under the assumption that the data are RMM, we can draw a probability tree showing the various mechanisms that can cause the missing data. From this, a set of required probabilities, which we denote $p_t(\cdot)$, can be estimated; for details of these in the current setting see Subsection 2.4.3 of Daniel and Kenward (2012). For the case of $T = 3$ observation times, these estimated probabilities are then used to estimate each of

$$\Pr(R_{i,1} = 1 \mid \mathbf{X}_i) = p_1(\mathbf{X}_i), \tag{12.7}$$

$$\Pr(R_{i,2} = 1 \mid \mathbf{X}_i, Y_{1,i}) = p_1(\mathbf{X}_i)p_2(\mathbf{X}_i, Y_{i,1}) + p_2(\mathbf{X}_i) \text{ and} \tag{12.8}$$

$$\Pr(R_{i,3} = 1 \mid \mathbf{X}_i, Y_{1,i}, Y_{2,i}) = p_1(\mathbf{X}_i)p_2(\mathbf{X}_i, Y_{i,1})p_3(\mathbf{X}_i, Y_{i,1}, Y_{i,2}) + p_1(\mathbf{X}_i)p_3(\mathbf{X}_i, Y_{i,1}) + p_2(\mathbf{X}_i)p_3(\mathbf{X}_i, Y_{i,2}) + p_3(\mathbf{X}_i). \tag{12.9}$$

Note that even in this nonmonotone setting, because the data are longitudinal, it remains the case that the missingness probabilities at each time-point depend only on past measurements of Y.

While (12.7) is always defined, for some subjects (12.8) and (12.9) are undefined. For example, if subject i has only Y_2 observed then $p_2(\mathbf{X}_i, Y_{i,1})$ cannot be calculated. Up to a function of the unknown $Y_{i,1}$, it can, however, be specified and in such cases (12.8) and (12.9) are specified as known functions of the unknown $Y_{i,1}$ or $Y_{i,2}$. This completes the description of the POM model.

We now use a modified form of MI using fully conditional specification. As with the monotone case, for each $t = 1, \ldots, T$, $\widehat{\pi}_{i,t}^{-1}$ is included as an additional covariate (additional to the specified POD model) when imputing $Y_{i,t}$. As noted above, $\widehat{\pi}_{i,t}^{-1}$ is, in general, missing for some subjects, and is therefore imputed (deterministically) as a function of the (possibly imputed) $\widetilde{Y}_{i,1}, \ldots, \widetilde{Y}_{i,t-1}$.

Although when generating such data, we only need to consider the distribution of each outcome variable Y_t conditional on the covariates and the previous $t-1$ outcome variables (since the future cannot determine the past), for the POD model it is necessary, in this nonmonotone case, to postulate the implied models for Y_t given all future outcome variables as well, and the future outcome variables must be included in the imputation models, *e.g.* Y_2 must be included in the imputation model for Y_1. Thus, the extended POD model in the nonmonotone case differs from that of the monotone case, since the imputation model for Y_t conditions on all past and future values of Y, as well as $\mathbf{X}$ and $\widehat{\pi}_t^{-1}$.

Finally, $\widehat{\mu}_{\mathrm{RMI}}$ is again calculated as the solution of

$$\sum_{k=1}^{K}\sum_{i=1}^{n}(\widetilde{Y}_{i,T,k} - \widehat{\mu}_{\mathrm{RMI}}) = 0 \tag{12.10}$$

and a variance estimate (subject to the same caveats as above) can be obtained from the MI variance formula.

It is conjectured in Daniel and Kenward (2012) that the estimator $\widehat{\mu}_{\mathrm{RMI}}$ defined in (12.10) is, at last approximately, DR. An outline argument for this is presented there, but we we note that, as we have seen in earlier chapters, the proposed procedure relies on multiple imputation by fully conditional specification, which itself is not theoretically justified away from the joint multivariate normal and the saturated log-linear model models. However, because of the inclusion of the weights, this DR setting cannot correspond to either of these models. Nevertheless, the FCS procedure has been extensively and very successfully used in practice, supported by simulation studies, beyond these models. Likewise, simulation studies (beyond those reported below) suggest that the proposed DR estimator behaves similarly well for a mixture of continuous, binary and categorical variables.

12.4 Simulation studies

12.4.1 Univariate MAR missing data

For comparison we first report results from a repeat of the first simulation study carried out by Bang and Robins (2005), adding the proposed RMI estimator as a fourth estimator to be compared with the IPW estimator, the OR estimator and the DR estimator.

In this part of the simulation study, $\mathbf{X} = (X_1, X_2, X_3)$ is always fully-observed with X_1, X_2, X_3 consists of three independent and identically distributed standard normal variables. Y is normally distributed with mean $s_{\text{true}}(\mathbf{X}, \boldsymbol{\beta})$ and unit variance, where $s_{\text{true}}(\mathbf{X}, \boldsymbol{\beta})$ is defined in Table 12.1, Section 1, where the POM model used to generate R is also described. To investigate the double robustness property, an incorrect POM model and an incorrect POD model are also specified as defined in Table 12.1, Section 1.

12.4.2 Longitudinal monotone MAR missing data

Next, we report results from a repeat of the longitudinal monotone simulation study carried out by Bang and Robins (2005), again with the addition of the RMI estimator as a fourth estimator to be compared with the IPW estimator, the OR estimator and the DR estimator.

As before, $\mathbf{X} = (X_1, X_2, X_3)$ is always fully-observed with X_1, X_2, X_3 independent and identically distributed standard normal variables. Y_1 is normally distributed with mean $\widetilde{s}^{(1)}_{\text{true}}(\mathbf{X}, \tilde{\boldsymbol{\beta}}_1)$ and unit variance, Y_2, conditional on Y_1, is normally distributed with mean $s^{(2)}_{\text{true}}(\mathbf{X}, Y_1, \boldsymbol{\beta}_2)$ and unit variance. Details are given in Table 12.1, Section 2.

One aspect not explained in Bang and Robins (2005) is that further calculation is needed to establish the implied form of the distribution of $Y_2 \mid \mathbf{X}$, which, using their notation, is $s^{(1)}_{\text{true}}(\mathbf{X}, \boldsymbol{\beta}_1)$. The conditional distribution of $Y_1 \mid \mathbf{X}$ is

$$\text{N}(3X_1 - 2X_1X_3, 1)$$

and the conditional distribution of $Y_2 \mid \mathbf{X}, Y_1$ is

$$\text{N}(-3X_1^2 + 3X_2 + Y_1^2 - 2X_2Y_1, 1).$$

The conditional expectation of $Y_2 \mid \mathbf{X}$ is therefore

$$\begin{aligned} &-3X_1^2 + 3X_2 + 1 + (3X_1 - 2X_1X_3)^2 - 2X_2(3X_1 - 2X_1X_3) \\ &= 1 + 3X_2 + 6X_1^2 - 6X_1X_2 - 12X_1^2X_3 + 4X_1X_2X_3 + 4X_1^2X_3^2. \end{aligned}$$

Thus, when carrying out the simulation study under the 'both models correct' scenario, the authors used $1, X_2, X_1^2, X_1X_2, X_1^2X_3, X_1X_2X_3, X_1^2X_3^2$ as the covariates for the second linear regression stage, as opposed to $1, X_1, X_1X_3$ as their paper suggests.

The implied $s^{(1)}_{\text{true}}(\mathbf{X}, \boldsymbol{\beta}_1)$ is given in Table 12.1, along with details of the correct POM model and the incorrect POM and POD models.

12.4.3 Longitudinal nonmonotone MAR missing data

Next, we report results from a longitudinal nonmonotone simulation study. In this case, neither the OR nor the DR estimator can be used and thus we compare

Table 12.1 Details of the simulation studies. I_l^Z stands for $I\left(Z_l > 0\right)$.

1. *Cross-sectional univariate*:	
True	$s_{\text{true}}(\mathbf{X}, \boldsymbol{\beta}) = \boldsymbol{\beta}\left(1, X_1^2, X_2, X_2X_3\right)^T, \boldsymbol{\beta} = (0, 1, 2.5, 3)$
	$\text{logit}\left\{\hat{\pi}_{\text{true}}(\mathbf{X}, \boldsymbol{\alpha})\right\} = \boldsymbol{\alpha}\left(1, I_1^X, I_2^X, I_3^X, I_1^X I_2^X\right)^T, \boldsymbol{\alpha} = (-1, 1, 0, 0, -1)$
False	$s_{\text{false}}(\mathbf{X}, \boldsymbol{\beta}) = \boldsymbol{\beta}\left(1, X_1, X_2^2\right)^T$
	$\text{logit}\left\{\hat{\pi}_{\text{false}}(\mathbf{X}, \boldsymbol{\alpha})\right\} = \boldsymbol{\alpha}\left(1, I_1^X, I_3^X\right)^T$
2. *Monotone longitudinal*:	
True	$\tilde{s}_1^{\text{true}}\left(\mathbf{X}, \boldsymbol{\beta}_1\right) = \tilde{\boldsymbol{\beta}}_1\left(1, X_1, X_1X_3\right)^T, \tilde{\boldsymbol{\beta}}_1 = (0, 3, -2)$
	$s_2^{\text{true}}\left(\mathbf{X}, Y_1, \boldsymbol{\beta}_2\right) = \boldsymbol{\beta}_2\left(1, X_1^2, X_2, Y_1^2, X_2Y_1\right)^T, \boldsymbol{\beta}_2 = (0, -3, 3, 1, -2)$
	$s_1^{\text{true}}\left(\mathbf{X}, \boldsymbol{\beta}_1\right) = \boldsymbol{\beta}_1\left(1, X_2, X_1^2, X_1X_2, X_1^2X_3, X_1X_2X_3, X_1^2X_3^2\right), \boldsymbol{\beta}_1 = (1, 3, 6, -6, -12, 4, 4)$
	$\text{logit}\left\{\hat{\pi}_1^{\text{true}}\left(\mathbf{X}, \boldsymbol{\alpha}_1\right)\right\} = \boldsymbol{\alpha}_1\left(1, I_1^X, I_2^X, I_3^X, I_1^X I_2^X\right)^T, \boldsymbol{\alpha}_1 = (1, -1, -1, 1, 1)$
	$\text{logit}\left\{\hat{\pi}_2^{\text{true}}\left(\mathbf{X}, Y_1, \boldsymbol{\alpha}_2\right)\right\} = \boldsymbol{\alpha}_2\left(1, I_1^X, I_2^X, I_3^X, I_1^X I_2^X, I_1^Y, I_3^X I_1^Y\right)^T, \boldsymbol{\alpha}_2 = (0, -1, -1, 0, 1, 0, 2)$
False	$s_1^{\text{false}}(\mathbf{X}, \boldsymbol{\beta}) = \boldsymbol{\beta}\left(1, X_1, X_2\right)^T$
	$s_2^{\text{false}}(\mathbf{X}, Y_1, \boldsymbol{\beta}) = \boldsymbol{\beta}\left(1, X_1, X_2^2, X_3^2, Y_1\right)^T$
	$\text{logit}\left\{\hat{\pi}_1^{\text{false}}(\mathbf{X}, \boldsymbol{\alpha})\right\} = \boldsymbol{\alpha}\left(1, I_2^X, I_3^X\right)^T$
	$\text{logit}\left\{\hat{\pi}_2^{\text{false}}(\mathbf{X}, \boldsymbol{\alpha})\right\} = \boldsymbol{\alpha}\left(1, I_1^Y\right)^T$

3. *Nonmonotone longitudinal*:	
True	$\tilde{s}_1^{\text{true}}\left(X, \tilde{\boldsymbol{\beta}}_1\right) = \tilde{\boldsymbol{\beta}}_1 \left(1, X^2\right)^T, \tilde{\boldsymbol{\beta}}_1 = (0, 1)$
	$s_2^{\text{true}}\left(X, Y_1, \boldsymbol{\beta}_2\right) = \boldsymbol{\beta}_2 \left(1, X, Y_1\right)^T, \boldsymbol{\beta}_2 = (0, -1, 2)$
	$s_1^{\text{true}}\left(X, Y_2, \boldsymbol{\beta}_1\right) = \boldsymbol{\beta}_1 \left(1, X, X^2, Y_2\right)$
	$p_1^{\text{true}}\left(X, \boldsymbol{\alpha}_{11}, \boldsymbol{\alpha}_{12}\right) = \dfrac{\exp\left\{\boldsymbol{\alpha}_{11}\left(1, \sqrt{\lvert X\rvert}\right)^T\right\}}{1 + \exp\left\{\boldsymbol{\alpha}_{11}\left(1, \sqrt{\lvert X\rvert}\right)^T\right\} + \exp\left\{\boldsymbol{\alpha}_{12}\left(1, \sqrt{\lvert X\rvert}\right)^T\right\}}$
	$p_2^{\text{true}}\left(X, \boldsymbol{\alpha}_{11}, \boldsymbol{\alpha}_{12}\right) = \dfrac{\exp\left\{\boldsymbol{\alpha}_{12}\left(1, \sqrt{\lvert X\rvert}\right)^T\right\}}{1 + \exp\left\{\boldsymbol{\alpha}_{11}\left(1, \sqrt{\lvert X\rvert}\right)^T\right\} + \exp\left\{\boldsymbol{\alpha}_{12}\left(1, \sqrt{\lvert X\rvert}\right)^T\right\}}$
	$\boldsymbol{\alpha}_{11} = (2, -1), \boldsymbol{\alpha}_{12} = (0, 0.5)$
	$\text{logit}\left\{p_2^{\text{true}}\left(X, Y_1, \boldsymbol{\alpha}_2\right)\right\} = \boldsymbol{\alpha}_2 \left(1, X, Y_1^2\right)^T, \boldsymbol{\alpha}_2 = (0, -2, 0.5)$
False	$s_1^{\text{false}}\left(X, Y_2, \boldsymbol{\beta}_1\right) = \boldsymbol{\beta}_1 \left(1, X, Y_2\right)^T$
	$s_2^{\text{false}}\left(X, Y_1, \boldsymbol{\beta}_2\right) = \boldsymbol{\beta}_2 \left(1, Y_1^2\right)^T$
	$p_1^{\text{false}}\left(X, \alpha_{11}, \alpha_{12}\right) = \dfrac{\exp\left(\alpha_{11}\right)}{1 + \exp\left(\alpha_{11}\right) + \exp\left(\alpha_{12}\right)}$
	$p_2^{\text{false}}\left(X, \alpha_{11}, \alpha_{12}\right) = \dfrac{\exp\left(\alpha_{12}\right)}{1 + \exp\left(\alpha_{11}\right) + \exp\left(\alpha_{12}\right)}$
	$\text{logit}\left\{p_2^{\text{true}}\left(X, Y_1, \boldsymbol{\alpha}_2\right)\right\} = \boldsymbol{\alpha}_2 \left(1, X, Y_1\right)^T$

(*continued overleaf*)

Table 12.1 (*continued*)

4. *Nonmonotone nonlongitudinal*:	
True	$\tilde{s}_1^{\text{true}}(X, \tilde{\boldsymbol{\beta}}_1) = \tilde{\boldsymbol{\beta}}_1 (1, X^2)^T, \tilde{\boldsymbol{\beta}}_1 = (0, 1)$
	$s_2^{\text{true}}(X, Y_1, \boldsymbol{\beta}_2) = \boldsymbol{\beta}_2 (1, X, Y_1)^T, \boldsymbol{\beta}_2 = (0, -1, 2)$
	$s_1^{\text{true}}(X, Y_2, \boldsymbol{\beta}_1) = \boldsymbol{\beta}_1 (1, X, X^2, Y_2)$
	$p_1^{\text{true}}(X, \boldsymbol{\alpha}_{11}, \boldsymbol{\alpha}_{12}) = \dfrac{\exp\left\{\boldsymbol{\alpha}_{11}(1, X, X^2)^T\right\}}{1 + \exp\left\{\boldsymbol{\alpha}_{11}(1, X, X^2)^T\right\} + \exp\left\{\boldsymbol{\alpha}_{12}(1, X, X^2)^T\right\}}$
	$p_2^{\text{true}}(X, \boldsymbol{\alpha}_{11}, \boldsymbol{\alpha}_{12}) = \dfrac{\exp\left\{\boldsymbol{\alpha}_{12}(1, X, X^2)^T\right\}}{1 + \exp\left\{\boldsymbol{\alpha}_{11}(1, X, X^2)^T\right\} + \exp\left\{\boldsymbol{\alpha}_{12}(1, X, X^2)^T\right\}}$
	$\boldsymbol{\alpha}_{11} = (1, -0.5, 0.2), \boldsymbol{\alpha}_{12} = (0, 0.5, -0.3)$
	$\text{logit}\left\{p_2^{\text{true}}(X, Y_1, \boldsymbol{\alpha}_{22})\right\} = \boldsymbol{\alpha}_{22}(1, X, Y_1)^T, \boldsymbol{\alpha}_{22} = (0, -1, 0.3)$
	$\text{logit}\left\{p_1^{\text{true}}(X, Y_2, \boldsymbol{\alpha}_{21})\right\} = \boldsymbol{\alpha}_{21}(1, X, Y_2)^T, \boldsymbol{\alpha}_{21} = (0, -1, 0.3)$
False	$s_1^{\text{false}}(X, Y_2, \boldsymbol{\beta}_1) = \boldsymbol{\beta}_1 (1, X^2, Y_2)^T$
	$s_2^{\text{false}}(X, Y_1, \boldsymbol{\beta}_2) = \boldsymbol{\beta}_2 (1, Y_1)^T$

the RMI estimator with the IPW estimator and an ordinary multiple imputation (MI) estimator, i.e. an estimator identical to the RMI estimator but without the inverse probability weights as additional covariates in the imputation model.

In this simulation study, X (univariate) is always observed and generated from a standard normal distribution. Y_1 and Y_2 are normally distributed with means $\widetilde{s}^{(1)}_{\text{true}}(x, \tilde{\boldsymbol{\beta}}_1)$ and $s^{(2)}_{\text{true}}(X, Y_1, \boldsymbol{\beta}_2)$, respectively (see Table 12.1, Section 3), and unit variance. The implied $s^{(1)}_{\text{true}}(X, Y_2, \boldsymbol{\beta}_1)$ is also given in the table.

Note that $s^{(1)}(\cdot)$ is now a function of Y_2. This is essential, since some subjects have Y_2 but not Y_1 observed. If Y_2 is omitted from the imputation model for Y_1, the resulting estimator is, in general, biased since the stationary distribution to which the Gibbs sampler in the FCS procedure converges is not the correct full-data distribution, even under MAR.

The POM model is defined by the multinomial logit model described in Table 12.1, Section 3, where the incorrect POM and POD models are also described.

12.4.4 Nonlongitudinal nonmonotone MAR missing data

Finally, we report results from a nonlongitudinal nonmonotone simulation study. Again, neither the OR nor the DR estimator can be used and thus we compare our RMI estimator with the IPW estimator and an ordinary MI estimator.

As in the previous simulation study, X (univariate) is always observed and generated from a standard normal distribution. Y_1 and Y_2 are normally distributed with means $\widetilde{s}^{(1)}_{\text{true}}(X, \tilde{\boldsymbol{\beta}}_1)$ and $s^{(2)}_{\text{true}}(X, Y_1, \boldsymbol{\beta}_2)$, respectively (see Table 12.1), and unit variance. The implied $s_1^{\text{true}}\left(X, Y_2, \boldsymbol{\beta}_1\right)$, the correct POM model and the incorrect POD model are given in of Table 12.1, Section 4.

Because of the difficulty associated with estimating the marginal weights in this setting (discussed briefly in Subsection 12.2.2 and at greater length in Subsection 2.4.3 of Daniel and Kenward, 2012), reliable estimates of all the required probabilities cannot be obtained, even for the complete records. Hence for this simulation study the true (known) weights have been used. As the true weights are used, no 'POM model' exists. To investigate the double robustness property, the following definitions are used: $\hat{\pi}_1^{\text{false}} = \sqrt{\hat{\pi}_1^{\text{true}}}$ and $\hat{\pi}_2^{\text{false}} = \sqrt{\hat{\pi}_2^{\text{true}}}$. There was no particular motivation for choosing this relationship between the correct and incorrect weights, except that it produced an appreciable, yet not too extreme, bias in the IPW estimator.

12.4.5 Results and discussion

The simulation studies were all based on a sample size of 500 with 1000 replicates, with the MI and robust MI procedures based on 10 imputations and 10 cycles of the FCS procedure. The results are shown in Table 12.2, where the bias of $\mathrm{E}(Y)$ is reported for the univariate setting, and the bias of $\mathrm{E}(Y_2)$ is reported for the remaining settings. The Monte-Carlo variance is the empirical variance of the estimator across the 1000 replicates, and the estimated variance for

Table 12.2 Results of simulation studies comparing the doubly robust multiple imputation (RMI) estimator with the inverse probability weighted complete records (IPW), outcome regression (OR) and multiple imputation (MI) estimators, together with the doubly robust (DR) estimator of Bang and Robins (2005). No subscript indicates correct specification of the relevant model(s). 'π – false' indicates that the estimator used an incorrectly specified POM model, 'y – false' indicates that the estimator used an incorrectly specified POD model and '$\pi \oplus y$ – false' indicates that both the POM and POD models were incorrectly specified.

Estimator	Bias	Monte-Carlo variance	Estimated variance	Coverage probability
1. *Cross-sectional univariate*:				
$\hat{\mu}_{\text{IPW}}$	−0.01	0.11	–	–
$\hat{\mu}_{\text{OR}}$	−0.00	0.04	–	–
$\hat{\mu}_{\text{DR}}$	−0.00	0.04	–	–
$\hat{\mu}_{\text{RMI}}$	−0.00	0.04	0.04	0.95
$\hat{\mu}_{\text{IPW}\cdot\pi-\text{false}}$	−0.36	0.13	–	–
$\hat{\mu}_{\text{DR}\cdot\pi-\text{false}}$	−0.00	0.04	–	–
$\hat{\mu}_{\text{RMI}\cdot\pi-\text{false}}$	−0.01	0.04	0.04	0.95
$\hat{\mu}_{\text{OR}\cdot y-\text{false}}$	−0.35	0.12	–	–
$\hat{\mu}_{\text{DR}\cdot y-\text{false}}$	−0.01	0.11	–	–
$\hat{\mu}_{\text{RMI}\cdot y-\text{false}}$	−0.02	0.12	0.12	0.93
$\hat{\mu}_{\text{DR}\cdot\pi\oplus y-\text{false}}$	−0.35	0.13	–	–
$\hat{\mu}_{\text{RMI}\cdot\pi\oplus y-\text{false}}$	−0.35	0.14	0.12	0.79
2. *Monotone longitudinal*:				
$\hat{\mu}_{\text{IPW}}$	−0.11	10.98	–	–
$\hat{\mu}_{\text{OR}}$	0.06	1.92	–	–
$\hat{\mu}_{\text{DR}}$	0.06	1.92	–	–
$\hat{\mu}_{\text{RMI}}$	0.07	1.91	1.83	0.94
$\hat{\mu}_{\text{IPW}\cdot\pi-\text{false}}$	−3.21	5.87	–	–
$\hat{\mu}_{\text{DR}\cdot\pi-\text{false}}$	0.06	1.92	–	–
$\hat{\mu}_{\text{RMI}\cdot\pi-\text{false}}$	0.08	1.92	1.83	0.93
$\hat{\mu}_{\text{OR}\cdot y-\text{false}}$	−4.99	3.51	–	–
$\hat{\mu}_{\text{DR}\cdot y-\text{false}}$	−0.36	10.51	–	–
$\hat{\mu}_{\text{RMI}\cdot y-\text{false}}$	−0.37	10.63	4.28	0.74
$\hat{\mu}_{\text{DR}\cdot\pi\oplus y-\text{false}}$	−2.35	8.13	–	–
$\hat{\mu}_{\text{RMI}\cdot\pi\oplus y-\text{false}}$	−2.37	7.38	3.67	0.57

(continued overleaf)

Table 12.2 (*continued*)

Estimator	Bias	Monte-Carlo variance	Estimated variance	Coverage probability
3. *Nonmonotone longitudinal*:				
$\hat{\mu}_{\text{IPW}}$	0.00	0.07	–	–
$\hat{\mu}_{\text{MI}}$	−0.01	0.03	–	–
$\hat{\mu}_{\text{RMI}}$	−0.02	0.03	0.03	0.95
$\hat{\mu}_{\text{IPW}\cdot\pi-\text{false}}$	−0.59	0.05	–	–
$\hat{\mu}_{\text{RMI}\cdot\pi-\text{false}}$	−0.03	0.03	0.03	0.94
$\hat{\mu}_{\text{MI}\cdot y-\text{false}}$	3.07×10^{31}	2.16×10^{65}	–	–
$\hat{\mu}_{\text{RMI}\cdot y-\text{false}}$	0.00	0.04	0.06	0.97
$\hat{\mu}_{\text{RMI}\cdot\pi\oplus y-\text{false}}$	2.32x	123.55	5.27×10^{8}	0.94
4. *Nonmonotone nonlongitudinal*:				
$\hat{\mu}_{\text{IPW}}$	0.01	0.07	–	–
$\hat{\mu}_{\text{MI}}$	0.00	0.03	–	–
$\hat{\mu}_{\text{RMI}}$	−0.00	0.03	0.03	0.95
$\hat{\mu}_{\text{IPW}\cdot\pi-\text{false}}$	0.25	0.06	–	–
$\hat{\mu}_{\text{RMI}\cdot\pi-\text{false}}$	0.00	0.03	0.03	0.95
$\hat{\mu}_{\text{MI}\cdot y-\text{false}}$	0.49	0.05	–	–
$\hat{\mu}_{\text{RMI}\cdot y-\text{false}}$	−0.04	0.03	0.03	0.95
$\hat{\mu}_{\text{RMI}\cdot\pi\oplus y-\text{false}}$	0.22	0.04	0.04	0.80

RMI is from Rubin's variance estimator. Kernel density plots for $E(Y)$, $E(Y_2)$ respectively, are given in Figure 12.1 and Figures 12.2–12.4.

It can be seen from Table 12.2 Sections 1 and 2, together with Figures 12.1 and 12.2, that in both the univariate cross-sectional and longitudinal monotone cases, for which the Bang and Robins (2005) method is applicable, its performance and that of the RMI method are very similar. In addition, the variance estimates obtained using Rubin's variance formula perform well when both models are correctly specified, although, as expected, they do not share the double robustness property possessed by the estimators themselves. Even though the proposed variance estimator does not take into account the variability of the estimated weights, at least in these simulations, the effect of this has proved negligible.

When the missing data are longitudinal but nonmonotone, the Bang and Robins (2005) method is no longer applicable, but the RMI procedure works very well: it exhibits the desired double robustness property as well as improved efficiency compared with IPW (see Section 3. of Table 12.2 and Figure 12.3). The loss of efficiency relative to OR and MI is negligible. We also see that RMI procedure again works well (Table 12.2 Section 4 and Figure 12.4) for nonlongitudinal nonmonotone data, when the true weights are used. □

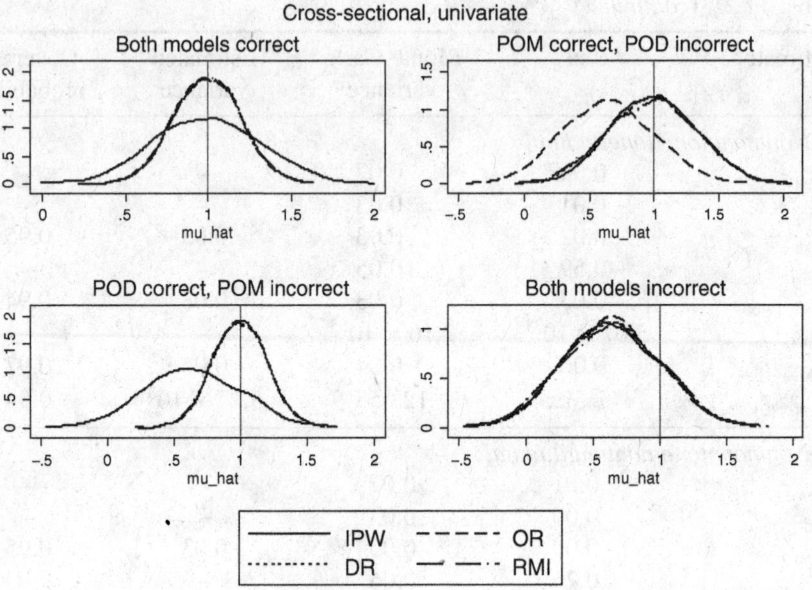

Figure 12.1 Kernel density plots for $\widehat{E(Y)}$ for the cross-sectional, univariate simulation study.

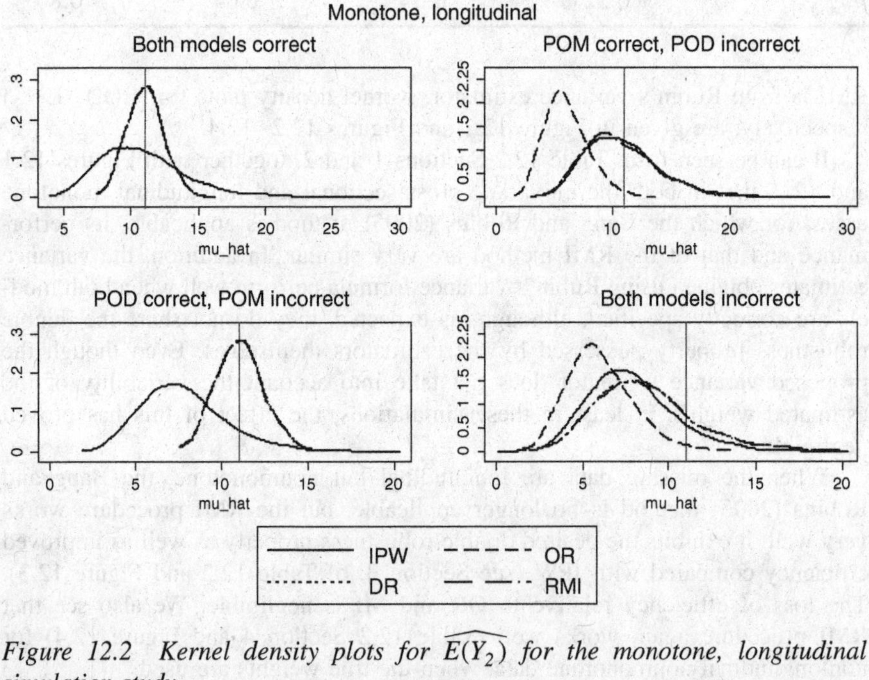

Figure 12.2 Kernel density plots for $\widehat{E(Y_2)}$ for the monotone, longitudinal simulation study.

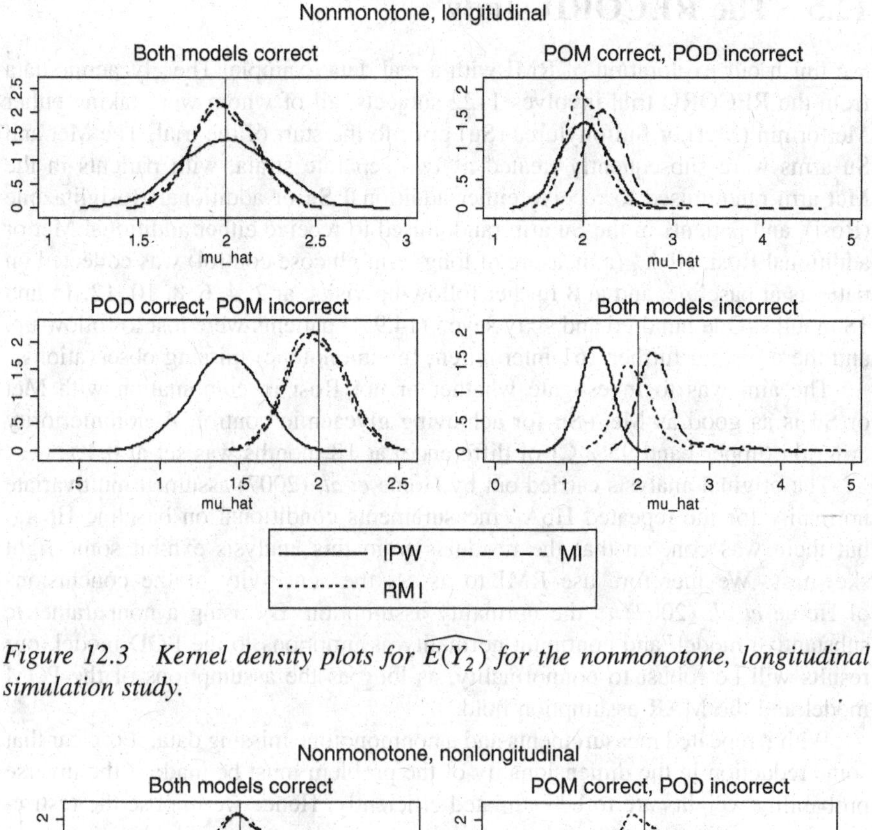

Figure 12.3 Kernel density plots for $\widehat{E(Y_2)}$ for the nonmonotone, longitudinal simulation study.

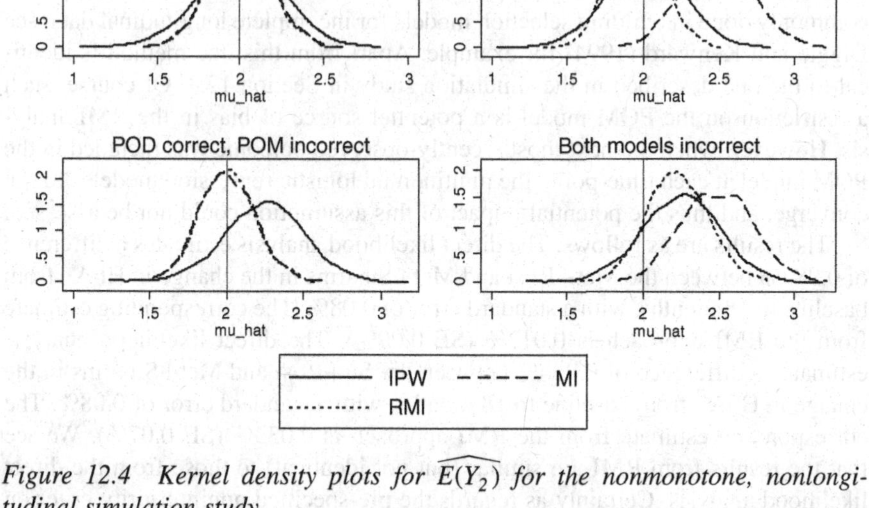

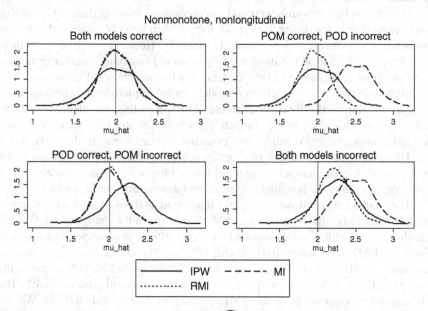

Figure 12.4 Kernel density plots for $\widehat{E(Y_2)}$ for the nonmonotone, nonlongitudinal simulation study.

12.5 The RECORD study

We finish our exploration of RMI with a real data example. The glycaemic data from the RECORD trial involves 1122 subjects, all of whom were taking either Metformin (Met) or Sulfonylurea (Su) prior to the start of the trial. The Met and Su arms were subsequently treated as two separate strata, with patients in the Met arm randomised to receive either additional Su or additional Rosiglitazone (Rosi), and patients in the Su arm randomised to receive either additional Met or additional Rosi. HbA_{1c} (a measure of long-term glucose control) was collected on patients at baseline, and at 8 further follow-up visits: at 2, 4, 6, 8, 10, 12, 15 and 18 months. One hundred and sixty seven (14.9%) patients were lost to follow-up, and there were a further 161 intermittent (nonmonotone) missing observations.

The aim was to investigate whether or not Rosi in combination with Met or Su is as good as Met+Su for achieving glycaemic control. A noninferiority criterion (upper band 95% CI of difference) at 18 months was set at 0.4%.

The original analysis carried out by Home *et al.* (2007) assumed multivariate normality for the repeated HbA_{1c} measurements conditional on baseline HbA_{1c}, but there was concern that the residuals from this analysis exhibit some right skewness. We therefore use RMI to assess the sensitivity of the conclusions of Home *et al.* (2007) to the normality assumption. By using a nonparametric substantive model, and confining normality assumptions to the POD model, our results will be robust to nonnormality, as long as the assumptions of the POM model and the MAR assumption hold.

With 8 repeated measurements and a nonmonotone missing data, it is clear that some reduction in the dimensionality of the problem must be made if the inverse probability weights are to be estimated efficiently. Hence we impose the restriction that, conditional on the most recently observed outcome, whether or not the next outcome is observed is independent of all other observed outcomes, as is commonly done in building selection models for incomplete longitudinal data, see Diggle and Kenward (1994) for example. Apart from this, the method is identical to the one described in the simulation study in Section 12.4. Of course, such a restriction on the POM model is a potential source of bias in the RMI analysis. However, when the next most recently-observed outcome was included in the POM model at each time-point, the multinomial logistic regression models did not converge, and thus the potential impact of this assumption could not be assessed.

The results are as follows. The direct likelihood analysis estimates a difference of 0.087% between the Met+Rosi and Met+Su arms in the change in HbA_{1c} from baseline to 18 months, with a standard error of 0.08%. The corresponding estimate from the RMI approach is 0.017% (SE 0.09%). The direct likelihood analysis estimates a difference of 0.066% between the Su+Rosi and Met+Su arms in the change in HbA_{1c} from baseline to 18 months, with a standard error of 0.08%. The corresponding estimate from the RMI approach is 0.033% (SE 0.07%). We see that the results from RMI are similar (but not identical) to those from the direct likelihood analysis. Certainly as regards the pre-specified noninferiority criterion of 0.4%, neither method supports the rejection of noninferiority.

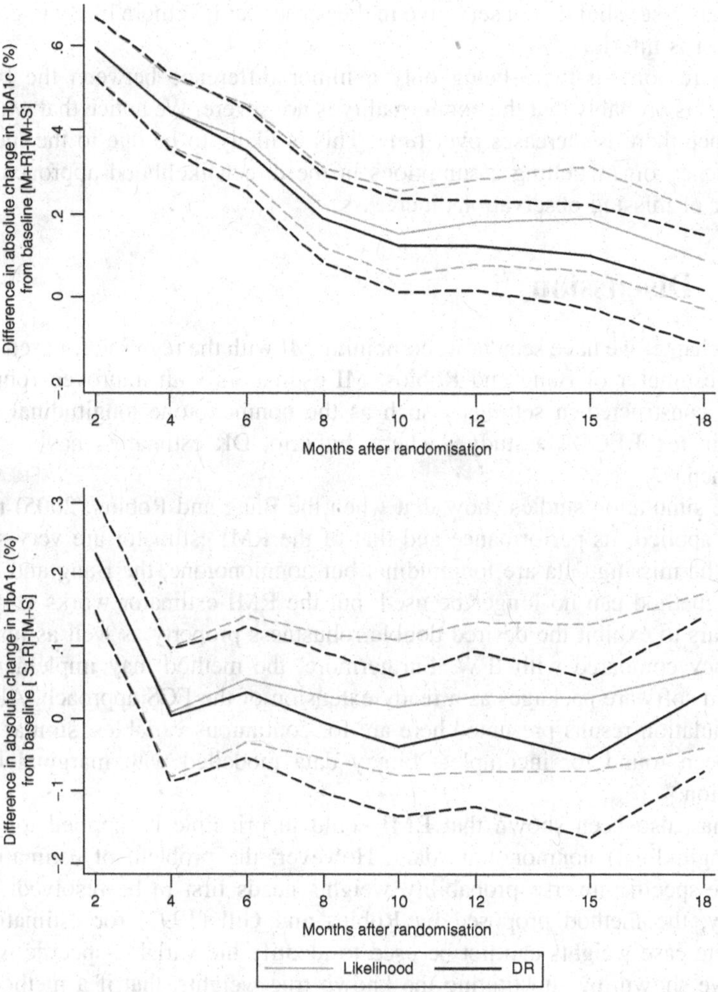

Figure 12.5 The differences between the HbA_{1c} profiles for the Met+Rosi and Met+Su arms (above) and for the Su+Rosi and Met+Su arms (below). The solid lines show the predicted differences, and the dotted lines show ± the pointwise standard errors for these differences.

Figure 12.5 shows the differences between these profiles for the two arms separately. Again it can be seen that the profiles are similar but not identical. The differences are substantively very small and unlikely to be important in practice. If anything, the RMI approach suggests a lower HbA_{1c} for the Rosi groups compared with the corresponding estimates from the direct likelihood method, whereas the estimates for the standard groups show less of a difference between the two methods. As a result, Rosi compared with standard looks to be slightly better under the RMI analysis suggesting that the direct likelihood analysis is (in this particular case) slightly conservative in the sense that it is more likely to conclude that Rosi is inferior.

The reason for there being only a minor difference between the two approaches is probably that the nonnormality is not severe. We notice that what little difference there is increases over time. This is likely to be due to the increased dependency on modelling assumptions in the direct likelihood approach as the number of missing observations increases.

12.6 Discussion

In this chapter we have seen how, combining MI with the regression-based doubly robust estimator of Bang and Robins, MI estimators with improved robustness can be constructed in settings – such as the nonmonotone longitudinal pattern found in the RECORD study – where, hitherto, DR estimators have not been implemented.

The simulation studies show that when the Bang and Robins (2005) method can be applied, its performance and that of the RMI estimator are very similar. When the missing data are longitudinal but nonmonotone, the Bang and Robins (2005) method can no longer be used, but the RMI estimator works very well: it appears to exhibit the desired double robustness property as well as improved efficiency compared with IPW. Furthermore, the method may implemented in standard software packages as a ready extension of the FCS approach. Although the simulation results presented here are for continuous variables, similar results have been found for incomplete binary data modelled with marginal logistic regression.

It has also been shown that RMI could in principle be applied to general (nonlongitudinal) nonmonotone data. However, the problem of estimating the variable-specific inverse probability weights needs first to be resolved. Unfortunately, the method proposed by Robins and Gill (1997) for estimating the complete case weights can not be used to identify the variable-specific weights. We have shown, by substituting the known true weights, that if a method were developed for estimating these probabilities, RMI could be used and would perform well.

Our focus has been on examples where the aim is to estimate the marginal mean of one of the variables. However, RMI can be used much more generally (for example to estimate the parameters of a regression of one variable on another) – and as easily – to obtain estimators with improved robustness, whenever ordinary MI is appropriate.

A criticism of DR methods has been their potential instability when the weights are too variable and their suboptimal performance when both the POD and POM models are misspecified (Kang and Schafer, 2007). These limitations apply equally to the RMI procedure described here. Recent work by Tan (2010); Vansteelandt *et al.* (2012); Tsiatis *et al.* (2011) has proposed improvements to the standard DR estimators with respect to these issues, and there does not appear to be major issues with applying these proposals within the RMI approach.

From a practical perspective we do not see this approach as being a general alternative to the conventional MI procedures explored in the rest of this book. Rather, as mentioned in the opening to this chapter, we expect its role to be more as part of a sensitivity analysis. In particular, it could be used to target certain incomplete variables which, for substantive reasons, might be thought to be particularly vulnerable to departures from underlying assumptions. If a robust version of MI, for such a variable, leads to notable changes in conclusions compared with conventional MI, then there are some grounds to suspect that there is indeed sensitivity associated the with this variable in the original MI analysis. The advantage of the approach is that when used in such a specific way, it requires very little additional work beyond a conventional MI analysis.

Appendix A

Markov Chain Monte Carlo

Here we briefly describe two Markov Chain Monte Carlo (MCMC) methods for drawing samples from a Bayesian posterior. For a detailed discussion of MCMC methods and their application, we refer the reader to Gilks *et al.* (1996) and Gelman *et al.* (1995).

Suppose we have observed data $\mathbf{Y}$, (typically n observations on q variables) and we have a statistical model which gives a likelihood for the data given parameter $\boldsymbol{\theta}$. In frequentist inference we typically write this $f(\mathbf{Y}; \boldsymbol{\theta})$, denoting the probability distribution of the data $\mathbf{Y}$ at the particular parameter value $\boldsymbol{\theta}$. However, in Bayesian inference the parameters themselves are random variables, so it is more convenient to write $f(\mathbf{Y}|\boldsymbol{\theta})$ when we are thinking about the distribution of $\mathbf{Y}$ given $\boldsymbol{\theta}$, and $f(\boldsymbol{\theta}|\mathbf{Y})$ when we are thinking about the distribution of $\boldsymbol{\theta}$ given $\mathbf{Y}$.

For example, if we have $Y_i \overset{i.i.d.}{\sim} N(\theta, 1)$, $i \in (1, \ldots, n)$ then $f(\mathbf{Y}|\theta) \sim N(\theta 1_n, I_n)$ and $f(\theta|\mathbf{Y}) \sim N(\bar{Y}, n^{-1})$. More generally, f is the multivariate normal model for $\mathbf{Y}$, with unstructured mean and covariance, as in (3.4).

Suppose we have a prior distribution for $\boldsymbol{\theta}$, denoted $f(\boldsymbol{\theta}|\boldsymbol{\gamma})$, where $\boldsymbol{\gamma}$ are the parameters of the prior distribution, chosen by the analyst. For simplicity we suppress these in the following, writing $f(\boldsymbol{\theta})$ for the prior.

Then, under Bayes theorem, the posterior distribution of the parameters given the data, $f(\boldsymbol{\theta}|\mathbf{Y})$, is given by

$$f(\boldsymbol{\theta}|\mathbf{Y}) = \frac{f(\mathbf{Y}|\boldsymbol{\theta}) f(\boldsymbol{\theta})}{\int f(\mathbf{Y}|\boldsymbol{\theta}) f(\boldsymbol{\theta})\, d\boldsymbol{\theta}} \propto f(\mathbf{Y}|\boldsymbol{\theta}) f(\boldsymbol{\theta}). \tag{A.1}$$

For certain choices of likelihood and prior, when $\mathbf{Y}$ is fully observed, the posterior distribution can be calculated exactly. More commonly, we will be unable to derive the posterior analytically. However, using a technique known

Multiple Imputation and its Application, First Edition. James R. Carpenter and Michael G. Kenward.

as Markov Chain Monte Carlo (MCMC), we can set up an iterative sampling algorithm to draw a sequence – known as a chain – of parameter values $\boldsymbol{\theta}^0, \boldsymbol{\theta}^1, \ldots, \boldsymbol{\theta}^r, \ldots$ whose stationary distribution is the posterior distribution (A.1). Thus, running this algorithm from initial values, after discarding the early values of the chain – known as the 'burn in' – we end up with a (correlated) sample from the posterior. We can use this sample to estimate aspects of the posterior distribution of interest (e.g. mean, mode, variance).

We now describe two algorithms for setting up the chain $\boldsymbol{\theta}^0, \boldsymbol{\theta}^1, \ldots, \boldsymbol{\theta}^r, \ldots$; a general algorithm, known as the Metropolis-Hastings sampler, and a special case called the Gibbs sampler.

Metropolis-Hastings sampler

Recall that the parameter vector is $\boldsymbol{\theta} = (\theta_1, \theta_2, \ldots, \theta_p)^T$. Let $\boldsymbol{\theta}_{-j} = (\theta_1, \ldots, \theta_{j-1}, \theta_{j+1}, \ldots, \theta_p)^T$, i.e. the parameter vector with parameter θ_j removed.

The algorithm proceeds as follows:

1. Choose initial values for each element of $\boldsymbol{\theta}$, and denote these $\boldsymbol{\theta}^0$.
2. At update step $r = 1, 2, \ldots$, initially set $\boldsymbol{\theta}^r = \boldsymbol{\theta}^{r-1}$. Then, for $j = 1, \ldots, p$ in turn:
   (a) Sample a proposed new value for θ_j^r from an appropriate proposal distribution, $\tilde{\theta}_j^r \sim f(\theta | \theta_j^r, \boldsymbol{\theta}_{-j}^r)$.
   (b) calculate the acceptance probability
   $$p = \min\left(1, \frac{\{f(\mathbf{Y}|\tilde{\theta}_j^r, \boldsymbol{\theta}_{-j}^r) f(\tilde{\theta}_j^r, \boldsymbol{\theta}_{-j}^r)\} f(\theta_j^r | \tilde{\theta}_j^r, \boldsymbol{\theta}_{-j}^r)}{\{f(\mathbf{Y}|\theta_j^r, \boldsymbol{\theta}_{-j}^r) f(\theta_j^r, \boldsymbol{\theta}_{-j}^r)\} f(\tilde{\theta}_j^r | \theta_j^r, \boldsymbol{\theta}_{-j}^r)}\right) \quad \text{(A.2)}$$
   then draw $u \sim$ uniform[0, 1] and accept $\tilde{\theta}$ if $u < p$, in other words accept the proposal with probability p.
   (c) If the proposal is accepted, replace the current value of θ_j^r in $\boldsymbol{\theta}^r$ with the proposal, $\tilde{\theta}_j^r$; otherwise retain the current value.
   (d) Return to step 2(a) to update the next element of the parameter vector.

The term

$$\frac{f(\theta_j^r | \tilde{\theta}_j^r, \boldsymbol{\theta}_{-j}^r)}{f(\tilde{\theta}_j^r | \theta_j^r, \boldsymbol{\theta}_{-j}^r)}$$

in (A.2) is known as the Hastings ratio.

Two kinds of proposal distribution are common in practice: (i) where the proposal distribution is a marginal distribution for θ_j, so that no conditioning is involved, and (ii) where the proposal distribution is symmetric, so that $f(\theta_j^r | \tilde{\theta}_j^r) = f(\tilde{\theta}_j^r | \theta_j^r)$. In the latter case the Hastings ratio is 1. In almost every setting in this book, we create proposals by drawing $\tilde{\Delta} \sim N(0, \sigma^2)$ and then setting $\tilde{\theta}_j^r = \theta_j^r + \tilde{\Delta}$. This means that $f(\tilde{\theta}_j^r|\theta_j^r) = f(\tilde{\Delta}) = f(-\tilde{\Delta}) = f(\theta_j^r|\tilde{\theta}_j^r)$, so that the Hastings ratio is 1.

In applications, it is good practice to plot θ_j^r against r for each parameter $j = 1, \ldots, p$ to check these the sampler has passed the 'burn in' phase and that it is 'mixing' (i.e. exploring the posterior distribution) well. If the sampler is still in the burn-in phase, that is, moving towards the stationary posterior distribution, then one or more of these will show a trend in the mean of θ_j^r with t. Once the stationary distribution has been reached, the graphs should show random variation but no trend.

If we have a good proposal distribution for a parameter, then it should update roughly 50% of the time, resulting in a chain with relatively low auto-correlation. If the proposal distribution has too great a variance, then the majority of the proposals will be rejected, and the chain will 'stick' and occasionally make larger jumps. Conversely if the proposal distribution has too small a variance, the posterior distribution will only be explored slowly.

It is important to realise that the algorithm above will update even if the underlying model, $f(\mathbf{Y}|\boldsymbol{\theta})f(\boldsymbol{\theta})$, is wrongly specified (for example, by having the same covariate included twice, or in a multivariate response model including the same response variable twice). This is another reason for monitoring the chains, which typically quickly reveal that something is wrong.

Most software packages, including `REALCOM-impute`, have options for displaying the chains, and a number allow more formal diagnostic checks of the convergence of the sampler.

To improve the mixing of the sampler, it is useful to standardise continuous variables to have mean zero and variance 1 before fitting the model. If this is done, we have found that a burn in of 1000 is typically sufficient, with updates of 500–1000 between drawing imputed data sets. Schafer (1997), p. 87 points out that slow convergence of the chains for one or more parameters when using the MCMC algorithm with missing data will likely indicate there is little information remaining in the observed data about that parameter. This in turn means that inference and imputed data are may be more dependent on the imputation model chosen. In practice it may be helpful to use an EM algorithm to find starting values for the MCMC sampler for the imputation model, or where possible a direct (restricted) maximum likelihood fit of the imputation model, to highlight any such problems. Schafer (1997) gives appropriate EM algorithms for the multivariate normal model, the log-linear model for categorical data and the general location model for a mix of categorical and multivariate normal data.

Gibbs sampler

If, in the update step, we are able to choose the proposal distribution for θ_j to be $f(\theta_j|\boldsymbol{\theta}_{-j}, \mathbf{Y})$, then the acceptance probability (A.2) is always 1. This special case of proposal distribution is known as the Gibbs sampler. Using the Gibbs sampler we do not have to be concerned about poor mixing due to the chain not updating, nor about the choice of variance for the proposal distribution. We therefore use this whenever possible.

Note that, while above we have updated each component, θ_j of the parameter vector $\boldsymbol{\theta}$ in turn, in practice we can update blocks of parameters together. For example, when fitting the multivariate normal model, we will see that we can update all elements of the covariance matrix together, and all elements of the mean vector together.

Missing data

Now suppose that we have missing data, and partition $\mathbf{Y} = (\mathbf{Y}_O, \mathbf{Y}_M)$. Assuming MAR, then modelling $f(\mathbf{Y}_O|\boldsymbol{\theta})$ gives valid inference for $\boldsymbol{\theta}$. However, this is typically awkward in practice, because we have to derive $f(\mathbf{Y}_O|\boldsymbol{\theta})$ from $f(\mathbf{Y}|\boldsymbol{\theta})$ by integrating out the missing data.

Fortunately, it turns out that using MCMC methods this is not necessary. We may simply regard the missing data as another set of parameters, and update these in their turn. Thus, under a Gibbs sampling approach we would first construct the conditional distributions $f(\mathbf{Y}_M|\mathbf{Y}_O, \boldsymbol{\theta})$, $f(\theta_j|\boldsymbol{\theta}_{-j}, \mathbf{Y})$, $j = 1, \ldots, p$ and then, having chosen starting values $\mathbf{Y}_M^0, \boldsymbol{\theta}^0$, at update r

1. draw $\boldsymbol{\theta}^r$ from $f(\boldsymbol{\theta}|\mathbf{Y}_O, \mathbf{Y}_M^{r-1})$, then

2. draw $\mathbf{Y}_M^r$ from $f(\mathbf{Y}_M|\mathbf{Y}_O, \boldsymbol{\theta}^r)$.

In practice, as discussed above, in step 1 it will often be convenient to subdivide step 1, updating subsets of the parameters conditional on the current draws of the remaining parameters and the missing data.

As an illustration of step 2, if the data follow a multivariate normal distribution, then for each unit with missing data, we calculate the conditional normal distribution of their missing data given their observed data and current draws of the parameters, $\boldsymbol{\theta}$. We then update their missing values with a draw from this distribution.

An advantage of using a MCMC approach for fitting imputation models is that we can use the same procedure for updating the parameters, in step 1, regardless of the pattern of missing data. In the context of MI, an MCMC approach also naturally incorporates the uncertainty in the parameter estimates, so that the between imputation variance is correctly incorporated.

The data augmentation algorithm (Tanner and Wong (1987), Schafer (1997), p. 71) is closely related to the Gibbs sampler. Essentially, instead of updating a single pair, $(\mathbf{Y}_M^r, \boldsymbol{\theta}^r)$, we update m pairs $(\mathbf{Y}_M^{r,1}, \boldsymbol{\theta}^{r,1}), \ldots, (\mathbf{Y}_M^{r,m}, \boldsymbol{\theta}^{r,m})$. This requires a minor modification to the update process. However, choosing $m = 1$ gives a valid data augmentation algorithm, which is then equivalent to a particular Gibbs sampler.

Appendix B

Probability distributions

Here we give the commonly used probability distribution functions (pdfs) in this book, and summarise some results for the multivariate normal distribution.

Univariate normal distribution

The univariate normal probability density function (pdf) of a random variable Y is

$$f(Y|\mu, \sigma^2) = \frac{1}{\sqrt{2\pi\sigma^2}} \exp\left\{-\frac{1}{2\sigma^2}(Y-\mu)^2\right\},$$

where Y, μ can take any real value and $\sigma^2 > 0$.

$E(Y) = \mu$ and $\text{Var}(Y) = \sigma^2$.

Multivariate normal distribution

The multivariate normal pdf of a $p \times 1$ vector of random variables $\mathbf{Y} = (Y_1, \ldots, Y_p)^T$ is

$$f(\mathbf{Y}|\boldsymbol{\mu}, \boldsymbol{\Omega}) = |2\pi\boldsymbol{\Omega}|^{-1/2} \exp\left\{-\frac{1}{2}(\mathbf{Y}-\boldsymbol{\mu})^T \boldsymbol{\Omega}^{-1}(\mathbf{Y}-\boldsymbol{\mu})\right\},$$

where elements of $\mathbf{Y}$ can take any real value, $\boldsymbol{\mu} = (\mu_1, \ldots, \mu_p)^T$ is a $p \times 1$ vector of real numbers with $E(Y_j) = \mu_j$, $j = 1, \ldots, p$, and $\boldsymbol{\Omega}$ a $p \times p$ positive definite matrix with $\text{Var}(\mathbf{Y}) = \boldsymbol{\Omega}$.

We may also write this density in terms of the precision matrix $\boldsymbol{\Lambda} = \boldsymbol{\Omega}^{-1}$ giving

$$f(\mathbf{Y}|\boldsymbol{\mu}, \boldsymbol{\Lambda}) = (2\pi)^{-p/2}|\boldsymbol{\Lambda}|^{1/2} \exp\left\{-\frac{1}{2}(\mathbf{Y}-\boldsymbol{\mu})^T \boldsymbol{\Lambda}(\mathbf{Y}-\boldsymbol{\mu})\right\},$$

Conditional normal distribution

Suppose $\mathbf{Y}$, of dimension $p \times 1$, follows a multivariate normal distribution with mean $\boldsymbol{\mu}$ and variance-covariance matrix $\boldsymbol{\Omega}$. Suppose we partition $\mathbf{Y} = (Y_1, \ldots, Y_p)^T$ into $\mathbf{Y}_q, \mathbf{Y}_r$ where $p = q + r$, $\mathbf{Y}_q = (Y_1, \ldots, Y_q)^T$ and $\mathbf{Y}_r = (Y_{q+1}, \ldots, Y_p)^T$. Thus $\mathbf{Y}^T = (\mathbf{Y}_q^T, \mathbf{Y}_r^T)$.

Partition the mean $\boldsymbol{\mu}$ in the same way into $\boldsymbol{\mu}_p$, $\boldsymbol{\mu}_r$, and partition the $p \times p$ variance-covariance matrix as

$$\boldsymbol{\Omega} = \begin{pmatrix} \boldsymbol{\Omega}_q & \boldsymbol{\Omega}_{qr} \\ \boldsymbol{\Omega}_{rq} & \boldsymbol{\Omega}_r \end{pmatrix},$$

where $\boldsymbol{\Omega}_q$ has dimension $q \times q$, $\boldsymbol{\Omega}_r$ dimension $r \times r$, $\boldsymbol{\Omega}_{qr}$ dimension $q \times r$, $\boldsymbol{\Omega}_{rq}$ dimension $r \times q$ and $\boldsymbol{\Omega}_{rq}^T = \boldsymbol{\Omega}_{qr}$.

Then $\mathbf{Y}_q$ has a multivariate normal distribution with mean $\boldsymbol{\mu}_q$ and variance $\boldsymbol{\Omega}_q$, and the conditional distribution $f(\mathbf{Y}_r|\mathbf{Y}_q)$ is multivariate normal with mean

$$\boldsymbol{\mu}_r + (\mathbf{Y}_q - \boldsymbol{\mu}_q)\boldsymbol{\Omega}_{qq}^{-1}\boldsymbol{\Omega}_{qr}$$

and variance

$$\boldsymbol{\Omega}_r - \boldsymbol{\Omega}_{rq}\boldsymbol{\Omega}_{qq}^{-1}\boldsymbol{\Omega}_{qr}.$$

Gamma distribution

The gamma pdf of a random variable $Y > 0$ is

$$f(Y|\alpha, r) = \frac{\alpha}{\Gamma(r)}(\alpha Y)^{r-1}e^{-\alpha Y},$$

where $r > 0$, $\alpha > 0$ and $Y > 0$.

Here, the gamma function, $\Gamma(r)$ is defined, for $r > 0$, as

$$\Gamma(r) = \int_0^\infty x^{r-1}e^{-x}\,dx.$$

For integer r, $\Gamma(r) = (r-1)(r-2), \ldots, 1 = (r-1)!$

Then $\mathrm{E}(Y) = r/\alpha$ and $\mathrm{Var}(Y) = r/\alpha^2$.

In the special case that $r = 1$ Y follows an exponential distribution.

χ^2 distribution

In the definition of the gamma distribution, if $\alpha = 1/2$ and $r = n/2$ then we say Y follows a χ_n^2 distribution, with mean n and variance $2n$.

t-distribution

If $X \sim N(0, 1)$ and independently $Y \sim \chi^2_n$, then

$$\frac{X}{\sqrt{Y/n}}$$

follows a t distribution with n degrees of freedom, denoted t_n.

The probability density function is

$$f(Y) = \frac{\Gamma\left(\frac{n+1}{2}\right)}{\sqrt{n\pi}\,\Gamma\left(\frac{n}{2}\right)}\left(1 + \frac{Y^2}{n}\right)^{-\frac{n+1}{2}}.$$

The t_n distribution has mean 0 and variance $n/(n-2)$ for $n > 2$. For $n = 1, 2$ the variance is undefined.

F-distribution

If $X \sim \chi^2_p$ and independently $Y \sim \chi^2_q$ then

$$\frac{X/p}{Y/q}$$

follows and F distribution on p and q degrees of freedom.

This has mean $q/(q-2)$ for $q > 2$ and variance

$$\frac{2q^2(p+q-2)}{p(q-2)^2(q-4)}$$

for $q > 4$.

Wishart distribution

The Wishart distribution of a positive definite matrix $\mathbf{W}$ has probability density function

$$\mathrm{W}(n, \mathbf{\Lambda}) = f(\mathbf{W}|n, \mathbf{\Lambda}) = \frac{|\mathbf{W}|^{(n-p-1)/2}}{2^{(np)/2}|\mathbf{\Lambda}|^{n/2}\Gamma_p\left(\frac{n}{2}\right)} \exp\left\{-\frac{1}{2}\mathrm{tr}(\mathbf{\Lambda}^{-1}\mathbf{W})\right\},$$

where p is the dimension of $\mathbf{W}$, $n > (p-1)$ is the degrees of freedom (which is not restricted to being integer), and $\mathbf{\Lambda}$ is a positive definite matrix.

Here tr means the trace of the matrix, defined as the sum of its diagonal elements. $\Gamma_p(n/2)$ is the multivariate gamma function, defined as

$$\Gamma_p\left(\frac{n}{2}\right) = \pi^{\frac{p(p-1)}{4}} \prod_{j=1}^{p} \Gamma\left(\frac{n+(1-j)}{2}\right).$$

The Wishart distribution has mean $n\mathbf{\Lambda}$ and variance $\text{Var}(\mathbf{W}_{ij}) = n(\mathbf{\Lambda}_{ij}^2 + \mathbf{\Lambda}_{ii}\mathbf{\Lambda}_{jj})$.

The χ_n^2 distribution is the special case of the Wishart distribution with $p = 1$, $\Lambda = 1$.

Inverse gamma distribution

The inverse gamma pdf of a random variable $Y > 0$ is

$$f(Y|\alpha, r) = \frac{\alpha}{\Gamma(r)}\alpha^{r-1}Y^{-(r+1)}e^{-\alpha/Y},$$

where $r > 0$, $\alpha > 0$ and $Y > 0$.

Then $\text{E}(Y) = \alpha/(r-1)$ and $\text{Var}(Y) = \alpha^2/(r-1)^2(r-2)$ for $r > 2$.

Inverse Wishart distribution

If the matrix $\mathbf{W}$ has a $\text{W}(n, \mathbf{\Lambda})$ distribution then its inverse $\mathbf{V} = \mathbf{W}^{-1}$ has an inverse Wishart $\text{W}^{-1}(n, \mathbf{\Lambda}^{-1})$ distribution with probability density function

$$f(\mathbf{V}|n, \mathbf{\Lambda}) = \frac{|\mathbf{V}|^{-(n+p+1)/2}}{2^{(np)/2}|\mathbf{\Lambda}|^{n/2}\Gamma_p(\frac{n}{2})} \exp\left\{-\frac{1}{2}\text{tr}(\mathbf{\Lambda}^{-1}\mathbf{V}^{-1})\right\}.$$

Under the inverse Wishart distribution,

$$E(\mathbf{V}) = \frac{1}{n-p-1}\mathbf{\Lambda}^{-1}.$$

B.1 Posterior for the multivariate normal distribution

Suppose we have a sample of size n from the p-dimensional multivariate normal distribution, denoted $\mathbf{Y}_i = (Y_{i,1}, \ldots, Y_{i,p})^T$, $i \in (1, \ldots, n)$. If we parameterise this in terms of the mean, $\boldsymbol{\mu}$ and precision matrix $\mathbf{\Lambda}$, the likelihood of the parameters is

$$L(\boldsymbol{\mu}, \mathbf{\Lambda}|\mathbf{Y}) = \prod_{i=1}^{n} \frac{|\mathbf{\Lambda}|^{1/2}}{(2\pi)^{p/2}} \exp\left\{-\frac{1}{2}(\mathbf{Y}_i - \boldsymbol{\mu})^T\mathbf{\Lambda}(\mathbf{Y}_i - \boldsymbol{\mu})\right\}$$

$$\propto |\mathbf{\Lambda}|^{n/2} \exp\left\{-\frac{1}{2}\sum_{i=1}^{n}(\mathbf{Y}_i - \boldsymbol{\mu})^T \mathbf{\Lambda}(\mathbf{Y}_i - \boldsymbol{\mu})\right\}$$

$$= |\mathbf{\Lambda}|^{n/2} \exp\left\{-\frac{1}{2}\mathrm{tr}(\mathbf{S\Lambda}) - \frac{n}{2}(\bar{\mathbf{Y}} - \boldsymbol{\mu})^T \mathbf{\Lambda}(\bar{\mathbf{Y}} - \boldsymbol{\mu})\right\}. \qquad \text{(B.1)}$$

Here $\bar{\mathbf{Y}} = \sum_{i=1}^{n} \mathbf{Y}_i/n$,

$$\mathbf{S} = \sum_{i=1}^{n}(\mathbf{Y}_i - \bar{\mathbf{Y}})(\mathbf{Y}_i - \bar{\mathbf{Y}})^T,$$

and the last equality can be derived by noting that, for example,

$$\mathbf{Y}_i^T \mathbf{\Lambda} \mathbf{Y}_i = \mathrm{tr}\{\mathbf{\Lambda}(\mathbf{Y}_i\mathbf{Y}_i^T)\}$$
$$= \mathrm{tr}\{(\mathbf{Y}_i\mathbf{Y}_i^T)\mathbf{\Lambda}\} \text{ for symmetric matrices } \mathbf{\Lambda}, (\mathbf{YY}^T).$$

Suppose we choose priors for $\boldsymbol{\mu}$, $\mathbf{\Lambda}$ as $\boldsymbol{\mu} \sim \mathrm{N}_p\{\mathbf{0}, (\lambda\mathbf{\Lambda})^{-1}\}$, and $\mathbf{\Lambda} \sim \mathrm{W}(\nu, \mathbf{S}_p)$. Then the prior for $(\boldsymbol{\mu}, \mathbf{\Lambda})$ is proportional to

$$|\lambda\mathbf{\Lambda}|^{1/2}|\mathbf{\Lambda}|^{(\nu-p-1)/2} \exp\left\{-\frac{1}{2}\mathrm{tr}(\mathbf{S}_p^{-1}\mathbf{\Lambda}) - \frac{1}{2}\boldsymbol{\mu}^T(\lambda\mathbf{\Lambda})\boldsymbol{\mu}\right\}.$$

It follows that the posterior is

$$f(\boldsymbol{\mu}, \mathbf{\Lambda}|\mathbf{Y}) \propto |\lambda\mathbf{\Lambda}|^{1/2} \exp\left\{-\frac{n}{2}(\bar{\mathbf{Y}} - \boldsymbol{\mu})^T \mathbf{\Lambda}(\bar{\mathbf{Y}} - \boldsymbol{\mu}) - \frac{\lambda}{2}\boldsymbol{\mu}^T \mathbf{\Lambda}\boldsymbol{\mu}\right\}$$
$$\times |\mathbf{\Lambda}|^{(n+\nu-p-1)/2} \exp\left\{-\frac{1}{2}\mathrm{tr}[(\mathbf{S}_p^{-1} + \mathbf{S})\mathbf{\Lambda}]\right\}$$
$$\propto f(\boldsymbol{\mu}|\mathbf{\Lambda}, \mathbf{Y}) f(\mathbf{\Lambda}|\mathbf{Y})$$

where

(a) $f(\boldsymbol{\mu}|\mathbf{\Lambda}, \mathbf{Y})$ is $N_p\{\boldsymbol{\mu}^\star, (\mathbf{\Lambda}^\star)^{-1}\}$ with

$$\boldsymbol{\mu}^\star = \bar{\mathbf{Y}}\left(\frac{n}{n+\lambda}\right), \quad \text{and} \quad \mathbf{\Lambda}^\star = (n+\lambda)\mathbf{\Lambda};$$

(b) $f(\mathbf{\Lambda}|\mathbf{Y})$ is $\mathrm{W}\{N + \nu, [\mathbf{S}_p^{-1} + \mathbf{S} + \bar{\mathbf{Y}}\bar{\mathbf{Y}}^T(n\lambda)/(\lambda + n)]^{-1}\}$.

If we make the prior for the mean, $\boldsymbol{\mu}$ less and less informative by letting $\lambda \to 0$, then the $f(\boldsymbol{\mu}|\mathbf{\Lambda}, \mathbf{Y}) \to \mathrm{N}_p\{\bar{\mathbf{Y}}, (n\mathbf{\Lambda})^{-1}\}$.

We note that in the case $p = 1$, this corresponds to $\mu \sim \mathrm{N}(\bar{Y}, \sigma^2/n)$ and $\sigma^2 \sim \{S_p^{-1} + \sum(Y_i - \bar{Y})^2\}/\chi^2_{n+\nu}$.

It remains to choose the parameters of the Wishart prior, ν, $\mathbf{S}_p$. One option is to chose $\mathbf{S}_p = \mathbf{S}$, with $\mathbf{S}$ estimated from the observed data, and ν_p just greater than its minimum permissible value of $(p - 1)$. In other words the smallest possible degrees of freedom (representing the greatest uncertainty) about an estimate of S based on the observed data.

An alternative arises if we note that, when looking at the posterior for $\boldsymbol{\mu}, \boldsymbol{\Sigma}$, we may relax the constraints on the parameters required for the prior to be a proper probability distribution, provided the posterior remains a proper probability distribution. Thus we may allow $\mathbf{S}_p^{-1} \to 0$. In the univariate case this now gives

$$\sigma^2 \sim \sum (Y_i - \bar{Y})^2 / \chi^2_{n+\nu}.$$

Applying the same argument to ν, we let $\nu \to -1$, so that the posterior for σ^2 tends to the sampling distribution for σ^2,

$$\sigma^2 \sim \sum (Y_i - \bar{Y})^2 / \chi^2_{n-1}.$$

Bringing all this together, letting $\lambda \to 0$, $\mathbf{S}_p^{-1} \to 0$ and $\nu \to -1$ gives:

$$\boldsymbol{\mu} \sim N\{\bar{\mathbf{Y}}, (n\Lambda)^{-1}\}$$

$$\boldsymbol{\Lambda} \sim \mathrm{W}(n-1, S^{-1}). \quad \text{(B.2)}$$

Schafer (1997), pp. 154–5 discuss this in more detail, noting that posterior (B.2) can be derived from the Jeffreys invariance principle.

In MI, especially if the mean (or more generally regression parameters) are the focus of inferential interest, provided the degrees of freedom of the Wishart prior are kept low, precise choices are unlikely to have a substantive impact on the results.

Bibliography

Afifi, A. and Elashoff, R. (1966) Missing observations in multivariate statistics I: Review of the literature. *Journal of the American Statistical Association*, **61**, 595–604.

Aitchison, J. and Bennett, J. A. (1970) Polychotomous quantal response by maximum indicant. *Biometrika*, **57**, 253–262.

Albert, J. H. and Chib, S. (1993) Bayesian analysis of binary and polychotomous response data. *Journal of the American Statistical Association*, **88**, 669–679.

Albert, P. S. and Follman, D. A. (2009) Shared parameter models. In *Longitudinal Data Analysis: A Handbook of Modern Statistical Methods* (Eds M. Davidian, G. Fitzmaurice, G. Molenberghs and G. Verbeke), pp. 433–452. Chapman & Hall/CRC.

Allison, P. D. (2002) *Missing Data*. Thousand Oaks, CA: Sage.

Andridge, R. R. and Little, R. J. A. (2010) A review of hot deck imputation for survey non-response. *International Statistical Review*, **78**, 40–64.

Ayieko, P., Ntoburi, S., Wagai, J., Opondo, C., Opiyo, N., Migiro, S., Wamae, A., Mogoa, W., Were, F., Wasunna, A., Fegan, G., Irimu, G. and English, M. (2011) A multifaceted intervention to implement guidelines and improve admission paediatric care in Kenyan district hospitals: a cluster randomised trial. *PLOS Medicine*, **8**, e1001018.

Bahadur, R. R. (1961) A representation of the joint distribution of responses to *n* dichotomous items. In *Studies in Item Analysis and Prediction* (Ed. H. Solomon). Stanford, CA: Stanford University Press.

Bang, H. and Robins, J. M. (2005) Doubly robust estimation in missing data and causal inference models. *Biometrics*, **61**, 962–973.

Barnard, J. and Rubin, D. B. (1999) Small-sample degrees of freedom with multiple imputation. *Biometrika*, **86**, 948–955.

Bartlett, J. A. and Shao, J. F. (2009) Successes, challenges, and limitations of current antiretroviral therapy in low-income and middle-income countries. *Lanced Infectious Diseases*, **9**, 637–649.

Bartlett, J. W. (2011) Personal communication.

Bartlett, J. W., Seaman, S., White, I. R. and Carpenter, J. R. (2012) Accommodating the model of interest within the fully conditional specification multiple imputation framework. *Submitted*.

Bernaards, C. A., Belin, T. R. and Schafer, J. L. (2007) Robustness of a multivariate normal approximation for imputation of incomplete binary data. *Statistics in Medicine*, **26**, 1368–1382.

Blatchford, P., Goldstein, H., Martin, C. and Browne, W. (2002) A study of class size effects in English school reception year classes. *British Educational Research Journal*, **28**, 169–185.

Boulle, A., Bock, P., Osler, M., Cohen, K., Channing, L., Hilderbrand, K., Mothibi, E., Zweigenthal, V., Slingers, N., Cloete, K. and Abdullah, F. (2008) Antiretroviral therapy and early mortality in South Africa. *Bulletin of the World Health Organization*, **86**, 657–736.

Bousquet, A. H., Desenclos, J. C., Larsen, C., Le Strat, Y. and Carpenter, J. R. (2012) Practical considerations for sensitivity analysis after multiple imputation applied to epidemiological studies with incomplete data. *BMC Medical Research Methodology*, **12**, 73.

Bowman, D. and George, E. O. (1995) A saturated model for analyzing exchangeable binary data: applications to clinical and developmental toxicity studies. *Journal of the American Statistical Association*, **90**, 871–879.

Brinkhof, M. W. G., Dabis, F., Myer, L., Bangsberg, D. R., Boulle, A., Nash, D., Schechter, M., Laurent, C., Keiser, O., May, M., Sprinz, E. and Egger, M. for the ART-LINC of IeDEA collaboration, X. A. (2008) Early loss of HIV-infected patients on potent antiretroviral therapy programmes in lower-income countries. *Bulletin of the World Health Organization*, **86**, 497–576.

Brinkhof, M. W. G., Pujades-Rodreguez, M. and Egger, M. (2009) Lost to follow-up in antiretroviral treatment programmes in resource-limited settings: systematic review and meta-analysis. *PLOS ONE*, **4**, e5790.

Brinkhof, M. W. G., Spycher, B. D., Yiannoutsos, C., Weigel, R., Wood, R., Messou, E., Boulle, A., Egger, M. and Sterne, J. A. C. (2010) Adjusting mortality for loss to follow-up: analysis of five ART programmes in sub-Saharan Africa. *PLOS ONE*, **5**, e14149.

Browne, W. J. (2006) MCMC algorithms for constrained variance matrices. *Computational Statistics and Data Analysis*, **50**, 1655–1677.

Busse, W. W., Chervinsky, P., Condemi, J., Lumry, W. R., Petty, T. L., Rennard, S. and Townley, R. G. (1998) Budesonide delivered by Turbuhaler is effective in a dose-dependent fashion when used in the treatment of adult patients with chronic asthma. *Journal of Allergy and Clinical Immunology*, **101**, 457–463.

Carpenter, J. R., Goldstein, H. and Kenward, M. G. (2011a) REALCOM-IMPUTE software for multilevel multiple imputation with mixed response types. *Journal of Statistical Software*, **45**(4), 1–14.

Carpenter, J. R. and Kenward, M. G. (2008) *Missing Data in Clinical trials – A Practical Guide*. Birmingham: National Health Service Co-ordinating Centre for Research Methodology.

Carpenter, J. R., Kenward, M. G. and Goldstein, H. (2012) Statistical modelling of partially observed data using multiple imputation: principles and practice. In *Modern Methods for Epidemiology* (Eds Y. Tu and D. Greenwood), pp. 15–31. New York: Springer.

Carpenter, J. R., Kenward, M. G. and Vansteelandt, S. (2006) A comparison of multiple imputation and inverse probability weighting for analyses with missing data. *Journal of the Royal Statistical Society, Series A (Statistics in Society)*, **169**, 571–584.

Carpenter, J. R., Kenward, M. G. and White, I. R. (2007) Sensitivity analysis after multiple imputation under missing at random – a weighting approach. *Statistical Methods in Medical Research*, **16**, 259–275.

Carpenter, J. R. and Plewis, I. (2011) Analysing longitudinal studies with non-response: issues and statistical methods. In *The SAGE Handbook of Innovation in Social Research Methods* (Eds M. Williams and P. Vogt), London: SAGE.

Carpenter, J. R., Pocock, S. and Lamm, C. J. (2002) Coping with missing data in clinical trials: a model based approach applied to asthma trials. *Statistics in Medicine*, **21**, 1043–1066.

Carpenter, J. R., Roger, J. H. and Kenward, M. G. (2013) Analysis of longitudinal trials with missing data: a framework for relevant accessible assumptions and inference via multiple imputation. *Journal of Biopharmaceutical Statistics*, in press.

Carpenter, J. R., Rücker, G. and Schwarzer, G. (2011b) Assessing the sensitivity of meta-analysis to selection bias: a multiple imputation approach. *Biometrics*, **67**, 1066–1072.

Chib, S. and Greenburg, E. (1998) Analysis of multivariate probit models. *Biometrika*, **85**, 347–361.

Clark, D. (2004) Practical introduction to record linkage for injury research. *Injury Prevention*, **10**, 186–191.

Clayton, D. G., Spiegelhalter, D., Dunn, G. and Pickles, A. (1998) Analysis of longitudinal binary data from multi-phase sampling (with discussion). *Journal of the Royal Statistical Society, Series B (statistical methodology)*, **60**, 71–87.

Clayton, D. G. (1991) A Monte Carlo method for Bayesian inference in frailty models. *Biometrics*, **47**, 467–485.

Cole, S. R., Chu, H. and Greenland, S. (2006) Multiple imputation for measurement error correction. *International Journal of Epidemiology*, **35**, 1074–1081.

Collins, L. M., Schafer, J. L. and Kam, C. M. (2001) A comparison of inclusive and restrictive strategies in modern missing data procedures. *Psychological Methods*, **6**, 330–351.

Committee for Medicinal Products for Human Use (2010) *Guideline on Missing Data in Confirmatory Clinical Trials*. London: European Medicines Agency.

Copas, J. B. and Shi, J. Q. (2000) Meta-analysis, funnel plots and sensitivity analysis. *Biostatistics*, **1**, 247–262.

Cowles, M. K. (1996) Accelerating Monte Carlo Markov chain convergence for cumulative-link generalized linear models. *Statistics and Computing*, **6**, 101–110.

Croxford, L., Ianelli, C. and Shapira, M. (2007) Documentation of the Youth Cohort Time-Series Datasets, UK Data Archive Study Number 5765, Economic and Social Data Service.

Daniel, R. M. and Kenward, M. G. (2012) A method for increasing the robustness of multiple imputation. *Computational Statistics and Data Analysis*, **56**, 1624–1643.

Daniel, R. M., Kenward, M. G., Cousens, S. N. and Stavola, B. L. D. (2012) Using causal diagrams to guide analysis in missing data problems. *Statistical Methods in Medical Research*, **21**, 243–256.

Daniels, M. J. and Hogan, J. W. (2000) Reparameterizing the pattern mixture model for sensitivity analysis under informative dropout. *Biometrics*, **56**, 1241–1248.

Daniels, M. J. and Hogan, J. W. (2008) *Missing Data in Longitudinal Studies*. London: Chapman & Hall.

Demirtas, H. and Schafer, J. L. (2003) On the performance of random coefficient pattern mixture models for non-ignorable dropout. *Statistics in Medicine*, **22**, 2553–2575.

Demirtas, H., Freels, S. A. and Yucel, R. M. (2008) Plausibility of multivariate normality assumption when multiply imputing non-Gaussain continuous outcomes: a simulation assessment. *Journal of Statistical Computation and Simulation*, **78**, 69–84.

Dempster, A. P., Laird, N. M. and Rubin, D. B. (1977) Maximum likelihood from incomplete data via the EM algorithm (with discussion). *Journal of the Royal Statistical Society Series B (Statistical Methodology)*, **39**, 1–38.

Diggle, P. J. and Kenward, M. G. (1994) Informative dropout in longitudinal data analysis (with discussion). *Journal of the Royal Statistical Society Series C (Applied Statistics)*, **43**, 49–94.

Drechsler, J. (2011) Multiple imputation in practice: a case study using a complex German establishment survey. *Advances in Statistical Analysis*, **95**, 1–26.

Fay, R. E. (1992) When are inferences from multiple imputation valid? *Proceedings of the Survey Research Methodology Section of the American Statistical Association*, pp. 227–232.

Fay, R. E. (1993) Valid inferences from imputed survey data. *Proceedings of the Survey Research Methodology Section of the American Statistical Association*, pp. 41–48.

Firth, D. (1993) Bias reduction of maximum likelihood estimates. *Biometrika*, **80**, 27–38.

Gelman, A., Carlin, J. B., Stern, H. S. and Rubin, D. B. (1995) *Bayesian Data Analaysis*. Florida: CRC press.

Gelman, A. G., Roberts, G. O. and Gilks, W. R. (1996) Efficient Metropolis jumping rules. In *Bayesian Statistics V* (Eds J. M. Bernardo, J. O. Berger, A. F. Dawid and A. F. M. Smith), pp. 599–608. Oxford: Oxford University Press.

Ghosh-Dastidar, B. and Schafer, J. L. (2003) Multiple edit/multiple imputation for multivariate continuous data. *Journal of the American Statistical Association*, **98**, 807–817.

Gilks, W. R., Richardson, S. and Spiegelhalter, D. J. (1996) *Markov chain Monte-Carlo in Practice*. London: Chapman and Hall.

Gill, R. and Robins, J. (1997) Sequential models for coarsening and missingness. In *Proceedings of the First Seattle Symposium in Biostatistics: Survival Analysis*. (Eds D. Y. Lin and T. R. Fleming), pp. 295–305. Berlin: Springer.

Goldstein, H. (2010) *Multilevel Statistical Models (4th edition)*. Chichester: John Wiley & Sons, Ltd.

Goldstein, H., Carpenter, J. R., Kenward, M. G. and Levin, K. (2009) Multilevel models with multivariate mixed response types. *Statistical Modelling*, **9**, 173–197.

Goldstein, H., Carpenter, J. R. and Browne, W. (2012a) Fitting multilevel multivariate models with missing data in responses and covariates, which may include interactions and non-linear terms. *Submitted*.

Goldstein, H., Harron, K. and Wade, A. (2012b) The analysis of record-linked data using multiple imputation with data value priors. *Statistics in Medicine* doi: 10.1002/sim.5508.

Hansen, P. C. (1998) *Rank-deficient and Discrete Ill-posed Problems*. Society for Industrial and Applied Mathematics, Philadelphia.

Harel, O. (2003) *Strategies for data analysis with two types of missing values*. Ph.D. thesis, Department of Statistics, The Pennsylvania State University, University Park, PA.

Harel, O. (2007) Inferences on missing information under multiple imputation and two-stage multiple imputation. *Statistical Methodology*, **4**, 75–79.

Harel, O. (2009) *Strategies for Data Analysis with Two Types of Missing Values*. Lambert Academic Publishing.

Harel, O. and Carpenter, J. R. (2012) Complete records regression with missing data: relating bias in coefficient estimates to the missingness mechanism, in preparation.

Harel, O. and Schafer, J. L. (2003) Multiple imputation in two stages. In *Proceedings of Federal Committee on Statistical Methodology Conference*. Available from http://www.fcsm.gov/03papers/Harel.pdf, accessed April 2012.

Harel, O. and Schafer, J. L. (2009) Partial and latent ignorability in missing data problems. *Biometrika*, **96**, 37–50.

He, Y., Zaslavsky, A. M., Harrington, D. P., Catalano, P. and Landrum, M. B. (2010) Multiple imputation in a large-scale complex survey: a practical guide. *Statistical Methods in Medical Research*, **19**, 653–670.

Healy, M. J. R. and Westmacott, M. (1956) Missing values in experiments analyzed on automatic computers. *Applied Statistics*, **5**, 203–206.

Higgins, J. P. T., White, I. R. and Wood, A. (2006) Missing outcome data in meta-analysis of clinical trials: development and comparison of methods, with recommendations for practice. *Technical report, MRC Biostatistcs Unit, Cambridge UK*.

Hippisley-Cox, J., Coupland, C., Vinogradova, Y., Robson, J., May, M. and Brindle, P. (2007) Derivation and validation of QRISK, a new cardiovascular disease risk score for the United Kingdom: prospective open cohort study. *British Medical Journal*, **335**, 7611–7623.

Hoerl, A. E. and Kennard, R. W. (1970) Ridge regression: biased estimation for nonorthogonal problems. *Technometrics*, **42**, 80–86.

Hollis, S. and Campbell, F. (1999) What is meant by intention to treat analysis? Survey of published randomised controlled trials. *British Medical Journal*, **319**, 670–674.

Home, P. D., Jones, N. P., Pocock, S. J., Beck-Nielsen, H., Gomis, R., and Komajda, M. H. and Curtis, P. (2007) Rosiglitazone record study: glucose control outcomes at 18 months. *Diabetic Medicine*, **24**, 626–634.

Horton, N. J., Lipsitz, S. R. and Parzen, M. (2003) A potential for bias when rounding in multiple imputation. *The American Statistician*, **57**, 229–232.

Horvitz, D. G. and Thompson, D. J. (1952) A generalisation of sampling without replacement from a finite universe. *Journal of the American Statistical Association*, **47**, 663–685.

Hsu, C.-H., Taylor, J. M. G., Murray, S. and Commenges, D. (2006) Survival analysis using auxiliary variables via nonparametric multiple imputation. *Statistics in Medicine*, **25**, 3503–3517.

Hsu, C.-H., Taylor, J. M. G., Murray, S. and Commenges, D. (2007) Multiple imputation for interval censored data with auxiliary variables. *Statistics in Medicine*, **26**, 769–781.

Hsu, C.-H., and Taylor, J. M. G. (2009) Nonparametric comparison of two survival functions with dependent censoring via nonparametric multiple imputation. *Statistics in Medicine*, **28**, 462–475.

Hughes, R., White, I. R., Carpenter, J. R., Tilling, K. and Sterne, J. A. C. (2012a) Joint modelling rationale for chained equations imputation. *Technical report*, University of Bristol, Department of Social Medicine.

Hughes, R. A., Sterne, J. A. C. and Tilling, K. (2012b) Comparison of imputation variance estimators. *Technical report*, University of Bristol, Department of Social Medicine.

Jaro, M. (1995) Probabilistic linkage of large public health data files. *Statistics in Medicine*, **14**, 491–498.

Kang, J. D. Y. and Schafer, J. L. (2007) Demystifying double robustness: A comparison of alternative strategies for estimating a population mean from incomplete data (with discussion). *Statistical Science*, **22**, 523–539.

Kenward, M. G. (1998) Selection models for repeated measurements with non-random dropout: an illustration of sensitivity. *Statistics in Medicine*, **17**, 2723–2732.

Kenward, M. G. and Carpenter, J. R. (2007) Multiple imputation: current perspectives. *Statistical Methods in Medical Research*, **16**, 199–218.

Kenward, M. G. and Carpenter, J. R. (2009) Multiple imputation. In *Longitudinal Data Analysis: A Handbook of Modern Statistical Methods* (Eds M. Davidian, G. Fitzmaurice, G. Molenberghs and G. Verbeke), pp. 477–500. London: Chapman & Hall/CRC.

Kenward, M. G. and Molenberghs, G. (1998) Likelihood based frequentist inference when data are missing at random. *Statistical Science*, **13**, 236–247.

Kenward, M. G. and Rosenkranz, G. (2011) Joint modelling of outcome, observation time and missingness. *Journal of Biopharmaceutical Statistics*, **21**, 252–262.

Kenward, M. G., Molenberghs, G. and Thijs, H. (2003) Pattern-mixture models with proper time dependence. *Biometrika*, **90**, 53–71.

Kim, J. K. (2002) A note on approximate Bayesian boostrap imputation. *Biometrika*, **89**, 470–477.

Kim, J. K., Brick, J. M., Fuller, W. A. and Kalton, G. (2006) On the bias of the multiple-imputation variance estimator in a survey setting. *Journal of the Royal Statistical Society, Series B (Statistical Methodology)*, **68**, 509–522.

Klebanoff, M. A. and Cole, S. R. (2008) Use of multiple imputation in the epidemiologic literature. *American Journal of Epidemiology*, **168**, 355–357.

Kott, P. (1995) A paradox of multiple imputation. *Proceedings of the Survey Research Methodology Section of the American Statistical Association*, pp. 380–383.

Lavori, P. W., Dawson, R. and Shera, D. (1995) A multiple imputation strategy for clinical trials with trunction of patient data. *Statistics in Medicine*, **14**, 1913–1925.

Lee, K. J. and Carlin, J. B. (2010) Multiple imputation for missing data: fully conditional specification versus multivariate normal imputation. *American Journal of Epidemiology*, **171**, 624–632.

Li, K. H., Raghunathan, T. E. and Rubin, D. B. (1991) Large-sample significance levels from multiply-imputed data using moment-based statistics and an F reference distribution. *Journal of the American Statistical Association*, **86**, 1065–1073.

Little, R. J. A. (1993) Statistical analysis of masked data. *Journal of Official Statistics*, **9**, 407–426.

Little, R. J. A. (1994) A class of pattern-mixture models for multivariate incomplete data. *Biometrika*, **81**, 471–483.

Little, R. J. A. and Rubin, D. B. (1987) *Statistical Analysis with Missing Data*. Chichester: John Wiley & Sons, Ltd.

Little, R. J. A. and Rubin, D. B. (2002) *Statistical Analysis with Missing Data (Second Edition)*. Chichester: John Wiley Sons, Ltd.

Little, R. J. A. and Yau, L. (1996) Intent-to-treat analysis for longitudinal studies with dropouts. *Biometrics*, **52**, 471–483.

Little, R. J. A. and Zhang, N. (2011) Subsample ignorable likelihood for regression analysis with missing data. *Journal of the Royal Statistical Society, Series C, Applied Statistics*, **60**, 591–605.

Lo, A. Y. (1986) Bayesian statistical inference for sampling from a finite population. *Annals of Statistics*, **14**, 1226–1233.

Louis, T. (1982) Finding the observed information matrix when using the EM algorithm. *Journal of the Royal Statistical Society, Series B (Statistical Methodology)*, **44**, 226–233.

Magder, L. S. (2003) Simple approaches to assess the possible impact of missing outcome information on estimates of risk ratios, odds ratios, and risk differences. *Controlled Clinical Trials*, **24**.

Mardia, K. V., Kent, J. T. and Bibby, J. M. (1979) *Multivariate Analysis*. Waltham, Massachusetts: Academic Press.

McCullagh, P. (1980) Regression models for ordinal data (with discussion). *Journal of the Royal Statistical Society, Series B (Statistical Methodology)*, **42**, 109–142.

Meng, X. L. (1994) Multiple-imputation inferences with uncongenial sources of input (with discussion). *Statistical Science*, **10**, 538–573.

Meng, X. L. and Romero, M. (2003) Discussion: Efficiency and self-efficiency with multiple imputation inference. *International Statistical Review*, **71**, 607–618.

Meng, X. L. and Rubin, D. B. (1992) Performing likelihood ratio tests with multiply-imputed data sets. *Biometrika*, **89**, 267–278.

Molenberghs, G. and Kenward, M. G. (2007) *Missing Data in Clinical Studies*. Chichester: John Wiley & Sons, Ltd.

Molenberghs, G., Michiels, B., Kenward, M. G. and Diggle, P. J. (1998) Monotone missing data and pattern-mixture models. *Statistica Neerlandica*, **52**, 153–161.

National Institute for Clinical Excellence (NICE) (2011) Glossary *accessed 17 October 2011 at* http://www.nice.org.uk/website/glossary/glossary.jsp.

National Research Council (2010) *The Prevention and Treatment of Missing Data in Clinical Trials*. Panel on Handling Missing Data in Clinical Trials. Committee on National Statistics, Division of Behavioral and Social Sciences and Education. Washington, DC: The National Academies Press.

Nevalainen, J., Kenward, M. G. and Virtanen, S. M. (2009) Missing values in longitudinal dietary data: a multiple imputation approach based on a fully conditional specification. *Statistics in Medicine*, **28**, 3657–3669.

Nielsen, S. F. (2003) Proper and improper multiple imputation. *International Statistical Review*, **71**, 593–627.

Nur, U., Shack, L. G., Rachet, B., Carpenter, J. R. and Coleman, M. P. (2010) Modelling relative survival in the presence of incomplete data: a tutorial. *International Journal of Epidemiology*, **39**, 118–128.

Olkin, I. and Tate, R. F. (1961) Multivariate correlation models with mixed discrete and continuous variables. *Annals of Mathematical Statistics*, **32**, 448–465.

Orchard, T. and Woodbury, M. (1972) A missing information principle: theory and applications. In *Proceedings of the Sixth Berkeley Symposium on Mathematics, Statistics and Probability, Volume 1*. (Eds L. M. Le Cam, J. Neyman and E. L. Scott), pp. 697–715. Berkeley: University of California Press.

Peto, R. (1973) Experimental survival curves for interval-censored data. *Journal of the Royal Statistical Society, Series C (Applied Statistics)*, **22**, 86–91.

Plewis, I., Calderwood, L., Hawkes, D. and Nathan, G. (2004) National Child Development Study and 1970 British Cohort Study Technical Report: Changes in the NCDS and BCS70 populations and samples over time. London: Institute of Education, University of London.

Raghunathan, T. E. (2006) Combining information from multiple surveys for assessing health disparities. *Allgemeines Statistisches Archiv*, **90**, 515–526.

Raghunathan, T. E., Lepkowski, J. M., Van Hoewyk, J. and Solenberger, P. (2001) A multivariate technique for multiply imputing missing values using a sequence of regression models. *Survey Methodology*, **27**, 85–95.

Rao, J. N. K. and Shao, J. (1992) Jackknife variance estimation with survey data under hot-deck imputation. *Biometrika*, **79**, 811–822.

Rao, J. N. K. and Wu, C. F. J. (1988) Resampling inference with complex survey data. *Journal of the American Statistical Association*, **83**, 231–241.

Reiter, J. P. (2007) Small-sample degrees of freedom for multi-component significance tests with multiple imputation for missing data. *Biometrika*, **92**, 502–508.

Reiter, J. P. and Raghunathan, T. E. (2007) The multiple adaptations of multiple imputation. *Journal of the American Statistical Association*, **102**, 1462–1471.

Ripley, B. D. (1987) *Stochastic Simulation*. New York: John Wiley & Sons, Inc.

Robins, J. M. and Gill, R. (1997) Non-response models for the analysis of non-monotone ignorable missing data. *Statistics in Medicine*, **16**, 39–56.

Robins, J. M. and Wang, N. (2000) Inference for imputation estimators. *Biometrika*, **85**, 113–124.

Robins, J. M., Mark, S. D. and Newey, W. K. (1992) Estimating exposure effects by modelling the expectation of exposure conditional on confounders. *Biometrics*, **48**, 479–495.

Robins, J. M., Rotnitzky, A. and Zhao, L. P. (1994) Estimation of regression coefficients when some regressors are not always observed. *Journal of the American Statistical Association*, **89**, 846–866.

Robins, J. M., Rotnitzky, A. and Zhao, L. P. (1995) Analysis of semiparametric regression models for repeated outcomes in the presence of missing data. *Journal of the American Statistical Association*, **90**, 106–121.

Rosenbaum, P. R. and Rubin, D. B. (1983) The central role of the propensity score in observational studies for causal effects. *Biometrika*, **70**, 41–55.

Royall, R. M. (1992) The model based (prediction) approach to finite population sampling theory. In *Current Issues in Statistial Inference: Essays in Honor of D Basu* (Eds M. Ghosh and P. K. Patahak), pp. 225–240. Institute of Mathematical Statistics.

Royston, P. (2007) Multiple imputation of missing values: further update of ice with emphasis on interval censoring. *The Stata Journal*, **7**, 445–464.

Royston, P. and Sauerbrei, W. (2008) *Multivariable Model-building*. Chichester: John Wiley & Sons, Ltd.

Rubin, D. B. (1976) Inference and missing data. *Biometrika*, **63**, 581–592.

Rubin, D. B. (1981) The Bayesian bootstrap. *Annals of Statistics*, **9**, 130–134.

Rubin, D. B. (1987) *Multiple Imputation for Nonresponse in Surveys*. New York: Wiley.

Rubin, D. B. (1996) Multiple imputation after 18 years. *Journal of the American Statistical Association*, **91**, 473–490.

Rubin, D. B. (2003) Discussion on multiple imputation. *International Statistical Review*, **71**, 619–625.

Rubin, D. B. and Schenker, N. (1986) Multiple imputation for interval estimation from simple random samples with ignorable nonresponse. *Journal of the American Statistical Association*, **81**, 366–374.

Särndal, C. E., Swensson, B. and Wretman, J. (1992) *Model Assisted Survey Sampling*. New York: Springer.

Schafer, J. L. (1997) *Analysis of incomplete multivariate data*. London: Chapman & Hall.

Schafer, J. L. (1999a) `MIX` software for multiple imputation of a mix of categorical and continuous data in S+. http://www.stat.psu.edu/~jls/misoftwa.html, accessed 27 July 2011.

Schafer, J. L. (1999b) Multiple imputation: a primer. *Statistical Methods in Medical Research*, **8**, 3–15.

Scharfstein, D. O., Rotnitzky, A. and Robins, J. M. (1999) Adjusting for nonignorable drop-out using semi-parametric nonresponse models (with comments). *Journal of the American Statistical Association*, **94**, 1096–1146.

Schott, J. M., Abartlett, J. W., Fox, N. C. and Barnes, J. for the Alzheimer's Disease Neuroimaging Initiative Investigators (2010) Increased brain atrophy rates in cognitively normal adults with lower cerebrosphinal fluid Aβ_{1-42}. *Annals of Neurology*, **31**, 1452–1462.

Schroter, S., Black, N., Evans, S., Carpenter, J., Godlee, F. and Smith, R. (2004) Effects of training on quality of peer review: randomised controlled trial. *British Medical Journal*, **328**, 673–675.

Seaman, S. R., Bartlett, J. W. and White, I. R. (2012a) Multiple imputation of missing covariates with non-linear effects and interactions: evaluation of statistical methods. *BMC Methodology*, **12**, 46.

Seaman, S. R., White, I. R., Copas, A. J. and Li, L. (2012b) Combining multiple imputation and inverse-probability weighting. *Biometrics*, **68**, 129–137.

Shen, Z. J. (2000) *Nested multiple imputation*. Ph.D. thesis, Department of Statistics, Harvard University, Cambridge, MA.

Siddique, J. and Belin, T. R. (2008) Using an approximate Bayesian bootstrap to multiply impute nonignorable missing data. *Computational Statistics and Data Analysis*, **53**, 405–415.

Spiegelhalter, D., Best, N., Carlin, B. P. and Van der Linde, A. (2002) Bayesian measures of model complexity and fit (with discussion). *Journal of the Royal Statistical Society, Series B (Statistical Methodology)*, **64**, 583–640.

Spiegelman, D., Rosner, B. and Logan, R. (2000) Estimation and inference for logistic regression with covariate misclassification and measurement error, in main study/validation study designs. *Journal of the American Statistical Association*, **95**, 51–61.

Steele, F., Goldstein, H. and Browne, W. (2004) A general multilevel multistate competing risks model for event history data, with an application to a study of contraceptive use dynamics. *Statistical Modelling*, **4**, 145–159.

Sterne, J. A. C., White, I. R., Carlin, J. B., Spratt, M., Royston, P., Kenward, M. G., Wood, A. M. and Carpenter, J. R. (2009) Multiple imputation for missing data in epidemiological and clinical research: potential and pitfalls. *British Medical Journal*, **339**, 157–160.

Su, Y., Gelmand, A., Hill, J. and Yajima, M. (2011) Multiple imputation with diagnostics (mi) in R: opening windows into the black box. *Journal of Statistical Software*, **45**, 1–31.

Tan, Z. (2010) Bounded, efficient and doubly robust estimation with inverse weighting. *Biometrics*, **97**, 661–682.

Tanner, M. and Wong, W. (1987) The calculation of posterior distributions by Data Augmentation (with discussion). *Journal of the American Statistical Association*, **82**, 528–550.

Tanner, M. A. (1996) *Tools for Statistical Inference*. Third Edition. New York: Springer.

Taylor, J. M. G., Murray, S. and Hsu, C. (2002) Survival estimation and testing via multiple imputation. *Statistics and Probability Letters*, **58**, 221–232.

Thijs, H., Molenberghs, G., Michiels, B., Verbeke, G. and Curran, D. (2002) Strategies to fit pattern-mixture models. *Biostatistics*, **3**, 245–265.

Tilling, K., Spratt, M., Sterne, J. A. C. and Carpenter, J. R. (2012) Dealing with interactions in analyses based on multiple imputation: a simulation study. *Technical Report, Department of Social Medicine, University of Bristol*.

Tsiatis, A. A. (2006) *Semiparametric Theory and Missing Data*. Springer, New York.

Tsiatis, A. A., Davidian, M. and Cao, W. (2011) Improved doubly robust estimation when data are monotonely coarsened, with application to longitudinal studies with dropout. *Biometrics*, **67**, 536–545.

UK Data Archive (2007) Youth Cohort Time Series for England, Wales and Scotland, 1984–2002 (computer file SN 5765). First Edition, Colchester, Essex: UK Data Archive, November 2007.

van Buuren, S. (2007) Multiple imputation of discrete and continuous data by fully conditional specification. *Statistical Methods in Medical Research*, **16**, 219–242.

van Buuren, S., Boshuizen, H. C. and Knook, D. L. (1999) Multiple imputation of missing blood presure covariates in survival analysis. *Statistics in Medicine*, **18**, 681–694.

Vansteelandt, S., Rotnitzky, A. and Robins, J. M. (2007) Estimation of regression models for the mean of repeated outcomes under nonignorable nonmonotone nonresponse. *Biometrika*, **94**, 841–860.

Vansteelandt, S., Carpenter, J. R. and Kenward, M. G. (2009) Analysis of incomplete data using inverse probability weighting and doubly robust estimators. *European Journal of Research Methods for the Behavioral and Social Sciences*, **6**, 37–48.

Vansteelandt, S., Bekaert, M. and Claeskens, G. (2012) On model selection and model misspecification in causal inference. *Statistical Methods in Medical Research*, **21**, 7–30.

Verbyla, A. P., Cullis, B. R., Kenward, M. G. and Welham, S. J, (1999) The analysis of designed experiments and longitudinal data by using smoothing splines. *Journal of the Royal Statistical Society, Series C (Applied Statistics)*, **48**, 269–311.

Verzilli, C. and Carpenter, J. R. (2002) A Monte Carlo EM algorithm for random coefficient-based dropout models. *Journal of Applied Statistics*, **29**, 1011–1021.

Von Hippel, P. T. (2009) How to impute interactions, squares and other transformed variables. *Sociological Methodology*, **39**, 265–291.

Wagai, J., Ntoburi, S., Irimu, G., Opiyo, N., Ayieko, P., Opondo, C., Carpenter, J. R. and English, M. (2012) Improving medical records: examining factors associated with better documentation of paediatric admissions to eight Kenyan hospitals enrolled in a cluster randomised trial. In preparation.

Wang, N. and Robins, J. M. (1998) Large-sample theory for parametric multiple imputation procedures. *Biometrika*, **85**, 935–948.

Welch, C., Petersen, I. and Carpenter, J. R. (2012) Multiple imputation for general practice records: application of 'forwards-backwards' algorithm. Forthcoming.

Welham, S. (2010) Smoothing spline models for longitudinal data. In *Longitudinal Data Analysis: A Handbook of Modern Statistical Methods* (Eds M. Davidian, G. Fitzmaurice, G. Molenberghs and G. Verbeke), pp. 253–290. Chichester: John Wiley & Sons, Ltd.

White, I., Carpenter, J. R., Evans, S. and Schroter, S. (2007) Eliciting and using expert opinions about non-response bias in randomised controlled trials. *Clinical Trials*, **4**, 125–139.

White, I. R. (2006) Commentary: dealing with measurement error: multiple imputation or regression calibration. *International Journal of Edpidemiology*, **35**, 1081–1082.

White, I. R. and Royston, P. (2009) Imputing missing covariate values for the Cox model. *Statistics in Medicine*, **28**, 1982–1998.

White, I. R., Daniel, R. and Royston, P. (2010) Avoiding bias due to perfect prediction in multiple imputation of incompete categorical variables. *Computational Statistics and Data Analysis*, **54**, 2267–2275.

Wood, A., Burgess, S. and White, I. R. (2012) Strategies for multiple imputation in individual patient data meta-analysis. *Submitted for publication*.

Yu, L. M., Burton, A. and Revero-Arias, O. (2007) Evaluation of software for multiple imputation of semi-continuous data. *Statistical Methods in Medical Research*, **16**, 243–258.

Yucel, R. M. (2011) Random covariances and mixed-effects models for imputing multivariate multilevel continuous data. *Statistical Modelling*, **11**, 351–370.

Yucel, R. M. and Zaslavsky, A. M. (2005) Imputation of binary treatment variables with measurement error in administrative data. *Journal of the American Statistical Association*, **100**, 1123–1132.

Zaslavsky, A. (1994) Comment on Meng, X-L., 'Multiple-imputation inferences with uncongenial sources of input'. *Statistical Science*, **9**, 563–566.

Zimmerman, D. L. and Núnez-Antón, V. A. (2010) *Antedependence Models for Longitudinal Data*. Chapman & Hall/CRC.

Index of Authors

Index of Examples

Index

Statistics in Practice

Human and Biological Sciences

Berger – Selection Bias and Covariate Imbalances in Randomized Clinical Trials
Berger and Wong – An Introduction to Optimal Designs for Social and Biomedical Research
Brown and Prescott – Applied Mixed Models in Medicine, Second Edition
Carpenter and Kenward – Multiple Imputation and its Application
Carstensen – Comparing Clinical Measurement Methods
Chevret (Ed) – Statistical Methods for Dose-Finding Experiments
Ellenberg, Fleming and DeMets – Data Monitoring Committees in Clinical Trials: A Practical Perspective
Hauschke, Steinijans & Pigeot – Bioequivalence Studies in Drug Development: Methods and Applications
Källén – Understanding Biostatistics
Lawson, Browne and Vidal Rodeiro – Disease Mapping with Win-BUGS and MLwiN
Lesaffre, Feine, Leroux & Declerck – Statistical and Methodological Aspects of Oral Health Research
Lui – Statistical Estimation of Epidemiological Risk
Marubini and Valsecchi – Analysing Survival Data from Clinical Trials and Observation Studies
Millar – Maximum Likelihood Estimation and Inference: With Examples in R, SAS and ADMB
Molenberghs and Kenward – Missing Data in Clinical Studies
O'Hagan, Buck, Daneshkhah, Eiser, Garthwaite, Jenkinson, Oakley & Rakow – Uncertain Judgements: Eliciting Expert's Probabilities
Parmigiani – Modeling in Medical Decision Making: A Bayesian Approach
Pintilie – Competing Risks: A Practical Perspective
Senn – Cross-over Trials in Clinical Research, Second Edition
Senn – Statistical Issues in Drug Development, Second Edition
Spiegelhalter, Abrams and Myles – Bayesian Approaches to Clinical Trials and Health-Care Evaluation

Walters – Quality of Life Outcomes in Clinical Trials and Health-Care Evaluation
Welton, Sutton, Cooper and Ades – Evidence Synthesis for Decision Making in Healthcare
Whitehead – Design and Analysis of Sequential Clinical Trials, Revised Second Edition
Whitehead – Meta-Analysis of Controlled Clinical Trials
Willan and Briggs – Statistical Analysis of Cost Effectiveness Data
Winkel and Zhang – Statistical Development of Quality in Medicine

Earth and Environmental Sciences

Buck, Cavanagh and Litton – Bayesian Approach to Interpreting Archaeological Data
Chandler and Scott – Statistical Methods for Trend Detection and Analysis in the Environmental Statistics
Glasbey and Horgan – Image Analysis in the Biological Sciences
Haas – Improving Natural Resource Management: Ecological and Political Models
Helsel – Nondetects and Data Analysis: Statistics for Censored Environmental Data
Illian, Penttinen, Stoyan, H and Stoyan D-Statistical Analysis and Modelling of Spatial Point Patterns
McBride – Using Statistical Methods for Water Quality Management
Webster and Oliver – Geostatistics for Environmental Scientists, Second Edition
Wymer (Ed) – Statistical Framework for Recreational Water Quality Criteria and Monitoring

Industry, Commerce and Finance

Aitken – Statistics and the Evaluation of Evidence for Forensic Scientists, Second Edition
Balding – Weight-of-evidence for Forensic DNA Profiles
Brandimarte – Numerical Methods in Finance and Economics: A MATLAB-Based Introduction, Second Edition
Brandimarte and Zotteri – Introduction to Distribution Logistics
Chan – Simulation Techniques in Financial Risk Management
Coleman, Greenfield, Stewardson and Montgomery (Eds) – Statistical Practice in Business and Industry

Frisen (Ed) – Financial Surveillance
Fung and Hu – Statistical DNA Forensics
Gusti Ngurah Agung – Time Series Data Analysis Using EViews
Kenett (Eds) – Operational Risk Management: A Practical Approach to Intelligent Data Analysis
Kenett (Eds) – Modern Analysis of Customer Surveys: With Applications using R
Kruger and Xie – Statistical Monitoring of Complex Multivariate Processes: With Applications in Industrial Process Control
Jank and Shmueli (Ed.) – Statistical Methods in e-Commerce Research
Lehtonen and Pahkinen – Practical Methods for Design and Analysis of Complex Surveys, Second Edition
Ohser and Mücklich – Statistical Analysis of Microstructures in Materials Science
Pourret, Naim & Marcot (Eds) – Bayesian Networks: A Practical Guide to Applications
Taroni, Aitken, Garbolino and Biedermann – Bayesian Networks and Probabilistic Inference in Forensic Science
Taroni, Bozza, Biedermann, Garbolino and Aitken – Data Analysis in Forensic Science